Living Well with Chronic Asthma, Bronchitis, and Emphysema

LIVING WELL WITH CHRONIC ASTHMA, BRONCHITIS, AND EMPHYSEMA

Myra B. Shayevitz, M.D.,
Berton R. Shayevitz, M.D., and
the Editors of Consumer Reports Books

CONSUMER REPORTS BOOKS

A DIVISION OF CONSUMERS UNION

YONKERS, NEW YORK

Library of Congress Cataloging-in-Publication Data

Shayevitz, Myra B., 1934–
    Living well with chronic asthma, bronchitis, and emphysema / by Myra B. Shayevitz, Berton R. Shayevitz, and the editors of Consumer Reports Books.
    p.   cm.
    Includes bibliographical references and index.
    ISBN 0-89043-416-6
    1. Lungs—Diseases, Obstructive—Popular works. I. Shayevitz, Berton R., 1931–   . II. Consumer Reports Books. III. Title.
RC776.03S52   1991
616.2′4—dc20

                                                        91-22642
                                                           CIP

Published previously as *Living Well with Emphysema and Bronchitis* (Doubleday)

Design and Composition by The Sarabande Press

Drawings by Michael Goldberg

First printing, October 1991

Manufactured in the United States of America

*We dedicate this book to all our patients
and those who love them*

CONTENTS

Contents

Contents

Contents

ACKNOWLEDGMENTS

A very special note of thanks to James R. McCormick, M.D., F.C.C.P., Associate Professor of Medicine, Medical College of Georgia, who critically reviewed the entire manuscript with such care.

Our own program was in large part inspired by the ideas of the farseeing Dr. Thomas L. Petty, M.D., F.C.C.P., Professor of Medicine, University of Colorado School of Medicine, pioneer in the field of pulmonary rehabilitation.

We especially wish to thank Antonios P. Stathatos, M.D., Chief, Medical Service, Veterans Administration Medical Center, Northampton, Massachusetts, who inspired our best efforts. In fact, the staff and administration of the Veterans Administration Medical Center in Northampton have helped us in many ways and have provided an environment for professional growth.

Sushma Palmer, D.Sc., Executive Director, Food and Nutrition Board, National Research Council, critically reviewed Chapter 5 in the original edition.

We thank Charles H. Nightingale, Ph.D., Director, Department of Pharmacy Service, Hartford Hospital, Hartford, Connecticut, and Research Professor, University of Connecticut School of Pharmacy, and his staff for reviewing the prescribed medications chart in the first edition.

Acknowledgments

Our appreciation and thanks to Robert Kellman, M.D., Assistant Professor of Otolaryngology, SUNY Health Science Center, Syracuse, New York, for reviewing the sections on rhinitis and sinusitis.

A special thank-you to Robin Solomon, R.N., M.S., for invaluable assistance in the section on home ventilators.

We also thank Donald Davis, Ph.D., of the University of Texas for his help in updating the chapter on nutrition.

A very special thank-you to Consumer Reports Books' Executive Editor, Sarah Uman.

INTRODUCTION

Have you given up a great deal in life because of chronic asthma, bronchitis, or emphysema, also known as chronic obstructive pulmonary disease, or COPD? Do you sit idly most of the day, bored? If you work, is it getting harder and harder? Do you spend a good portion of the day afraid—not understanding your disease or what to do about it? If this is so, we say, "Enough!" You can live a full life in spite of COPD. In fact, you can "live well" with a wide range of activities. Chances are you can exercise actively, eat well, have sex, participate in recreational activities, and enjoy life again.

If you are using this book in conjunction with an established pulmonary rehabilitation program, you are very fortunate indeed, for pulmonary rehabilitation centers can improve functioning by a full 50 percent, and this book should provide valuable supplemental guidance and information.

If not, use this book in conjunction with your own physician to create your own individual rehabilitation program.

We assume in each chapter (except the one on sex) that you are alone and must function entirely independently. If, however, you are lucky enough to have a partner to assist you, use your new knowledge to become a true helpmate.

Although we will remind you of this from time to time throughout the book, please remember that all the suggestions herein are subject to your doctor's approval.

Read carefully and thoughtfully. You are about to become a member of your own health care team.

Chapter 1

COPD: Chronic Asthma, Bronchitis, and Emphysema Explained

Have you been diagnosed as having COPD—chronic bronchitis, emphysema, or asthma?

Have you a full understanding of these diseases and their relationship to each other?

Do you want to know exactly what these terms mean and have a full comprehension of their effects on you and your family? If so, read on.

COPD, an abbreviation for chronic obstructive pulmonary disease, usually refers to chronic bronchitis and emphysema, which affect at least 16 million people in the United States and together constitute one of the fastest-growing health problems in this country. Chronic bronchitis and emphysema are responsible for at least 50,000 deaths a year in the United States alone. In men over the age of 40, COPD is second only to coronary disease as a cause of disability. With the increase in the incidence of smoking among women in the past few years has come a concomitant increase in deaths from COPD in women. In fact, cancer of the lung, an almost completely preventable disease, now kills more women than cancer of the breast. Moreover, dying is only part of the problem. It is the long years of disability, joblessness, loss of income, depression, repeated hospitalization, loss of family and other normal activities that give life meaning (such as recreation, sex, and work) that make chronic bronchitis and emphysema frightening problems.

At least 6 million people in the United States, and more than 5 percent of the population in industrialized countries, are affected by asthma, a disease that frequently begins in childhood but which may have its onset quite late in life. Asthma is not caused by smoking cigarettes. Asthma beginning early in life is usually associated with an allergy and tends to disappear with adulthood, whereas the asthma of adults is frequently chronic and followed by permanent remission in less than 25 percent of cases. Although the causes of chronic bronchitis, emphysema, and asthma are completely different, the symptoms, medications, problems, and sometimes the lifelong course are similar. In addition, these diseases often coexist in the same person, with each one contributing to the affected individual's symptoms. Before we describe the individual disorders and their similarities, we need to study some basic anatomy and physiology. One thing is certain: You owe it to yourself, to the one life on earth that you have, to know all about these diseases.

ANATOMY AND PHYSIOLOGY LESSONS

Air, smoke, germs, allergens, and pollutants pass from the nose and mouth into a large central duct called the *trachea*. The trachea branches into smaller ducts, the *bronchi* and *bronchioles*, which lead to the *alveoli* (Fig. 1.1). These latter are the air sacs—tiny, delicate, balloonlike structures composed of blood vessels (capillaries) supported by connecting tissue and enclosed in a gossamer-thin membrane. The respiratory system is like an upside-down tree: The trachea is the trunk, and the bronchi and bronchioles are the branches. This is known as the *bronchial tree*, a term we'll use from now on. The alveoli are the leaves. The blood vessels of the alveoli carry the red blood cells, which pick up oxygen and transport it to the rest of the body. Carbon dioxide, a cellular waste product, is released to the alveoli from the bloodstream and exhaled. The tiny alveoli, supported by a framework of delicate elastic fibers, give the lung a very distensible quality and the ability to "snap back" like a stretched rubber band when distended by air. This is called *elastic recoil*.

2

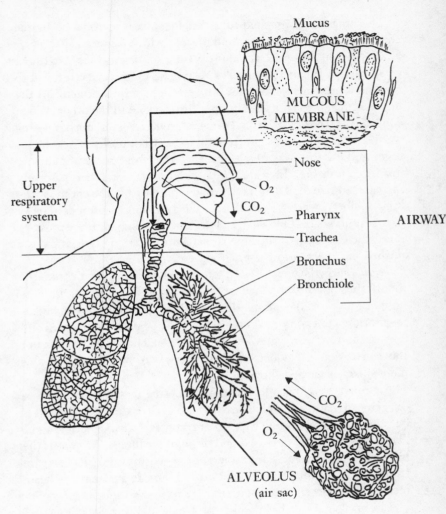

Figure 1.1 Anatomy of the Respiratory System. Note the similarity to an upside-down tree. The trachea is the trunk, the bronchi and bronchioles are the branches, and the alveoli are the leaves. Oxygen enters and carbon dioxide exits the bloodstream via the alveoli. The mucous membrane contains mucus-producing and ciliated cells.

The lungs and bronchial tubes are like a tree surrounded by the chest wall, composed of bone and muscle, which functions like a bellows. The muscles contract and in doing so increase the size of the chest cavity. When the muscles relax, the chest cavity returns to normal. The principal muscles of inspiration, or breathing in, are the diaphragm and the muscles linking the ribs one to the other. When contracting, the dome-shaped diaphragm flattens and pushes downward. At the same time, contraction of the rib muscles raises the rib cage, and in this way the volume of the chest increases during inspiration, or breathing in. The lung is elastic, and so it passively increases in size to fill this newly made space within the chest. As the lung, including the alveoli, enlarges, air from our environment flows in to fill this space. During exhalation, or breathing out, the muscles relax, the elasticity of the lung returns it to a resting size, and air is pushed out, back into the environment.

Ventilation is the term used to refer to the transport of air from the mouth through the bronchial tree to the alveoli and back through the nose or mouth to the outside air. Ventilation, as you can see, equals inspiration and expiration combined. Air is 80 percent nitrogen and 20 percent oxygen; oxygen is vital for the metabolism of our cells and the conversion of foodstuffs into energy. A by-product of this metabolism is carbon dioxide.

Air must pass through the bronchial tree to the alveoli before oxygen can get *into* the bloodstream and carbon dioxide can get *out* because it is the alveoli that are in contact with blood vessels. *Perfusion* refers to the flow of blood through the lungs. *Diffusion* is the term used to describe the passage of oxygen into the bloodstream from the alveoli and the return of carbon dioxide across the delicate membrane between the blood vessels and the alveoli.

The bronchial tree has two kinds of special lining cells. The first type can secrete mucus as a protection against injury and irritation. The second, present from the largest branch (the trachea) down to the smallest branches (the bronchioles), are covered with fine, hair-like structures called *cilia*. The surface of each of these cells contains 200 cilia. In a normal lung, lining cells covered with cilia stand like an army at attention. These cells are supported by smooth muscle cells and elastic and collagen fibers. The cilia wave in the direction of the mouth and act as a vital defense system, physically removing germs and irritating substances. The cilia are covered with fine islands of mucus. The mucus helps trap irritants and germs.

SUMMARY During inspiration, what you breathe leaves the mouth, the nose, and the back of the throat and is swept down into the bronchial tree. Because this is the way air flows, it is called the *airway*. Covering cells lining the bronchial tree, cilia, are constantly beating with an upward motion in your defense. Other cells secrete mucus to entrap unwanted particulates as another defense mechanism. From the bronchial tree air passes into the alveoli, where oxygen then diffuses into the blood perfusing the lungs to participate in vital cell functions. Carbon dioxide diffuses into the alveoli from the blood and leaves the body during exhalation.

CHRONIC BRONCHITIS

This is a disease characterized by a daily cough productive of sputum for at least three months each year for two consecutive years when no other disease is present to account for these symptoms. A rattling cough or frequent clearing of the throat may have the same significance as a productive cough. The diagnosis of chronic bronchitis is made by this history, rather than by any abnormalities found on a chest X ray or even through a pulmonary function test.

As the result of cigarette smoking (or, rarely, other irritants), the mucous cells of the bronchial tree respond by excessive production of their product. The first sign of excessive production of mucus is usually morning cough. As cigarette smoking continues over the years, the irritation increases, and coughing continues throughout the day. The excess mucus provides food for bacteria. Now infection is added to irritation. Mucus changes from clear to yellow, since it now contains white blood cells (*polymorphonuclear leukocytes*, hereafter referred to as *PMNs*), defense cells to fight off the infecting organisms by engulfing them. When the bacteria win, the infection becomes deep enough to cause actual destruction of the bronchial wall. Scar tissue replaces the fine cells lining the bronchial tree, and scars give rise to areas of narrowing. Some bronchioles become totally obliterated. *Bronchospasm,* or tightening of the muscles of the bronchial tree, occurs. Other bronchioles become dilated or enlarged. The mucus stagnates, and bacteria grow. How can we paint this picture vividly? It's like plugged plumbing. So far, we've only discussed your mucus-producing cells. What about your army, the ciliated cells?

Exposure to cigarette smoke for as little as 30 seconds paralyzes cilia for a minimum of 15 minutes. Continued exposure to cigarette smoke permanently damages the cilia and their ability to beat and to remove mucus, bacteria, and other irritants. This can occur after as little as one year of smoking. Finally, the ciliated cells fall out, leaving you with bald spots. They are replaced with cells that have no defensive properties.

As bacteria, no longer cleared by cilia and multiplying in excess mucus, grow, PMNs are called into the area as another line of defense. They produce enzymes—chemical substances—to destroy the bacteria, but these enzymes can also damage or destroy the delicate supporting structures of the cells lining the bronchial tree as well as the membranes of the alveoli. In effect, these now become killer enzymes. Unfortunately, they kill the good as well as the bad.

EMPHYSEMA

When the air sacs are exposed to cigarette smoke and other respiratory irritants, they also produce a defensive cell called an *alveolar macrophage* (hereafter referred to as AM). AMs engulf irritants and bacteria and call for more PMNs to come into the lungs. The lung tissue, so delicate, flexible, and so important for the passage of oxygen into the bloodstream, with its network of elastins and collagens, also becomes the target for the enzyme *elastase* and other chemical substances produced by the PMNs and the AMs. There are natural defense systems that inhibit the enzymes released by AMs and PMNs,

6

specifically *alpha-1-antitrypsin* (AAT), but it appears that this inhibiting function is impaired in smokers. Its primary function is to inhibit elastase. It is therefore an antielastase. Emphysema results from an imbalance between the neutrophil elastase in the lungs, which destroys elastin and other connective tissue components, and the antielastases that are responsible for deficiency states. (Those with severe AAT deficiency should register with the National Heart, Lung, and Blood Institute, Pulmonary Branch, 9000 Rockville Pike, Building 10, Room 6D06, Bethesda, MD 20892, Tel: 301-496-1597.)

In all types of emphysema, elastin and collagen fibers are destroyed. The lung loses its elastic recoil, like a rubber band that can't snap back; air sacs and blood vessels are irreversibly damaged.

WHEN EMPHYSEMA AND CHRONIC BRONCHITIS MEET

Here's where emphysema and chronic bronchitis get together. After reading this you'll readily see why these two diseases have been lumped under the name chronic obstructive pulmonary disease. As described above, the bronchi are weakened and narrowed by chronic bronchitis. During inspiration, as we told you, respiratory muscles actively contract and keep the airways open. During expiration, when the muscles relax, the air flows rapidly and the pressure in the bronchial tree drops below that of the surrounding lung. The lungs, partially destroyed, are no longer able to put traction on the bronchi to keep them open. Weakened bronchial walls then collapse, choking off the vital flow of air. This is called *airway collapse and air trapping*. Weakened by enzymes, the walls of the alveoli rupture, blood vessels die, and lung tissue is replaced with scar tissue, leaving areas of destroyed alveoli like "sinkholes," the smaller ones called *blebs* and the larger ones called *bullae*. The end result is a set of big, over-expanded lungs with a weakened, partially plugged bronchial tree subject to airway collapse and air trapping with blebs and bullae; and breathing, particularly exhalation, becomes a slow, difficult process. Do you have a big "barrel chest"? Now you know why.

Can anything else go wrong? Absolutely. Next comes mismatched mates (Fig. 1.2). Just as each branch of a tree ultimately leads to a leaf, so in the normal lung each final branch of the bronchial tree leads to an alveolus, which is surrounded by blood vessels. In the lung with COPD some of the branches of the bronchial tree become partially or totally blocked by mucus. Blood can easily get to the alveolus but air cannot. The blood leaves the alveolus and returns to the heart and the rest of the body without oxygen.

In other areas of the lung, the bronchial tree may have escaped excessive mucus and be able to transport air. However, the tiny air sacs are now ruptured, and the number of blood vessels is greatly reduced. Therefore, when air arrives in the alveolus, there are no blood vessels there to transport their vital cargo to the cells. In other areas of the bronchial tree, alveolar walls and blood vessels may be totally obliterated. This is called *ventilation to perfusion imbalance.*

These mismatched mates, coupled with collapsed airways and plugged plumbing attacked by killer enzymes and defended by a paralyzed army, all paint the picture of COPD. To varying degrees, the person with COPD has a tree with a narrow, defective trunk and sparse leaves.

Is this your medical history?

You were probably well as a child, with no evidence of respiratory problems. You started smoking in your early teens. After a few years you noticed you had more colds than your nonsmoking friends. After about 10 years of smoking, every time you got a cold or upper respiratory infection (URI), it went into your chest. At first, these chest colds would last about two weeks, then about four to six weeks (cilia impaired, mucous glands overproducing in response to irritation). Finally, you were left with a morning cough every day, which you called a cigarette cough (cilia impaired and ciliated cells beginning to fall out, glands overproducing). Your cough went from morning cough to the ability to bring up sputum any time of the day. Respiratory infections became more frequent and lasted longer. You

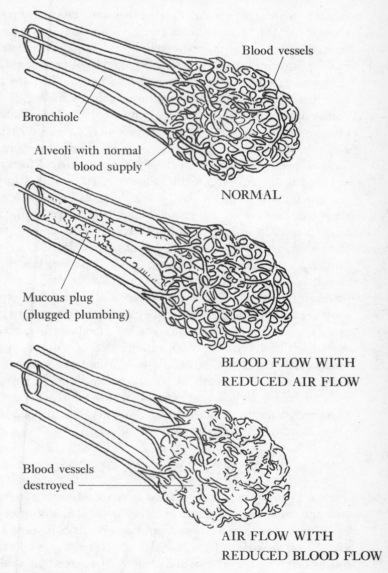

Blood vessels

Bronchiole

Alveoli with normal
blood supply

NORMAL

Mucous plug
(plugged plumbing)

BLOOD FLOW WITH
REDUCED AIR FLOW

Blood vessels
destroyed

AIR FLOW WITH
REDUCED BLOOD FLOW

Figure 1.2   Mismatched Mates

began to notice that you tired easily, that some tasks were no longer pleasurable. You began to be short of breath when hurrying up a hill or walking up a few flights of stairs (cilia impaired, ciliated cells missing, overproduction of mucus, plugging of bronchial tree, air trapping, causing increased work of breathing). Then any type of hurrying frequently began to produce a choking feeling, as though your wind was being cut off (cilia impaired, ciliated cells missing, overproduction of mucus, plugging of bronchial tree, air trapping, airway collapse). With acute infections you began to wheeze or to have bronchospasm in which the air was extremely difficult to get out. Finally, it became difficult to hurry, even on a level surface. It became difficult to get a day's work done, to perform sex, to do shopping, cooking, cleaning, walking, to care for yourself—and no amount of deep or hard breathing seemed to make any difference (cilia impaired, ciliated cells missing, overproduction of mucus, plugging of bronchi, air trapping, airway collapse, loss of elastic recoil, ruptured alveoli [blebs and perhaps bullae], mismatched mating). Periods of breathlessness increased in intensity, especially associated with acute infections (e.g., viruses, pneumonia) or exposure to irritants (air pollutants, smoke), high humidity, or cold air. At these times you may have experienced confusion, insomnia, restlessness, headaches, either a fast, slow, or irregular heart rate, marked shortness of breath, and/or rapid breathing. Intensive therapy may have been necessary, often in a hospital. If you were unable to compensate with usual treatments, you may have needed artificial ventilation.

WHERE ASTHMA FITS IN

Asthma is a disease of intermittent airway obstruction from irritation and inflammation of the bronchial wall. Bouts of wheezing (a sound resulting from air moving through partially blocked air passages) due to spasm of the muscles of the airways, and excessive mucus secretion occur. The bronchial tree becomes "plugged" with thick secretions. It is now known that, just as in bronchitis, PMNs also infiltrate the walls of the bronchial tree, and that areas of the lining cells may actually shed. Contact with allergens, infections, and chemical sensitizers may all cause airway inflammation. When this happens, there is a release of chemical substances leading to swelling, increased secretions, and then "hyperresponsiveness," or narrowing of the bronchial tree. After exposure to the trigger stimulus, the bout of airway hyperresponsiveness—that is, spasm of the bronchial muscles—may last anywhere from hours to weeks to months. Sometimes, the asthmatic attack (hyperresponsiveness) occurs immediately after contact with the offending substance. Other times, wheezing may occur eight hours or more after the challenge period. Asthmatic symptoms may also occur with physical exercise and exposure to cold air.

Unfortunately, in the asthma of adults the exact cause is very seldom known. Asthma may be caused by a variety of things ranging from being upset, or getting a virus or some other respiratory infection, to changes in the barometric pressure or changes in temperature, to exposure to a large number of airborne or ingested allergens or fumes. Triggers for asthma may include common household cleaning agents, polishes, waxes, scented toiletries, exercise, molds, animal danders, house dust mites, yeasts, industrial chemicals, foods and food additives such as MSG, or even aspirin and related compounds (the nonsteroidal antiinflammatory drugs).

During an acute attack of asthma over a period ranging from a few minutes to a few hours or days, wheezing and excessive mucus production increases. If the attack does not resolve itself spontaneously or with medication, severe distress may occur with air trapping, blueness (cyanosis) around the mouth, anxiety, a fast heart rate, and the need for hospitalization. If the attack is prolonged, it is called *status asthmaticus*. If wheezing is most severe at night, it is called *nocturnal asthma*.

Fortunately, there are few deaths from acute asthma attacks, but they can be dangerous and should be treated as soon as possible.

Two diseases may be contributing factors to asthma, so we will mention them here. The first is *sinusitis*. The nose and sinuses are

11

lined, just as is the lower respiratory tract described earlier, with ciliated cells and mucus-secreting cells. The nose and sinuses are highly susceptible to allergens and irritants. Upon their inhalation, excessive swelling occurs. The sinuses, which are thin-walled cavities in the bones of the skull, secrete over one quart of fluid per day, which is usually swallowed. When the nasal passages swell, the openings to the sinuses may become blocked. These openings, by the way, are no bigger than the point of a ballpoint pen. The nose is filled with organisms. The sinuses are sterile, but when the nose becomes inflamed and the openings to the sinuses are blocked, the sinuses may become infected and drainage of the mucus can be severely impeded. This condition may exacerbate asthma. The most common symptom associated with sinusitis is facial pain and pressure sensation located over the cheeks and upper teeth, in the forehead above the eyes, in the back of the skull, and on the sides of the skull. If you suffer from any of these symptoms or prolonged continuation of nasal swelling, you should bring this to the attention of your doctor.

The second disorder is *gastroesophageal reflux*. In this syndrome, sour stomach contents back up into the lower part of the esophagus, the tubelike structure that spans the area from the mouth to the stomach. When this happens, it may "trigger" bronchospasm of a significant degree. The most common symptom of gastroesophageal reflux is burning in the chest, or heartburn. Sometimes, gastroesophageal reflux produces nocturnal, or nighttime, asthma. If you are frequently awakened with wheezing and shortness of breath, the possibility of gastroesophageal reflux should be investigated.

There are many similarities between chronic bronchitis, emphysema, and adult asthma. During bouts of bronchospasm excess mucus production occurs, leading to plugging of the airways and mismatched mating (ventilation/perfusion inequality). There is evidence now that the cilia are impaired in asthmatics, making asthmatics more prone to frequent infection. In adults asthma and wheezing may occur every day and lead to chronic airway trapping and a syndrome of persistent, irreversible obstruction of the bronchial tree. The exact relationship between asthma, chronic bronchitis, and emphysema still remains somewhat uncertain. Chronic asthma has been classified under chronic obstructive pulmonary disease, although doctors usually refer to the combination of emphysema and bronchitis as COPD. The long-term course is much more variable and has not been well studied. Because of the natural history of asthma, patients with chronic asthma, chronic bronchitis, and emphysema have much the same needs in terms of dealing with physical disability and relapses. They also take many of the same medications and should practice the same self-protection techniques that we describe in this book.

AN ENDING WITH A NEW BEGINNING

By following our strategy, you can reverse some aspects of your problem, prevent many new problems, and slow progression of your illness. Some things cannot be changed. We cannot repair the sinkholes in your lungs or get you new cilia or strong bronchial walls; we *can* increase your overall respiratory muscle strength and improve the efficiency of your heart and lungs. You'll always be more prone to infections than the next person, but we *can* show you how to protect yourself from *becoming* infected and how to keep the side effects of a relapse or an attack to a minimum. We cannot promise you a life free from medicines and supplemental oxygen, but we *can* teach you how to use your medication and oxygen effectively to minimize the side effects and maximize the benefits.

Your figure may not become that of a bathing beauty or a weight lifter; we *can* try to help you increase your muscle mass, which translates into increased strength, and to normalize your fat content.

We cannot promise you will never land in the hospital, but if admitted you should be well informed and capable of cooperating. Your knowledge should lessen fears and hasten recovery.

We cannot fashion you into a superathlete or keep your energy at a high level all day. We *can* show you how to be athletic and at the same time conserve energy, to do all the tasks you need to do and have energy left over for those you *want* to do.

This book will also discuss having fun, eating well, enjoying sex, working (or working longer), and elevating your mood.

This book is meant to supplement and not to substitute for a good physician, but a knowledgeable patient who takes care of himself or herself may well need fewer visits to the doctor. And the patient who tries hard to do right by himself or herself is a pleasure for any physician. With increased comprehension comes appreciation—you and your doctor should both think more of each other. Your functional capacity can improve. We can prove to you that you are a whole, precious person able to take control of your life—and a full one at that. We cannot cure your disease, but we *can* help to arrest or stabilize it.

It's time to get back some of what you've given up, and perhaps find new worlds you never dreamed of. It's time to make your move, *now*, before you have to give up even more. One thing is certain: The old way didn't work. That's why you're reading this book. Try this new way.

Chapter 2

SMOKING AND LIFE EXPECTANCY

AN ASSASSIN EXPOSED

M ake no mistake about it: If you smoke, cigarettes are killing you. The U.S. surgeon general reports that cigarette smoking is the "single greatest preventable cause of death and disability in the United States today." Smoking is the major cause of chronic bronchitis and emphysema. Fifty thousand people will die yearly of these two diseases. If what we told you in Chapter 1 about COPD and smoking interested you but didn't convince you, read on.

Cigarette smokers have approximately double the death rate from heart disease of nonsmokers. Recent evidence suggests that smoking adversely affects the concentration of the "good" cholesterol (see Chapter 5), decreasing its production. About one in 500 cigarette smokers dies from lung cancer each year. This translates to 120,000 people in the United States in 1988. Twenty-two thousand will die from other tobacco-related cancers, and 130,000 will die from tobacco-related heart attacks and strokes. If you started smoking at the age of 15 and smoked the rest of your life, you would have half the chance of living to the age of 75 as compared with your friend who never smoked.

New evidence shows that sidestream smoke—the smoke given off between puffs—contains several thousand chemicals. Sidestream smoke has higher concentrations of noxious compounds than the mainstream smoke inhaled by the smoker, including twice as much tar and nicotine and three times as much 3-4 benzopyrene and five times as much ammonia. New evidence shows that those who regularly inhale sidestream smoke have an increased incidence of coughs, bronchitis, and cancer of the lung.

Don't try to tell yourself that when you smoke, you feel better. You only *think* you smoke to feel good. There is every reason to suggest that you are seriously dependent. In between cigarettes your nicotine level drops, and you feel better when you bring the level back up. No person who coughs up sputum all day, suffers from shortness of breath, easy fatigability, and decreased enjoyment from life smokes for the fun of it. You smoke because you can't help it. What else could that mean but addiction?

The original report of the surgeon general's advisory committee in 1964 stated that smoking had an adverse effect on health but also alleged that smoking did not fulfill the criteria for addiction for the following reasons: (1) no tolerance developed; (2) there were no withdrawal symptoms; (3) antisocial behavior was not elicited when cigarettes were not available. Now we know better! In 1977 the Royal College of Physicians in London in its report "Smoking and Health" described the nicotine withdrawal syndrome in which there is intense craving, anxiety, irritability, restlessness, depression, inability to sleep, changes in the gastrointestinal system including constipation, and impaired performance when doing such tasks as driving.

As for tolerance, we now know it develops rapidly. By the time you are finished with one pack of cigarettes, you have 200 jolts of nicotine. This happened with the first pack you ever smoked. At first, perhaps, you were sick when you smoked. You felt dizzy, your heart beat fast, or you were nauseated. Of course, this all went away very rapidly. You began smoking more to get a sense of well-being; you told yourself cigarettes made you less irritable. It was insufficient nicotine, for which you developed a tolerance, that made you irritable. This is what was relieved by a cigarette. Feeding your addiction makes you feel good.

Violent outbursts have occurred in public places when smokers have been denied access to cigarettes. There it is—antisocial behavior, the last criterion for addiction.

Have you any idea of the effects of smoking on those around you? Researchers recently found actual damage in the airways of children from hundreds of families who had smoking parents as compared with children whose parents did not smoke. Also, the children of smokers have abnormal pulmonary function studies and an increased incidence of infected ears. Nonsmokers who are exposed to cigarette smoke at work might have the same defects as those people who smoke 10 cigarettes a day.

A SMOKER'S RISK/BENEFIT RATIO

Take a piece of paper and in the left-hand column write down all the benefits you receive from smoking. Here are the risks for the right-hand column:

    chronic obstructive pulmonary disease
    heart attack
    cancer of the lung
    cancer of the throat and esophagus
    stroke
    long-term disability as a respiratory or cardiac cripple
    injuring others by direct contact with your cigarette smoke

Is smoking worth it? How many thousands of dollars have you spent on cigarettes? Don't forget to add in the bills for your medical care. Each time you want to smoke a cigarette, think of that risk/benefit ratio. You can *live well* and have a full life. There is only one way to treat smoking—*stop!*

A ONE-SECOND TEST TO DETERMINE YOUR LIFE EXPECTANCY

A one-second test to determine your life expectancy is the *forced expiratory volume at one second*, known for short as the FEV_1, done after inhaling a bronchodilator. Here's how this simple test works. The *vital capacity*, or *VC*, is defined as the maximum amount of air that can be exhaled after maximal inspiration. Ordinarily, this test is done on a recording device that measures not only the volume of air but the speed at which it is exhaled. The portion of the vital capacity exhaled in one second is known as the FEV_1. If you inhale a bronchodilator prior to doing the vital capacity, then the FEV_1 after bronchodilators is thus defined. The vital capacity itself, a simple test available in most physicians' offices, is predicted by height and age. The normal FEV_1 is 75 percent or more of the total normal vital capacity.

This test determines life expectancy *based on your present condition*. No attempt to predict the outcome in any single person can be made because there is much room for change—for better or worse. We have summarized some test results in a simple graph, and we ask you to look at where you *might* stand now (see Fig. 2.1).

Here is how to understand the graph. Take the results of your postbronchodilator FEV_1 and determine into which of the four lines labeled "% Predicted FEV_1" it fits. You can then plot the percent of survival at two, five, 10, and 15 years. For instance, approximately 55 percent of those who have an FEV_1 of 50 percent of predicted are alive at 10 years.

A FORMULA TO CHANGE RESULTS OF THE ONE-SECOND TEST

Here is a simple formula to help you change the results of the one-second test: $SS + PD + E = ILE$. Does that sound more complicated than Einstein's $E = mc^2$? The formula stands for Stop Smoking + Proper Diet + Exercise = Increased Life Expectancy. You will learn all the latest information on diet, exercise, and self-care in this book.

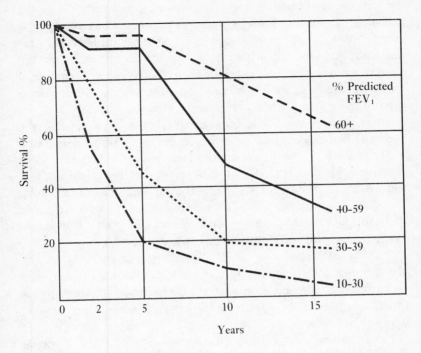

Figure 2.1 Relationship of Survival to Percent of Predicted Post-bronchodilator Forced Expiratory Volume at 1 Second (FEV_1)

CALLING IT QUITS—HERE'S HOW

Basically, there are two ways to stop smoking: tapering and quitting. Try quitting first. We believe that quitting absolutely and completely is the single most effective way to successfully stop smoking. There are several medical aids for those who can't quit without a crutch. The first is the use of a chewing gum containing nicotine polacrilex, available by prescription only. Once you quit smoking, you must then quit using the gum. Slowly chew the gum until your tongue tingles or you feel as though the nicotine is now in your body and you are satisfied. You can also chew the nicotine gum in advance of the time that you know you will have an urge to smoke. Once you feel the effect, "park" the gum in your mouth in the pocket between your cheek and your teeth, leaving it ready for the next time you get the urge to smoke. A second possible helper is the use of clonidine, a medicine ordinarily used to lower blood pressure. You might wish to discuss these two methods of quitting with your doctor.

If you use the alternative route of tapering, make a schedule for yourself. Remember, you are trying to cut down on your nicotine intake each day. You will have a natural tendency to hold the smoke in your lungs longer than before and to smoke the cigarette down to a shorter butt. If you cut down on the tar and nicotine in your cigarettes or on the number of cigarettes smoked, be knowledgeable about this fact and don't fool yourself. Remember, even if you choose to taper, you still must stop completely someday.

You can use some simple tools to help you stop smoking. Try chewing gum, nibbling on carrots, or having a friend or mate provide a pleasing alternate sensation, such as a back rub when the going gets tough. Read books about quitting smoking and invent some of your own simple tools.

Here is some advice from a pamphlet issued by the National Cancer Institute entitled *Clearing the Air*:

Before quitting:

1. Have a friend quit with you.
2. Switch to a brand that you find distasteful.
3. Smoke only half of each cigarette, and postpone lighting your first cigarette of the day by one hour each day.
4. Decide in which hours—odd or even—of the day you will smoke.
5. Buy only one pack of cigarettes at a time.
6. Don't smoke under pleasurable circumstances. If you like to smoke in company, smoke only when you are alone.

7. Try to break the "automatic" habit by smoking at odd times of the day and using a different hand to hold your cigarette.
8. Frequent places where smoking is prohibited, such as libraries.
9. Set the date, and then *quit!*

Immediately after quitting:

1. Continue to visit places where smoking is prohibited.
2. If you miss the sensation of cigarettes, munch on raw carrot sticks or hold a pencil in your hand to fiddle with.
3. Avoid all situations that you associate with smoking, such as watching television or sitting in a special place.
4. Talk to people who don't smoke, and avoid your smoking friends for now.
5. Try to change your daily routine.
6. Note your progress on a calendar, especially for the first three months.
7. Drinking large quantities of water and fruit juices may be of help.

Make a regular daily schedule for yourself that does not include cigarettes, and *stick to it!*

Chapter 3

THERAPY

HELPING YOUR DOCTOR MANAGE
YOUR CASE

We hope that after reading the first chapter of this book you realize that COPD is characterized by ups, downs, and relapses. You should aim to minimize relapses on the one hand and improve your daily functioning on the other. Early and proper use of medication is an important key to successful treatment of COPD relapses. Unchecked relapses result in bouts of severe bronchitis, wheezing, pneumonia, respiratory failure, hospitalization, and increasing disability and loss of function.

Your doctor is not with you on a daily basis. You have to be the one to know when you are beginning a relapse. The doctor will be delighted to hear that you want to be a member of your own health care team, armed with a sound knowledge of your disease. It's important that you have a frank talk with your doctor and explain right away that you have a better understanding of the disease process.

We hope you're going to say that you've stopped smoking (if, of course, you were a smoker), and that you intend to embark on a daily regimen of self-improvement, physical examination, good eating habits, exercise, and healthy thoughts and contacts.

You may be sure the doctor wants a knowledgeable partner helping to handle your case. He or she wants you to know what you are doing; know all the names of your medications, their side effects, and perhaps how to manipulate them yourself in certain specific instances; and when to call early in a relapse. The doctor would rather treat you at the beginning of an infection than see you lying blue *in extremis* in a hospital bed. Explain that you want to be an effective partner, and that you'll know when to call and that your conversations will be intelligent, well informed, and right to the point. You'll be using his or her time more effectively. Communicate your urgent desire to get your physician's help in your new program to help yourself.

USE OF SPRAYS AND PRESCRIBED DEVICES

Inhalation therapy equipment such as the *updraft nebulizer* is usually used to facilitate the delivery of a bronchodilator as deep as possible into the respiratory tract. An updraft nebulizer also can instill mucus-thinning agents, antiinflammatory agents, antiasthmatic drugs, and sometimes antibiotics. This equipment is usually driven by an oilless air compressor and is lightweight and convenient to use. In using an updraft nebulizer, merely breathe slowly and comfortably. Try to prolong inspiration by silently counting "one one-thousand, two one-thousand" at the end of inspiration. It's imperative that you keep your equipment clean. Cleaning and sterilization instructions reproduced by permission of the American College of Chest Physicians are as follows:

Cleaning and Sterilization of Inhalation Therapy Equipment*

1. Each night wash manifold, tubing, mouthpiece, nebulizer, etc., in mild detergent. (Equipment should be scrubbed thoroughly.)

---

*Statement by the Committee on Therapy, American Thoracic Society. *American Review of Respiratory Disease* 98:521–22, 1968. As published in John E. Hodgkin,

2. Rinse the equipment well, making sure all soap is removed.
3. Soak equipment in vinegar solution containing 2 parts of white distilled vinegar with 3 parts distilled water. Soak for 20 minutes.
4. Rinse after soaking in vinegar solution.
5. Let drain dry on *clean* towel (do not wipe or dry with towel).
6. REMEMBER: All water must be removed from the tubing.
7. After equipment is dry, reassemble, ready for use, or store in plastic bag or dust-free area.

NOTE: The Loma Linda University Medical Center has a protocol for the cleaning of home respiratory therapy equipment which varies from the above statement in the following points:

1. After each use, the manifold, mouthpiece, nebulizer, etc., should be disassembled and rinsed thoroughly in hot running water. The parts should be allowed to air dry on a paper towel.
2. Only the mouthpiece need be washed in mild detergent each night.
3. The disinfecting procedure described in the above statement is performed twice a week rather than nightly.
4. The detachable parts are immersed in a white vinegar solution (1 part vinegar, 2 parts water) and allowed to soak for 30 minutes.
5. Hang tubing over a towel rack or shower rod to drain off excess water while drying.

---

ed., *Chronic Obstructive Pulmonary Disease: Current Concepts in Diagnosis and Comprehensive Care* (Park Ridge, IL: American College of Chest Physicians, 1979), p. 65.

TABLE 3.1

The Most Commonly Prescribed Medications and Their Principal Uses and Side Effects

The information in this chart covers the principal uses and side effects of medications discussed but not every possible use or side effect. Know the indications, dosage, and side effects of any other medicines you take. Drugs are divided by category according to their uses. Each drug has both a chemical or generic name and a trade or company name. In the text a trade name is always enclosed in parentheses. In the chart a trade name is always capitalized, while a generic name is not. Please note the key at the end of the chart.

Drug	Why Used	Dosage	Side Effects	Report to the Doctor Immediately
I. BRONCHODILATORS[a]	to relieve bronchospasm, reduce wheezing and shortness of breath, improve function of respiratory muscles			
A. *Xanthines*[b]			1. nausea	1–3
Theophylline (Choledyl, Theolair, Theo-Dur, Quibron, et al.)		0.5–0.7 mg/kg of normal body weight per 24 hr.—usually about 500–800 mg/day in divided doses	2. stomach pain 3. vomiting 4. trouble sleeping 5. fast or irregular heartbeat 6. confusion 7. vomiting blood 8. loss of appetite 9. irritability, restlessness	5–8
(Uniphyl)		400–800 mg once daily		
B. *Beta-adrenergic stimulants*			1. nervousness	3, 4, 7, 8
1. Metaproterenol (Alupent)			2. shaking 3. headache	

Drug	Why Used	Dosage	Side Effects	Report to the Doctor Immediately
liquid		0.2–0.3 ml diluted in 2.5 ml saline or water	4. rapid or irregular heartbeat	
tablets		20 mg 3–4 times a day	5. nausea	
metered dose inhaler		2–3 inhalations every 4–6 hr., not more than 12 per day	6. muscle cramps 7. chest pain	
Repetabs		4 mg every 12 hr.	8. vomiting 9. weakness	
2. Terbutaline (Brethine, Bricanyl) tablets		2.5–5 mg 3–4 times daily		
metered dose inhaler		2 inhalations 3–4 times daily, not more than 20 per day		

26

Drug	Why Used	Dosage	Side Effects	Report to the Doctor Immediately
3. Isoetharine (Bronkosol) liquid		1/2 ml diluted with 3 parts saline or water, 4 times a day or every 4 hr.		
metered dose inhaler		2 inhalations 4 times a day or every 4 hr., not more than 12 per 24 hr.		
4. Albuterol (Ventolin[a], Proventil) tablets		2–4 mg 3–4 times a day		
metered dose inhaler		1–2 inhalations every 4–6 hr., not more than 12 per day		
5. Pibuterol acetate (Maxair)		2 inhalations 3–4 times daily, not more than 20 per day		

Drug	Why Used	Dosage	Side Effects	Report to the Doctor Immediately
II. ANTIBIOTICS[a]	to combat bacterial infection			
A. *Tetracyclines*			1. burning in stomach 2. vomiting 3. diarrhea 4. increased sensitivity of skin to sunlight 5. rash 6. itching 7. nausea 8. sore mouth and tongue	1–3, 5–8
1. (Sumycin, Tetrex[c,d], others)		250–500 mg every 6 hr.		
2. Doxycycline (Vibramycin)[d]		100 mg every 12 hr. for one day, then 100 mg daily or 100 mg every 12 hr.		
B. *Penicillins*[c]			1. fever 2. hives 3. itching, rash 4. nausea 5. diarrhea 6. wheezing 7. sore mouth and tongue 8. mild stomach upset	1–7
1. Ampicillin (Omnipen, Polycillin, Principen, others)		250–500 mg every 6 hr.		
2. Amoxicillin (Amoxil, Polymox, Trimox, others)		250–500 mg every 8 hr.		
3. Amoxicillin/Clavulanate (Augmentin)		250–500 mg every 8 hr.		

28

Drug	Why Used	Dosage	Side Effects	Report to the Doctor Immediately
C. *Cephalosporins*				
1. Cephradine (Keflex, Velosef, Anspor)		250–500 mg every 6 hr.	1. nausea, vomiting 2. skin rash, hives 3. severe abdominal pain	1–6, 9
2. Cefaclor (Ceclor)		250–500 mg every 8 hr.	4. fever 5. severe or persistent diarrhea	
3. Cefuroxime (Ceftin)		250–500 mg every 12 hr.	6. weakness 7. itching (rectal or genital)	
4. Cefixime (Suprax)		400 mg every 24 hr.	8. mild diarrhea 9. sore tongue and mouth	
D. *Erythromycin*[c] (E.E.S.400, Erythrocin, others)		250–500 mg every 6 hr.	1. *fever* 2. hives 3. itching, rash 4. nausea and abdominal cramps 5. diarrhea 6. wheezing 7. sore mouth and tongue	1–7, 9

29

Drug	Why Used	Dosage	Side Effects	Report to the Doctor Immediately
			8. mild stomach upset	
			9. dark urine, pale stools, yellow eyes	
E. *Sulfa drugs*[c,e] Trimethoprim-sulfamethoxazole (Septra, Bactrim, regular or double-strength)		3 tablets every 12 hr. or one double-strength tablet (DS) every 12 hr.	1. paleness 2. black-and-blue spots 3. bleeding 4. redness of skin 5. weakness, fever 6. itching, rash, hives 7. peeling skin 8. light sensitivity 9. sore tongue 10. turn yellow 11. severe diarrhea 12. headache 13. joint pains 14. hallucinations 15. insomnia 16. pain when urinating	1–11, 13–16
F. Others				
1. Ciprofloxacin (Cipro)		500–750 mg every 12 hr.	1. restlessness 2. seizures 3. hallucinations 4. xanthine toxicity	2–4

30

Drug	Why Used	Dosage	Side Effects	Report to the Doctor Immediately
III. STEROID HORMONES[a]				1-7, 9
A. *Prednisone, Methylpred-nisolone, Dexamethasone* (Medrol, Decadron, others)	decrease bronchospasm, decrease swelling, decrease inflammation, relieve wheezing in bronchial tree	variable; as little as possible is used to relieve syptoms, but may vary from 1 to 10 or more tablets per day	1. blurred vision 2. frequent urination 3. increased thirst 4. bone pain 5. black stools 6. abdominal pain 7. new infection 8. mood change 9. swelling of feet 10. nervousness 11. thinness of skin, easy bruisability 12. facial puffiness 13. increased appetite 14. restlessness 15. weight gain 16. insomnia 17. muscle weakness	
B. *Beclomethasone*[g] (Vanceril, Beclovent) metered dose inhaler		8-20 inhalations per day	1. hoarseness 2. sore mouth	

Drug	Why Used	Dosage	Side Effects	Report to the Doctor Immediately
C. *Flunisolide* (AeroBid) metered dose inhaler		2–4 inhalations twice per day		
D. *Triamcinolone acetonide* (Azmacort)		2 inhalations 4 times per day, up to 16 inhalations per day		
IV. DIGITALIS AND ALLIED CARDIAC GLYCOSIDES A. *Digoxin* (Lanoxin)	to improve the strength of contractions of the heart, treat left heart failure, and treat disturbances of heart rythmn	0.125–0.25 mg daily (may be started with higher dose for a few days)	1. loss of appetite 2. abdominal pain 3. nausea, vomiting 4. very rapid, slow, or uneven pulse 5. weakness 6. blurred, yellow vision 7. diarrhea 8. mood changes 9. breast swelling	1–8

Drug	Why Used	Dosage	Side Effects	Report to the Doctor Immediately
V. DIURETICS[a]				
A. Loop diuretic (most potent)			1. loss of hearing	1–6, 9
1. Furosemide[f] (Lasix)	to prevent excessive fluid retention	20–40 mg 1–2 times a day, but very variable, up to 200 mg or more daily	2. skin rash, hives 3. bleeding, bruising 4. yellow eyes, skin 5. irregular or fast heartbeat 6. muscle cramps 7. decreased sexual ability (thiazide diuretic) 8. lightheadedness, dizziness 9. unusual weakness	
B. Thiazide diuretics (less potent)				
1. Hydrochlorothiazide[f] (HydroDIURIL)		25–100 mg a day		
2. Dyazide	combination of thiazide diuretic plus a chemical to prevent loss of potassium	1–2 capsules daily		
3. Aldactazide		1–2 tablets daily		
4. Moduretic		1–2 tablets daily		

33

Drug	Why Used	Dosage	Side Effects	Report to the Doctor Immediately
VI. MAST CELL INHIBITORS[a]				
Cromolyn sodium (Intal)	a unique category that inhibits the release of chemicals that cause wheezing and bronchospasm		1. weakness 2. nosebleed 3. wheezing 4. nasal congestion	3
liquid		ampules, 1–4 times a day, inhaled from a power-driven nebulizer		
powder		capsules, 1–4 times a day, inhaled through a special device called a Spinhaler®		
metered dose inhaler		2 separate sprays, 4 times per day or 2 sprays 15 min. prior to exercise		
VII. EXPECTORANTS– MUCOLYTIC AGENTS[a]	to thin secretions			
Guaifenesin (Robitussin)		100–400 mg every 4–6 hr.	1. nausea 2. vomiting 3. drowsiness	
Iodinated glycerol (Organidin)		2 tablets 4 times a day		

Drug	Why Used	Dosage	Side Effects	Report to the Doctor Immediately
elixir solution		1 tsp. 4 times a day		
		20 drops 4 times a day		
VIII. PARASYMPATH-OLYTICS				
Ipratropium bromide (Atrovent) metered dose inhaler	to reduce wheezing	to reduce wheezing / 2 inhalations 4 times a day	1. exacerbation of glaucoma 2. difficulty with urination 3. dry mouth 4. tremor 5. palpitations	1 and 2
solution		1–2 ml every 4–6 hr. by inhalation		

Key: a Could be manipulated with doctor's permission (see later discussion).
b Take with food to avoid nausea.
c Take on an empty stomach with full glass of water; allow 1 hr. before and 2 hr. after meals.
d Do not take milk, dairy products, antacids, vitamin-mineral or iron preparations within 2 hr. of taking this medicine.
e Drink additional glasses of fluid unless otherwise directed.
f Medicine may result in loss of body potassium. Unless otherwise directed, eat foods high in potassium (e.g. citrus fruits, bananas).
g When inhaling steroids, always rinse mouth thoroughly after each treatment.

The proper use of *metered dose inhalers* (MDIs) was studied by Michael T. Newhouse, M.D., at the Regional Chest Unit, St. Joseph's Hospital, Hamilton, Ontario, Canada, and reported in *Bronkoscope*, vol. 2, no. 2, p. 6. Metered dose inhalers are the easiest and most efficient gadgets we now have to deliver aerosolized medication. Package instructions regarding assemblage and cleaning are very clear. Read them carefully. It behooves you to know the latest information on how to use MDIs with maximal efficiency. Dr. Newhouse's experiment was interesting. He made specially prepared inhalers containing radioactive material and then had volunteers hold them in various positions, inhaling and exhaling at various rates. Here's what he found: The single most important factor in efficient use of an inhaler is to keep the mouth open. The MDI should be held about one and a half inches from a wide-open mouth. Direct the nebulizer to the back of the mouth. Second, breathe out quietly just before releasing the dose and then breathe in as slowly as possible over five to six seconds, activating the nebulizer until you have reached the height of inspiration. Third, hold your breath as long as possible for a maximum of up to 10 seconds. Fourth, breathe out slowly.

Attachments called spacers are available for MDIs. They allow improved delivery of the medication by eliminating the necessity of synchronizing the discharge of aerosol with inspiration.

There are other new gadgets, such as the Ventolin Rotahaler, and some others we may have missed. Make sure that a knowledgeable person such as a respiratory therapist, your doctor, or his assistant shows you how to use each device correctly; and know exactly how to keep it clean and troubleshoot any minor problems.

As with any other medication, know exactly how much and how often when it comes to things you inhale.

OTHER IMPORTANT THERAPIES

Supplemental Oxygen

This is a wonderful drug and may be essential to your functioning. Some people worry about becoming addicted to oxygen. That can't happen. It is possible, however, for you to become extremely oxygen-sensitive and for too much oxygen to actually suppress your respirations. This will not happen if you follow your doctor's instructions. You should know about that in case your doctor wants a lower flow rate than you might like. In general, people use about one to two liters for sedentary activities and sleep, and three or four when moving vigorously. Some people need oxygen only at night, because they don't ventilate adequately during sleep; others need it only with exercise. Still others should use it continuously, because their oxygen level is always low.

One of the most exciting developments in the past few years has been the introduction of *trans-tracheal oxygen* (hereafter called TTO). In this method, oxygen is delivered directly into the trachea through a small catheter inserted in a series of steps. You might consider this opening similar to the tract made in an earlobe for pierced earrings.

The small catheter in the trachea delivers oxygen directly to the lungs, bypassing the nose and throat. No cannula need be worn on the face, and the tubing can be run under your clothing. It should be firmly attached to the belt with a clip, however. If the catheter does fall out by mistake and becomes contaminated, you need only return to an extra nasal cannula that you keep on your person until you can insert another trans-tracheal catheter. Two possible side effects of the trans-tracheal catheter are slight bleeding and "mucus balls." Mucus balls, although large and frightening in appearance, are usually benign and can be easily coughed up. With the TTO system, the oxygen dose may be cut by 50 percent at rest and 30 percent with effort. This means, in addition to the improved cosmetic appearance, there is improved mobility because of the chance to stay out longer.

Another system for delivery of oxygen is called the *implanted intratracheal catheter*. This catheter is similar to the trans-tracheal oxygen catheter in that it produces the same cost savings and longer-lasting benefits of low-flow oxygen. It has the additional advantage, however, of being completely invisible. In this procedure, the intratracheal catheter is implanted directly into the trachea after a small incision is made. The other end of the tube is then tunneled under the skin of the chest wall and exits the body, usually around the belt line. For the first three weeks after the oxygen catheter has been placed, you need to change the bandage at least every day, or whenever it becomes wet. Both trans-tracheal oxygen and intratracheal oxygen can produce improvements in cor pulmonale, the heart failure associated with COPD.

In addition to the TTO and intra-tracheal oxygen, there are delivery devices that synchronize oxygen delivery with inspiration. A synchronized canister may last as long as 17.2 hours at two liters per minute. The ability to stay out for 17 hours without a refill will greatly expand your horizons and improve your quality of life. Look for other pulsed oxygen-delivery conserving devices. Under the new federal regulations, your physician may designate pulsed delivery of oxygen.

Oxygen may be delivered from a central tank or from an oxygen enricher. Neither of these two devices is portable. There are, however, enrichers small enough to fit in the trunk of an automobile. The oxygen enricher contains no oxygen at all but extracts and concentrates oxygen from the air. You should get 50 feet of extra tubing to allow you extra mobility. If you are highly oxygen-dependent and using an enricher, you should have a small auxiliary tank in case of an electrical power failure.

In general, for people who desire mobility, we recommend the liquid oxygen system with a central tank and a portable auxiliary container, either with an over-the-shoulder strap or with a stroller, like a luggage carrier. The auxiliary tank contains up to eight hours of oxygen, depending on the liter flow you require.

When using oxygen, you should never be within five feet of a flame. Oxygen is *not* flammable, but it will greatly enhance the combustion of other substances. Follow the advice of your oxygen supplier.

Oxygen decreases the work of breathing and lessens the strain on your heart. It corrects a lack of blood oxygen that can otherwise occur when you don't breathe as deeply during sleep as you do during your waking hours. In addition, oxygen improves your ability to exercise, and more exercise means better muscle mass and more strength. The ability to exercise means a lot of other things, too. You'll read more about that in our special chapter covering the subject. Studies have shown that, when needed, the use of oxygen prolongs life; the more hours per day oxygen therapy is given, the better the survival.* As stated above, all patients with COPD, however, do not require supplementary oxygen. Your doctor is the best one to know whether you do or do not.

If you do require oxygen, make sure you know the exact liter flow required for sleep, sedentary activities, activities of daily living (including toileting), sex, and exercise.

Pursed-Lip Breathing

Pursed-lip breathing is a useful tool to keep your airways open. Breathe in through the nose and, on expiration, purse your lips, taking twice as long to breathe out, as though you were going to whistle. This does not allow the air to flow out of the bronchial tree as rapidly. Keeping the flow rate down keeps the pressure up, and this prevents airway collapse. Use pursed-lip breathing whenever you like, including during exercise. Do it if it makes you feel better, and disregard it if it doesn't.

*Increased survival has been demonstrated with greater than 14–16 hours of daily oxygen use when indicated.

Abdominal Breathing

By using pursed-lip breathing while doing abdominal breathing exercises, you can strengthen the function of the diaphragm and decrease the energy needed in breathing, reducing strain placed on the upper chest muscles. These relaxing exercises are easy to learn and don't take much energy. Begin by lying on your back with your hand on your abdomen. As you breathe in through the nose, you should feel your abdomen rise and then, as you exhale slowly through the mouth with pursed-lip breathing, the abdominal wall should relax and therefore fall. Another refinement is to place a small weight, such as two to 10 pounds, on the abdomen. Repeat the same exercises. You might repeat abdominal breathing while walking up stairs and while sitting. Breathing retraining, if it can be accomplished and incorporated into your daily life, may prove to be very helpful. You are aiming for slower and deeper, that is, abdominal, breathing. You want to pursue any course that will reduce the energy required to breathe effectively. Start by sitting in a chair and using abdominal breathing for five minutes twice a day.

Postural Drainage

Everything in this world runs better downhill than uphill, and with postural drainage you are trying to get your secretions to run downhill, to facilitate their removal. You should practice postural drainage right after you use your bronchodilator *if it is helpful* and results in increased clearing of secretions. If it does not, postural drainage is not necessary. Here are some simple postural drainage positions done in bed using two or three pillows (Fig. 3.1). Your doctor may prescribe others.

While you are doing postural drainage, if somebody is with you, cupping or vibration to the back may help to shake the secretions loose. In cupping, the fingers of the hands are held together like a cup and a gentle alternating tapping motion is made over the chest, or, alternatively, there are small, inexpensive back vibrators available. If cupping or vibration makes your ribs sore, desist—or modify so the motions are not as vigorous. Do cupping and vibration only on the rib cage. Avoid the spinal column, breast bone, and breasts. Do postural drainage on an empty stomach.

It is extremely important to clear the lungs of secretions effectively in order to reduce the volume of remaining secretions to the lowest possible amount. The use of bronchodilators, antibiotics, postural drainage, cupping, and vibration all aim to accomplish that end. With secretions out of the way, your passages are free to transport air. With secretions in the way, they're plugged up, just as we described in Chapter 1.

Fluids

Fluids, containing water, will help loosen secretions. Drinking six to eight glasses of water a day is generally acceptable and is thought to help thin out thick sputum. In some cases water restriction is necessary. It will then be prescribed by your doctor. Soda, tea, coffee, milk, and juices are predominantly water.

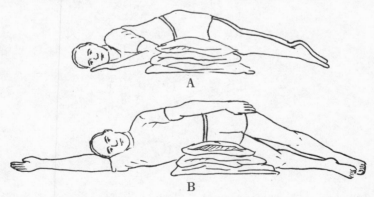

Figure 3.1   Postural Drainage. (A) First on your abdomen. (B) Then on each side. Remain in each position for five minutes and follow each position with a therapeutic cough.

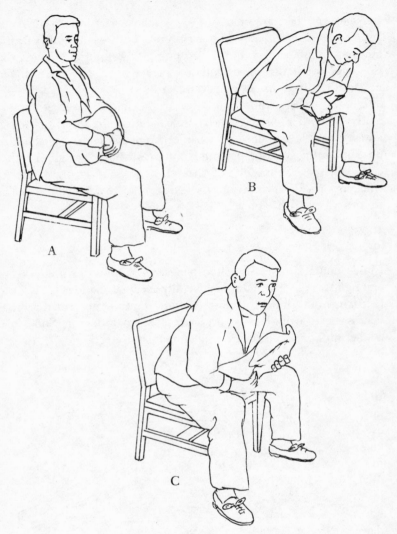

Figure 3.2   Therapeutic Cough: (A) Proper starting position, feet supported, shoulders relaxed, knees flexed. (B) Lean forward slowly, exhaling with pursed-lip breathing. (C) Final cough position, mouth open. See text for complete sequence.

Effective Coughing

A good therapeutic cough is another proven way to clear secretions (Fig. 3.2). Sit up, your head flexed forward, your shoulders relaxed in a slight forward position, your feet on the floor, a pillow held to your abdomen. Lean forward slowly, blowing out using pursed-lip breathing. Begin to sit up, and as you do so slowly "sniff" the air in, feeling your abdomen push out against the pillow. (Do not take fast breaths at this point. You want to get a nice column of air behind your mucus plugs to help push them out when you actually give your therapeutic cough.) Repeat three or four times, refraining from actually coughing. When you feel ready to cough, take a good, deep breath, pushing the pillow out, then lean forward once again, using gravity to help you. Begin your cough by making a false, stuttering (or staccato) cough, trying to get enough force present to maximize air flow and secretion outflow without causing airway collapse. Keep your mouth open while coughing (but please prevent infection of others by using a handkerchief). Do a therapeutic cough after completing each postural drainage position.

SELF-EVALUATION:
A THREE-MINUTE DAILY PHYSICAL EXAM

In addition to becoming fully informed about drugs and supplementary therapy, you have to be capable of performing a good physical examination on yourself for early detection of problems. You want to know exactly how you're doing and when additional therapy or a visit to the doctor might be important. With a little practice, three minutes or less a day will do it. You'll soon become an expert and pick up minor changes in yourself that could be significant long before you might be going to the doctor for your appointment. Here's your daily physical exam explained in detail. We'll follow it with an easy-to-record chart. Do your physical at the same time each day if you can.

1. Take your resting pulse (ideally, you should have been sitting for at least five minutes and not exercising for at least half an hour) for 30 seconds and multiply by two. (For how to take your pulse, see Chapter 6.)
2. Check your respiratory rate for 30 seconds and multiply by two. Respiratory rates vary widely, especially when you are concentrating on them. After doing this every day, you'll soon learn the variations that are acceptable for you.
3. Put your hand on the back of your neck and then on your forehead; learn to know when you feel hot. Take your temperature if you are uncertain or not feeling up to par.
4. Test your cough—that is, give a resounding cough and listen. Having no sputum is normal. You should know what your baseline cough is; only then can you determine if the volume of your secretions might be increasing. This is a critical part of your daily physical exam, for the increase in the volume of secretions heralds the onset of a relapse. Grade your test cough 0 to 4+.
5. Sputum check. As you cough, expectorate into a clear plastic or glass container. You will need to check three items. First, check the sputum volume. Grade 0 to 4+. Second, note sputum thickness and grade 0 to 4+, with 0 being none to extremely thin and 4+ being thick and sticky sputum that sticks to the bottom of the container when you turn it over. Last, check the sputum color, with 0 being virtually clear and 4+ being puslike, yellow, gray, or green. Two plus and 3+ indicate intermediate changes.

   An additional word about sputum volume: If you can't tell from your morning cough whether your volume is up or down, measure your full 24-hour sputum by coughing consistently into the same cup. Date the cup, cover well, and check your sputum volume from day to day. Make your own scale of 0 to 4+ based on these measurements. Keeping 24-hour sputums for four days will give you a good start.

6. Wheezing. This is a sound made by air usually in expiration moving through a partially blocked bronchial tube. Usually expiration becomes longer and more difficult and there may or may not be an actual audible sound. Grade wheezing or a wheezing sensation 0 to 4+.

7. Edema (fluid accumulation in the tissues) check. Press your thumb down into the skin over your lower shin or on the side of your ankle, holding while you count to three slowly, then release. Is there a depression or "pit"? If so, you are collecting water in your legs. Know how much edema you usually have (we all frequently have a slight amount if we look for it) on a good day. Grade 0 to 4+.

8. Weight. Step on the scale and record your weight at the same time dressed the same way each day. Know what is an allowable variation for you, usually within a three-pound shift up or down.

9. Measurement of peak flow. For this you will need a peak flow meter, an inexpensive simple device available from drug and medical supply stores that measures, in liters per minute, the maximum velocity of air leaving the lungs during one forced exhalation. Take a deep breath in and blow out into a home peak flow meter as hard and as fast as you can. Record the value on the chart. You might want to do your peak flow more than once, until you are sure you have a correct value.

10. Functional capacity. Walk rather briskly around the room. Stretch and think about yourself. How do you feel in an overall way? Is your chest tight and constricted? Are you mobilizing or producing secretions easily? Can you walk around the room without undue difficulty? Do you feel calm as opposed to tense and anxious? Do you have air hunger as opposed to what you consider to be "normal" respiration? Look at yourself critically. You will have ups and downs, and you must learn what minor variations require no change in your treatment and what changes in

your breathing pattern, respiratory rate, and functional capacity are significant. Call your functional capacity poor, good, or excellent, or perhaps you rate yourself fair. The use of the terms is flexible as long as you know what they mean.

SELF-EVALUATION DIARY

Here's a diary (see Table 3.2) to help you record your physical examination. Note that you may have to keep the diary for a whole week to be able to fill in columns one and two, "Examination Findings on a Good Day" and "Usual Variation." Also note that once you are used to keeping the diary you may "look back" at information in columns one and two, and in subsequent weeks you need only record the daily changes.

Another excellent method of self-evaluation is to keep a multiple peak flow chart. Let's say that on arising, at midday, and in the evening you measure your peak flow and chart it (see Fig. 3.3). Note that in the example we give, the peak flow is lowest in the morning and improves throughout the day. If this is so for you, could the environment in the bedroom or accumulated secretions be contributing to your symptoms?

Additionally, peak flows may drop abruptly before asthmatic attacks when there is no other symptomatology present. You and your physician may wish to utilize this early warning sign.

A DAILY THERAPEUTIC TECHNIQUE

Pulmonary toilette is a form of chest physical therapy coupled with the effective use of a bronchodilator. Its aim is to prevent or ameliorate bronchospasm and facilitate the removal of secretions. Begin with a hot drink, which helps loosen secretions.

Follow this by inhaling a bronchodilator and moisture (e.g., steam) if prescribed for you. Next comes postural drainage. Postural drainage is advisable when there are poorly produced secretions and

TABLE 3.2

Sample Self-evaluation Diary

Week of _____

		Examination Findings on a Good Day	Usual Variation	Mon	Tues	Wed	Thurs	Fri	Sat	Sun
Resting pulse		80	80-95	90						
Resting respiratory rate		20	16-24	18						
Temperature by touch		Normal	—	Norm.						
Test cough	0-4+	1+	0-2+	1+						
Sputum volume	0-4+	1+	1-2+	1+						
Sputum thickness	0-4+	1+	1-2+	2+						
Sputum color	0-4+	1+	1-2+	1+						
Wheezing	0-4+	0	0-1+	0						
Edema	0-4+	0	0	0						
Weight		160	157-160	158						
Measurement of peak flow		300 liters per minute	150-300	250						
Functional Capacity Poor Good Excellent		G	G-E	G						

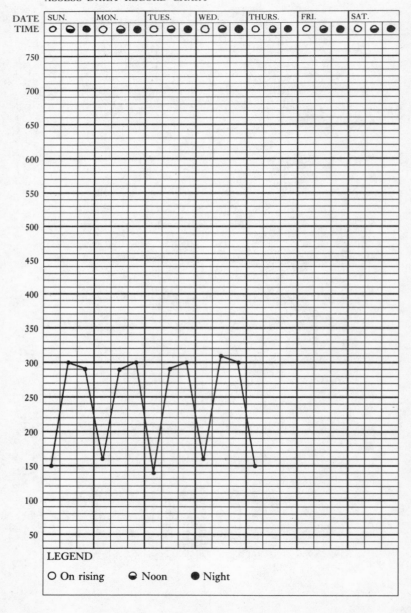

Figure 3.3 Multiple Peak Flow Chart

NAME:

DATE TIME	SUN.			MON.			TUES.			WED.			THURS.			FRI.			SAT.		

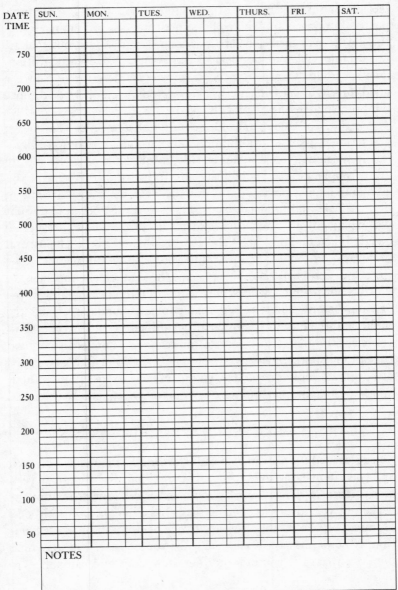

750
700
650
600
550
500
450
400
350
300
250
200
150
100
50

NOTES

when it helps you. If, after three days of postural drainage you do not feel better (i.e., clearer), it would probably be useless to continue postural drainage, but you could reinstitute postural drainage anytime, whenever secretions are increased. Use the positions that are most comfortable and practical for you. As you change each position, do a controlled therapeutic cough (previously described). Now is a good time to inhale beclomethasone or cromolyn if prescribed, since the bronchial tree is maximally cleared.

A regimen of pulmonary toilette is advised four times a day only if you have excessive sputum production (or mucus secretion). Practically speaking, you may not be able to squeeze it all in. If you are away from home, you should have an MDI with you. Wherever you are, go to a quiet place, even if it is the women's or men's room, sit down, inhale your bronchodilator, and at least put your head down if you have sputum production and try to give a good therapeutic cough. If you find that you feel exceptionally well after each postural drainage, you should try to commit yourself to a full regimen four times a day. If postural drainage helps, it is extremely important to do this full regimen at least in the morning on arising and in the evening before going to bed. Secretions accumulate during the night, and the morning is frequently a difficult time for you. Allow yourself 30 minutes to complete the regimen. This is also a good time to add another glass or cup of hot liquid. By drinking two cups of hot liquid four times a day, you fit in your extra ration without another thought. Do pulmonary toilette on an empty stomach.

MANIPULATING YOUR MEDICATIONS

You've learned the uses and side effects of all the medicines you take, and you can make an intelligent self-evaluation; now we can go yet a step further. *With your doctor's permission,* you can learn to manipulate certain of your drugs at specific times based on your own physical examination. To do this, you need your doctor's absolute cooperation. If he or she says it isn't right for you, it isn't. You may find, however, that once you indicate your knowledge and willingness to help in your care, the doctor is more than happy to allow you this latitude. Perhaps you already have a supply of antibiotics to take whenever the volume of your secretions increases. Here are some of the ways that medications can be manipulated safely and the specific times and the specific symptoms or physical findings that would warrant such changes.

1. You may not require full therapeutic doses of bronchodilators on a daily basis; during attacks of acute wheezing, you may be instructed to increase the number of tablets of your bronchodilator (e.g., Alupent, Ventolin, etc.) by one or two tablets a day, risking some nervousness or shakiness.

   Another way to maximize bronchodilator effect is to increase the number of inhalations a day from the metered dose inhaler (i.e., increase from two breaths four times a day to two breaths every four hours). You may not be at the maximum number of drops for the bronchodilator you use in the updraft nebulizer, and the frequency of use there might also be increased by your physician from four times a day to every four hours day and night. Pre-exercise use of inhaled bronchodilator may prevent or minimize exercise-induced wheezing.

2. Whenever the volume of your secretions increases significantly or whenever there is a consistency or color change you definitely associate with a relapse, you may be allowed to take antibiotics, which you keep on hand specifically for that purpose, for seven to 10 days.

3. Instructions to avoid a prolonged attack of wheezing may be, for example, to take six extra tablets of prednisone early on and then decrease the daily dose by one tablet every several days thereafter, providing you feel better, until you are back to your maintenance dose or off prednisone entirely.

4. Are you a person who gains water weight? You usually know this by a weight gain of more than three pounds or a

noticeable "pit" on self-examination. Doctors frequently allow patients to take an extra one to two tablets of diuretic on those days, along with an increase in supplemental potassium. If you do take supplemental potassium now, let's say 20–40 milliequivalents per day, here's an easy way to tell how much extra to take. Measure all your urine output for 12–24 hours after taking extra diuretics. For every quart of urine over two quarts (your usual daily output) you might require 20 extra milliequivalents of potassium.

5. Cromolyn sodium can be increased before and during your bad seasons if you have allergies. The number of puffs of beclomethasone can also be increased. Cromolyn sodium and inhaled steroids are not useful during acute attacks of wheezing. They prevent future attacks. They may also be used to prevent attacks of exertional asthma when taken in advance of the effort.

6. Expectorants such as guaifenesin can be increased or added to your daily regimen whenever your secretions thicken.

7. With an exacerbation of your illness you may require more oxygen. A typical regimen when you have increased difficulty in breathing might be: to sleep and sit, one to two liters; to eat and to walk slowly, three to four liters; to defecate and to perform activities of daily living, three to four liters.

Now it's time to have a talk with your doctor about this whole business of changing your medication during an acute exacerbation of your illness. For that, we've provided a sample chart called the Therapeutic Manipulation Chart (see Fig. 3.4). Really a detailed patient instruction form, it's purely optional between you and your doctor. Perhaps you already have instructions to change some drugs in case of a relapse or wheeze. The number and names of medications you manipulate may change at any time, depending on what works and what doesn't work for new changes in your condition. Use this chart to work out allowable changes in regimen with your physician.

To utilize the chart properly, fill in the names and usual doses of your medications in the first column. (We have completed column two for you.) Your doctor can then scan your drug regimen, checking yes or no and filling out the details on the "yes" drugs. This chart is a sample only and does not apply to any particular individual. *Your* chart should be developed with your physician.

RELAPSE AND PROGRESS— KEEPING TRACK

Shouldn't you let bygones be bygones and put relapses out of mind and concentrate on the good times? In spirit, yes; in documentation, no. You want to pin down exactly what happened before and during a relapse—what was done and what worked (and what didn't). You must be a good detective so that, when the same syndrome happens again, you can share with your physician the information you've got stashed away.

It's important to follow your progress toward recovery when you have a bad spell. Record events accurately in a Relapse Progress Diary (see Fig. 3.5). If you need to, keep an allergy record as well.

WHEN TO CALL THE DOCTOR

You know you should call the doctor when you are extremely short of breath, feel very ill, have a high temperature or chest pain, or cough up blood. What we're talking about here is calling the doctor *before* you become this ill, when the signs and symptoms are just beginning. Remember, early treatment of a true relapse is a key to successful therapy. You obviously have to make some choices; you can't call the doctor for every symptom or sign. However, after reading this chapter, you are in a position to make educated decisions. Let's say you have completed your physical exam for the day and note abnormalities that although perhaps not immediately alarming should now alert you to the fact that you may be suffering a relapse. Do you have any instructions on your therapeutic manip-

Date: _____

Patient please complete ▶

Doctor please complete ▶ ▶ ▶

Drugs Name/usual dose, if any	Reasons Why You Might Manipulate the Drug	Suggested Manipulation	No	Yes	(Dr. please elaborate if necessary)
Bronchodilator tablet: *theophylline* 250 mgs. 2x/day (fill in name/dose)	Increased wheezing and shortness of breath	__ extra tablets __ x per day	X		
Bronchodilator spray: *albuterol*, 2 inhalations every 6 hr. (fill in name/dose)	Increased wheezing and shortness of breath	Increase to 2 breaths every 4 hr.		X	while awake until improved and then reduce to usual dose. Stop and notify me if you notice a rapid or irregular heart action
Bronchodilator drops: (fill in name/dose)	Increased wheezing and shortness of breath	Increase by __ drop(s) and use every __ hr.			
Antibiotic: *doxycycline*, 100 mg. (fill in name/dose)	Increase in thickness or volume of sputum; significant color change; fever	1 tablet(s) every 12 hr. x 10 days		X	Call me y/no improvement within 36 hours
Steroid: *prednisone*, 5 mg 2x/day (fill in name/dose)	Increased wheezing and shortness of breath	Take 6 tablet(s) x 2 days, then decrease by 1 tablet(s) every 2 days until baseline dose		X	Divided into 2 daily doses if necessary—otherwise take in one dose before breakfast. Notify me within 14 hours of beginning this regimen

54

Drugs Name/usual dose, if any	Reasons Why You Might Manipulate the Drug	Suggested Manipulation	No	Yes	(Dr. please elaborate if necessary)
Diuretic: _furosemide,_ _40 mg/day_ (fill in name/dose)	Increased edema (water accumulation)	____ extra tablets daily x ____ days			_Call me if edema occurs or daily weight increases by 3 pounds_
Expectorant: _____ (fill in name/dose)	Increased thickness of sputum	____ tbsp./tablets ____ x per day x ____ days			
Other:					

Figure 3.4   Therapeutic Manipulation Chart

55

Figure 3.5

Relapse Progress Diary

Dates: _____ to _____

Changing Signs/Symptoms	Measures Taken	What Happened
Resting pulse 120	1) 3/4/91 postural drainage increased to every 4 hours.	3/4/91 chest tight but no severe distress
Respiratory rate 30	2) steam added	sputum greenish, large volume
Temperature 101	3) ampicillin, 500 mg every 6 hours	3/5/91 volume sputum less, color gray, less tightness
Test cough secretions 3+	4) increased fluids to 8 glasses per day.	P^a 115 R^b 24 T^c 98.6
Sputum volume 3+		
Sputum thickness 3+	5) albuterol spray increased to 2 inhalations every 4 hours	3/6/91 definitely better—secretions thinner—not so tight, no temp.
Sputum color change 2+		
Wheezing 2+		P 110 R 20 T 98.6
Edema 0	6) prednisone, 6 tabs 3/4/85 — then ↓ by 1 every 2 days	3/7/91 almost back to self P 100 R 16 T 98.6
Weight same	7) physician called 3/4/91, 3/5/91, 3/6/91, to call back if not back to baseline by 3/10	3/8/91 better P 90 R 16 T 98.6
Functional capacity poor		3/9/91 back to baseline P 85 R 16 T 98.6

^{a}P = pulse rate
^{b}R = respiratory rate
^{c}T = temperature

56

ulation chart? If so, follow them! Continue to assess your physical condition every few hours throughout the day if necessary.

Are things getting better, or worse? It takes 24 to 36 hours for sputum to begin to return to normal after an antibiotic is started. Temperature should abate within 24 to 36 hours. After a diuretic is taken, improvement in edema should occur within a few hours to a day. If your pulse is, for example, 10 beats above your normal variation, this may not come down until wheezing and shortness of breath lessen and your sputum returns to a more normal thickness, volume, and color. If your pulse remains persistently above its normal variation and you are feeling worse, let your doctor know.

If a positive finding on your physical exam indicates to you that you are on the verge of a significant relapse, or when, having manipulated your medications to the best of your ability, you realize that you are not getting better, your doctor should hear from you.

Perhaps you're not gasping, but you know you're not well either, and at the moment it's too complicated for you to figure out whether you should be increasing your diuretics, steroids, bronchodilator, or whatever else is on your instruction sheet. You can still call the doctor and explain your physical findings. Have your medication chart ready and any ideas that you might have as to what usually helps you when you have these physical findings. Your doctor's advice will be much more effective if you, or your spouse, call and clearly explain the problem: "Doctor, my overall functional capacity appears to be decreased. I have a thick cough, and my sputum has turned gray-green. My pulse is up over its usual level by 20 beats a minute, and my respiratory rate is higher by four breaths a minute. I have no fever. My weight is up by four pounds. What do you suggest? Do you think I should take an antibiotic and one extra tablet of my diuretic? Am I sick enough to come in for a visit?"

How can you be sure? Ask your doctor when you should call, and do this well in advance of any possible need for such a call. Show your doctor the physical exam checklist. He or she might want to add or subtract from it. If, for instance, you always have about 1+ or 2+ fluid in your legs, let's say, from chronic venous disease, you may not have to call him or do anything if the swelling in your legs increases a little bit. Your responsibility—and your doctor can share it with you—is to know when to call the doctor early in a relapse.

Chapter 4

Self-Protection

Prevention is the best treatment of all. Self-protection deserves a major commitment on your part. Here are some of the hazards to learn about so that you know how to cope with them or avoid them completely.

WEATHER CONDITIONS

Nature dictates that we maintain our body temperature at about 98.6°F. If body temperature rises above normal, heart work is increased and blood vessels in the skin dilate to eliminate the excess heat. If it is above 83° outside, no vigorous walking or exercising is advisable unless the humidity is very low. The body maintains normal temperature by evaporation of fluid or sweating; evaporation of sweat cools the body. When the air, however, is filled with water, it is much more difficult, and this process is less efficient. Therefore, before exercising outside, check the temperature and humidity (see Fig. 4.1).

From studying the chart you can see that when the temperature is 75° and the humidity is 60 percent, you are entering the danger zone. If you are like most of our patients with significant COPD, you should definitely not exercise outside. An air conditioner that reduces the surrounding temperature as well as the humidity is impor-

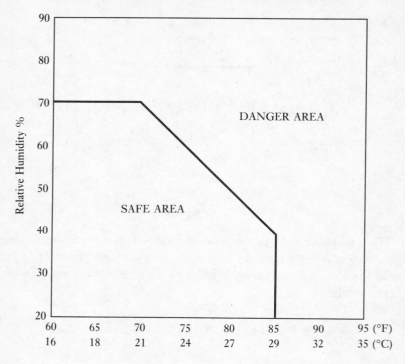

Fig 4.1 Air Temperature

tant for you. On the other hand, when the temperature is down around 70°, the ideal humidity is between 40 and 60 percent. You should try to keep your home at this temperature the year round. Your secretions will be the loosest, and your body will work efficiently.

Excessive cold stresses the body's ability to maintain its normal temperature. The older we get, the more difficult it is for us to keep our temperature at 98.6° when the environment is very cold. In addition, for many patients with COPD, cold air can induce an attack of bronchospasm. Do not go out for any length of time if the temperature is below 25°F. When exposing yourself to cold in the winter, make sure you're wearing a hat pulled down over the ears, since a great deal of circulation goes through the scalp. Use mittens instead of gloves, since one finger can warm the other. To warm inspired air, use a scarf over the face, tucked under the brim of your hat, or a cold-weather face mask, easily obtained at drugstores. Long underwear designed to wick away sweat is advisable, since sweating following exertion in a cold atmosphere results in an icelike fluid on your skin and you may become hypothermic. Dress in layers (see Chapter 6 for suggestions).

The windchill factor is announced throughout the day on radio and television and is a measure of the cooling effect of windy conditions. You lose more heat when the wind is blowing than when it is calm. Therefore, the windchill factor expresses the effective temperature for you in terms of the prevailing coldness as well as the speed of the wind. Consult the Windchill Chart (Fig. 4.2) to note when it's either safe or dangerous for prolonged time in the cold.

OUTDOOR POLLUTION

Smog and air pollution are very dangerous and can result in wheezing, airway injury, loss of precious functional capacity, and sometimes even death.

Beware of sulfur oxides in the air, especially near power plants, oil refineries, smelters, paper pulp mills, and wineries. Oxides of nitrogen pollute air near power plants and oil refineries and are extruded from automobile exhausts, which also produce ozone.

Exposure to grain dust (in the vicinity of grain elevators) and castor bean dust (near castor bean plants) has been known to result in asthma.

Pollens are important sources of air pollution. Hay fever, caused by ragweed, for instance, can affect up to 5 to 10 percent of the population of the United States. Ragweed is prevalent in the North Atlantic states from August through October, in the Great Plains from July to October, and in California from June to September. Know which trees, grasses, and weeds are prevalent at each season of the year in your area and protect yourself accordingly. In your "bad

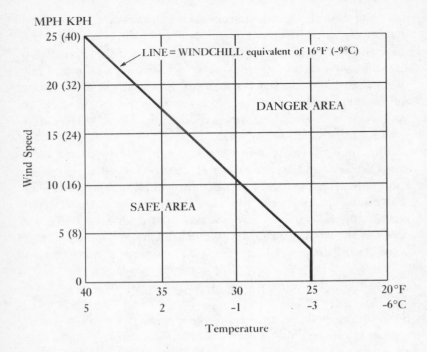

Figure 4.2   Windchill Chart

seasons," protect yourself by using pollen masks (available at drug-stores), air conditioners, and air filters and purifiers and by staying inside. A particularly good mask is one that contains a carbon shell. This mask has the advantage of protecting against low-level chemical exposures as well as the usual noxious dusts and pollens.

Do not go out in the smog, and avoid walking outside when the traffic is extremely heavy. In Dallas, for instance, the air may contain 248 tons of acetone, 8 tons of ammonia, 69 tons of freon, 5 tons of sodium bicarbonate, 102 tons of toluene, 189 tons of tri-chlorethylene, and 65 tons of xylene. Walk outdoors in the early morning, and avoid altogether any dusty outside atmosphere. The air quality index, issued by the Weather Bureau, is a composite of the national ambient air quality standard and measures ozone, carbon monoxide, sulfur dioxide, nitrogen oxide, particulates, and lead. No other substances are measured. An air quality index of 0–50 is good, 50–100 moderate, 100–200 unhealthy, 200–300 very unhealthy, and 300–500 hazardous. This measurement is based only on the substance with the highest level and does not measure the cumulative affect of all pollutants. Therefore, let your body be your guide.

The air quality index may be acceptable, but if you don't feel well outdoors, get indoors and into an air-conditioned and preferably air-filtered room.

Be advised that there is danger at gasoline pumps. Many of the most toxic chemicals in outdoor air can be traced to gasoline. Gasoline, which contains benzene and toluene, tends to vaporize at the pump. This is especially true of some self-serve stations. Benzene can be a potent carcinogen and has been implicated in causing leukemia and lymphoma, as well as irritation to the respiratory tract and asthma. Be sure to keep gasoline off your skin, stand upwind from the gas pump, roll up your windows, and choose stations that have vapor recovery lines. These appear to be accordionlike bellows on the nozzle.

Chemical sprays on your lawn or on your neighbor's may trigger attacks of COPD. Avoid chemical sprays on your own lawn and trees, and ask your neighbors to warn you before their property is sprayed with chemicals. If your area is undergoing aerial spraying with pesticides for any reason, such as fruit flies in California, try to leave the area. If you are housebound, close all windows and doors tightly, using duct tape to seal them if necessary, and stay in a room with an air purifier on maximum and an air conditioner. The air purifier should be designed to filter chemical fumes as well as dust and pollen. On your own lawn, we recommend using alternative nontoxic measures.

Do not allow leaves to accumulate in the fall, because they can decay and support growth of molds, which thrive on decaying leaves.

Wind conditions are important. The most healthful atmosphere is probably that in which there is a gentle breeze. When wind speed is less than five miles per hour, pollutants tend to accumulate and hover over the ground. Above 15 miles per hour there is an increased concentration of mold and dust in the air.

If you are a swimmer, take care around swimming pools, outdoor as well as indoor. Chlorine is an irritant to the lower respiratory tract and the nasal passages. If you have a sensitive respiratory tract, it may not be at all advisable for you to swim in a chlorinated pool, or even to sit by one. As always, you must be your own detective. Keep chlorine in mind. We'll have more to say about this potent and potentially sensitizing irritant in our section on indoor air pollution.

INDOOR POLLUTION

Beware of sulfur oxides, emitted in large amounts from kerosene space heaters, and nitrogen oxides emitted from kerosene heaters or stoves and stoves burning natural gas, wood, or coal. The indoor allergens, irritants, and triggering agents are many. Be aware that these include animal dander, house dust mite fecal antigens, common household cleaning chemicals such as those containing chlorine (bleach) or ammonia, perfumes, deodorants, hair sprays, detergents, scented soaps, scented toiletries, pesticide sprays, floor polishes and waxes, furniture polish and waxes, and all other household cleaning agents made from petroleum products or emitting irritant fumes. If you can smell it, the product may be causing or contributing to your respiratory problems.

Air pollution can also cause cancer if, for example, one inhales arsenic near sources such as smelters or polycyclic hydrocarbons, which are emitted from diesel engines and petroleum refineries. Arsenic, also present in tobacco smoke, is found in high concentrations indoors, along with radon daughters emitted from construction materials and asbestos from ceiling and floor tiles, sprayed-on insulation, and the insulation outside and at times inside boilers and heating ducts. The incidence of lung cancer is higher in families of asbestos workers and among nonsmoking spouses of smokers as opposed to spouses of nonsmokers.

Smoke—and by this we mean other people's smoking—is a hazard you *must* avoid. If a person sharing a home with you smokes, it's as though you were exposed to a minimum of 10 cigarettes a day. Do not stay in the same room with anyone smoking. Put up No Smoking signs in your home and throw out any ashtrays. If friends want to smoke, ask them to step outside. If your mate smokes, the same applies. Your atmosphere needs to be smoke-free.

Although the tight or sick building syndrome usually refers to illness at work, take care that your home in general is not making you sick. In recent years, coincident with the growth of the chemical industry and the need to economize on fuel costs, we all made our homes and office buildings as airtight as possible. In addition, many older buildings, especially older government buildings, have inadequate ventilation systems. A hospital, for instance, may have 800 chemicals present in the atmosphere in tiny amounts. This combination of increased volatile chemicals and poor or decreased ventilation may result in a number of symptoms including respiratory irritation. Other symptoms that have been described are irritation of the eyes, a tight feeling in the chest, unusual fatigue, depression, an inability to concentrate, joint and muscle pains, headache, itching ears, a feeling of claustrophobia, hives, and skin rashes. Even forgetfulness, diarrhea, irritability, and impaired reading comprehension have been described. The symptoms may vary from individual to individual, and only one person or whole groups may be affected, so if you don't feel well at work, think: "Could my workplace be contributing to my illness?" But if you don't feel good at home and feel good at work, you should think just the opposite: "Could my home be contributing to my illness?" So think about it. Do you feel better outdoors than indoors? If so, do you feel better indoors at home or indoors at work? How do you feel in your cellar? In your bedroom? Your kitchen? How about various buildings or rooms at work? Multiple peak flow measurements may be of great help in making a proper assessment not only of when, but also of where, you have the most difficulty.

Hobbies can be culprits. The list of arts and crafts materials that can cause lung damage is long. They include the following:

- solvents found in lacquers and other thinners, paint removers, cleaners, and other materials
- metals such as lead, cadmium, and uranium found in pigments, pottery glazes, solders, photochemicals, and alloys
- mineral dusts like crystalline silica and asbestos found in stones, clays, and pottery glazes
- gases such as chlorine, nitrogen dioxide, and sulfur dioxide produced as a by-product of welding, photo processing, kiln and foundry firings, and similar processes
- chemicals such as acids and alkalis used in a variety of arts and crafts processes, including etching, photography, and, textile dyeing*

If your hobby is important to you and you need to protect yourself, wear a protective mask. Masks can be purchased from industrial supply and safety firms.

Make sure ventilation is more than adequate when engaging in a hobby with even the slightest potential for lung damage.

Talcum powder and hairspray may be inhaled into the lungs. Forget hairsprays and body powders; they may aggravate your breathing difficulty.

OCCUPATIONAL HAZARDS

Your job could be adversely affecting your lungs, nose, or sinuses. Repetitive inhalation or absorption of any number of various chemicals or substances, even in extremely small amounts, may produce classic asthma or exacerbate your chronic COPD, sinusitis, or rhinitis, and, as we have said before, sinusitis and rhinitis can in itself exacerbate COPD. Failure to recognize occupational asthma may result in permanent disability. Check your occupation against the following causes of occupational asthma (see Table 4.1).

*Information reproduced from *American Lung Association Bulletin* 69, no. 3 (May/June 1983).

TABLE 4.1

Causes of Occupational Asthma

Agent	Occupation
Animal products, insects, others	
Laboratory animals (rats, mice, rabbits, guinea pigs)	laboratory worker, veterinarian, animal handler
Birds	
Pigeon, budgerigar	pigeon breeder
Chicken	poultry worker
	bird fancier
Insects	
Grain mite	grain worker
Locust	research laboratory worker
River fly	power plant crew along rivers
Screw worm fly	flight crew
Cockroach	laboratory worker
Cricket	field contact
Bee moth	fish bait breeder
Moth and butterfly	entomologist
Plants	
Grain dust	grain handler
Wheat/rye flour	baker, miller
Buckwheat	baker
Coffee beans	food processor
Castor bean	oil industry worker
Tea	tea worker
Tobacco leaf	tobacco manufacturing worker
Hops *(Humulus lupulus)*	brewery chemist
Biologic enzymes	
B. subtilis	detergent industry worker
Trypsin	plastic, pharmaceutical worker
Pancreatin	pharmaceutical worker
Papain	laboratory, packaging worker
Pepsin	pharmaceutical worker
Flaviastase	pharmaceutical worker
Bromelin	pharmaceutical worker
Fungal amylase	manufacturing worker, baker

Agent	Occupation
Vegetables	
Gums	
Gum acacia	printer
Gum tragacanth	gum manufacturing worker
Others	
Crab	crab processor
Prawns	prawn processor
Hoya	oyster farmer
Larva of silkworm	sericulturist
Diisocyanates	
Toluene diisocyanate	polyurethane industries, plastics, varnish worker
Diphenylmethane diisocyanate	foundry worker
Hexamethylene diisocyanate	automobile spray painter
Anhydrides	
Phthalic anhydride	epoxy resin, plastics worker
Trimellitic anhydride	epoxy resin, plastics worker
Tetrachlorophthalic anhydride	epoxy resin, plastics worker
Wood dust	
Western red cedar (*Thuja plicata*)	carpenter, construction worker, cabinet maker, sawmill worker
California redwood (*Sequoia sempervirens*)	
Cedar of Lebanon (*Cedra libani*)	
Cocabolla (*Dalbergia retusa*)	
Iroko (*Chlorophora excelsa*)	
Oak (*Quercus robur*)	
Mahogany (*Shoreal* sp)	
Abiruana (*Pouteria*)	
African maple (*Triplochiton scleroxylon*)	
Metals	
Platinum	platinum refinery worker
Nickel	metal plater
Chromium	tanner
Cobalt	hard metal industry worker
Vanadium	hard metal industry worker
Tungsten carbide	hard metal industry worker
Fluxes	
Aminoethyl ethanolamine	aluminum solderer
Colophony	electronics worker

Agent	Occupation
Drugs	
Penicillins	pharmaceutical worker
Cephalosporins	pharmaceutical worker
Phenylglycine acid chloride	pharmaceutical worker
Piperazine hydrochloride	chemist
Psyllium	laxative manufacturer
Methyldopa	pharmaceutical worker
Spiramycin	pharmaceutical worker
Salbutamol intermediate	pharmaceutical worker
Amprolium HCl	poultry feed mixer
Tetracycline	pharmaceutical worker
Sulphone chloramides	manufacturer, brewery worker
Other chemicals	
Dimethyl ethanolamine	spray painter
Persulphate salts and henna	hairdresser
Ethylene diamine	photographer
Azodicarbonamide	plastics and rubber worker
Dioazonium salt	photocopying and dye worker
Hexachlorophene (sterilizing agent)	hospital staff
Formalin	hospital staff
Urea formaldehyde	insulation, resin worker
Freon	refrigeration worker
Paraphenylene diamine	fur dyer
Furfuryl alcohol (furan-based resin)	foundry mold maker

CONTROLLING YOUR ENVIRONMENT

Home

You spend at least 10 hours a day at home (mostly in the bedroom). You may be sensitive or "allergic" to many more things than you ever realized. Sensitivities or allergies to foreign substances contribute to bronchospasm. Try to remove sources of dust, mold, feathers, animal dander, and other allergens and irritating substances from the environment. Here are some suggestions. Use the ones you believe are pertinent for you, and before you pass these suggestions off as unimportant and too much trouble, remember: House dust, scents, fumes from petroleum-based products, chlorine, pesticides, and other common household agents can be unexpected culprits in relapses of COPD. Remember, once again, your bedroom and bathroom should be your refuge. When you sleep at night, you should get the cleanest, purest, most unadulterated air possible. After you have had a hard day or been exposed to an irritating substance or substance to which you are allergic, you should be able to shower off, wash your hair, and go into your refuge. The following suggestions apply to your whole home, but especially to your refuge, your bedroom and bathroom.

BED.
1. Some authorities recommend using zippered, allergen-proof covers (usually plastic) on pillows, mattresses, and box springs and sealing the zippers with heavy tape. Plastic, however, may emit respiratory irritants. An alternate method is to cover the mattress with a cotton barrier cloth, putting a mattress pad over that, and washing the mattress pad every month. A word of caution about mattresses: New mattresses, especially, contain flame retardants and pesticide residues that may be disturbing to the respiratory tract. The true hypoallergenic mattress is made of washed organic cotton with 100-percent-cotton ticking and no added chemicals. To allow the manufacturer to omit chemicals from the mattress, you need a doctor's prescription.
2. Do not store anything under the bed.
3. Use blankets and pillows made of 100-percent cotton. Blankets should be washed to remove sizing. If you can smell any odor in the blanket at all, soak it overnight in the washing machine with some vinegar in the water and wash several times in a nontoxic fume-emitting detergent. The blankets may then be placed in a cotton duvet. Wash the duvet every month or so, and in that way your blankets will stay dust-free.
4. Use a short cotton comforter (no feathers) if needed for

extra warmth instead of a bedspread. Once again, take care that no odor is emitted from the comforter.
5. Use 100-percent cotton, preferably uncolored, sheets. Wash all sizing out with the method described for cotton blankets.
6. Do not sleep in a bedroom next to the garage.

WINDOWS. Buy only washable cotton curtains. Avoid venetian blinds and draperies.

FLOORS. Avoid shaggy carpets. House dust and house dust mites and their fecal particles, as well as mold, may abound in carpets, causing asthma and instability in chronic bronchitis sufferers. It is desirable to avoid *all* carpets. If, however, you already have a carpeted floor, try the following method to reduce house dust mites.

To test for the presence of house dust mites, use the Acarex test, available in drugstores. If the mites are present, spread Acarosan, also available from the druggist, on the carpet and leave it on overnight before vacuuming it off. Acarosan may keep the carpet free of the mites for months at a time, and you can check by doing the Acarex test.

Ordinary vacuum cleaners may actually stir dust up and help it spread throughout your home. There are also exceptionally efficient vacuum cleaners made especially for those people who need to have thorough removal of molds and dust. For everyday cleaning when dust is low, a lightweight electric broom may be adequate and a lot more portable. The ideal floor is made of natural stone, such as Mexican pavers, ceramic tile, or wood covered with a nontoxic fume-emitting sealer. Remember, a foam carpet backing may be hypoallergenic in the sense that it does not contain animal hair, but it may emit formaldehyde.

FURNITURE. Use 100-percent cotton canvas and avoid leather (especially new leather) upholstery. It's best to use older furniture in the bedroom and in your home in general. If you wish to refurbish the furniture, use nontoxic fume-emitting sealers.

71

MISCELLANEOUS.

1. Use washable paint or wallpaper on the walls.
2. Avoid pictures and wall hangings.
3. Keep closet doors shut. Do not hang recently dry-cleaned clothes in the closet. Dry-cleaned clothes should be placed elsewhere for a period of at least three months in a well-ventilated space away from living areas.
4. Keep dust catchers—such as books, knickknacks, stuffed animals, and toys—to a minimum.
5. Do not use aerosols anywhere in your house.
6. Eliminate perfumes, powders, all scented toiletries and soaps, detergents, softening agents, flowers, and plants. Use large coffee cans with tightly covered lids to store fume-emitting household items such as shoe polish, felt-tipped pens, and the like if you must have them in your house at all.
7. Keep pets out of your room.
8. Dust your room with a damp cloth every two weeks. Remember to wear a mask over your nose and mouth while dusting. Open the windows and ventilate the room adequately while cleaning. Do not enter a room that's just been dusted for several hours.
9. Remove plants from your bedroom or other rooms in which you spend a lot of time (they are dust catchers). Perhaps you can tolerate a spider plant, though, since it is said that spider plants remove formaldehyde and other noxious agents from the air along with carbon dioxide and, as all plants do, produce oxygen. However, remember not to let the spider plant get dusty, and don't ask too much of it. It is said that one plant per 100 square feet helps produce clean air.
10. Remove anything with any odor at all from the house, or cover the top, seal the item with aluminum foil, or store in a tightly sealed covered container. A good general rule is that if you can smell it, get rid of it.
11. Use safe, nontoxic fume-emitting household chemicals

and cleaners, and don't forget lemon juice, vinegar (in water it does a great job on glass), baking soda, and washing soda. We clean our silverware with toothpaste.

HEATING.
1. Electric heating or hot water is preferred over hot air ducts. If you have hot air heat, install an electrostatic filter.
2. Avoid electric fans (they stir up dust).
3. If you still wake up miserable in the morning, consider sealing the ducts tightly with aluminum foil and tape and using an electric heater in your bedroom. Filters, air conditioners, and air purifiers are very helpful. Investigate products carefully before purchasing to determine if they are truly effective. The air purifier should remove dust, mold, and noxious fumes such as formaldehyde.
4. Keep the temperature between 68° and 70°F and the humidity between 40 and 60 percent. When humidity is low, respiratory infections, airborne dust and allergens, and asthmatic symptoms are exacerbated. When humidity is above 60 percent, there is an increase in fungal growth and bacterial and viral life, dust mites and asthmatic symptoms are more common, and there is a greater tendency for outgassing of formaldehyde.

KITCHEN.
1. Keep well ventilated and as smoke-free as possible. Use microwave ovens and electric frying pans (see later section), avoid gas stoves and appliances, and clean out all the harsh-smelling chemicals and cleaning agents under the kitchen sink.

DAMP AREAS (BASEMENT, CELLAR, LAUNDRY AREAS).
1. Use a dehumidifier to help decrease mold growth.
2. Humidifiers and air conditioners can be a source of mold growth. For air conditioners, clean the coils and the drip

pan with a mixture of one cup of vinegar to one gallon of water. During the warm summer months, weekly cleaning is advisable. Both furnace and air-conditioning filters should be replaced every two months and vacuumed monthly. Electrostatic filters should be washed every 30 days. We do ours in our dishwashing machine. The fans and housings of air conditioners and furnaces should be vacuumed annually. Vacuum ducts annually, if possible. A professional will undoubtedly be needed for this task. Clean your humidifier weekly, whenever it is in use, with the same vinegar solution you use on the air conditioner.

3. For demolding your cellars and summer dwellings, use one half cup of borax to a quart of water and wear a mask while cleaning. If you can have someone else clean your basement and avoid the area altogether, that is much to be desired. A dehumidifier for the basement may be a good investment.

Crowds and Cars

When you are driving in your own car, turn the air-conditioning to maximum, even in the winter (of course while keeping the heat on), in order to reduce the intake of noxious outdoor fumes. If you can afford it or need it, consider an in-car air filter. Don'tdrive near other cars and don't tailgate, because you will be subjected to their fumes. Keep your car clean and dry and have your engine cleaned every year. Remember, air conditioners in cars can become moldy also.

If at all possible, stay away from anyone who is sneezing or coughing. If you do have to socialize with somebody with a respiratory infection, turn away quickly if that person begins to cough and, most of all, *do not shake hands with or touch the cougher.* If you are exposed to somebody who coughed, wash your hands, because the virus on your hands, which then may be lifted to the nose, eyes, or mouth, may infect you.

In a restaurant, sit in the no-smoking section. Ask your friends not to wear scented toiletries. If you are hugged by someone wearing perfume, cologne, or after-shave, step back as quickly as possible. Remember, if you get fumes on your clothes, leave them outside of your bedroom.

Pets

Pets are a joy and a commitment. You have to be careful with dander, feathers, and other allergens that are a part of being an owner of some birds and animals. A poodle grows wool, does not shed or have dander, and might be called nonallergenic. Make sure the dog can exercise outside the house. Perhaps you have a yard, a chain, or a run, or a neighborhood youngster who can walk the dog for you if you cannot fulfill that commitment. Tropical fish or goldfish make wonderful pets, but they don't provide the affection that a dog does. Cats are ideal in some ways because they need not go out; however, cat dander is too frequently an allergen for cats to be recommended.

MISCELLANEOUS HAZARDS

Choking

If you choke on food in public, put your hand to your throat in the international choking sign; give your best therapeutic cough. If obstruction is severe and you have no help, use the following self-save technique: Make a fist with one hand and push the fist with the other hand as hard as possible into the middle of the area between your belly button and rib cage. Push up and in sharply. Repeat if necessary.

Alternate technique: Bend over a high-backed chair, railing, or table edge. Press your abdomen into the edge with a quick movement. Repeat if necessary.

Influenza and Pneumonia

Take appropriate vaccines—the influenza vaccine yearly and Pneumovax, a protection against pneumococcal (a kind of bacteria) pneumonia, once.

Exercise

Exercise may induce asthma or wheezing. Try to avoid activities that definitely cause severe wheezing, no matter what you do. However, two inhalations of a bronchodilator spray just before exercise may end the entire problem. Cromolyn sodium inhalation ten minutes before exercise may also be helpful. If you have this problem, be sure to tell your doctor rather than becoming sedentary.

Aspirin and Nonsteroidals

Aspirin, aspirin-containing preparations (e.g., Alka-Seltzer, Anacin, Fiorinal), and aspirin's cousins (the nonsteroidal antiinflammatory drugs (e.g., Motrin, Advil, Tolectin, Feldene, Indocin) may, especially in individuals with nasal polyps, induce asthmatic episodes that may be life threatening. Use aspirin substitutes, such as acetaminophen. People with aspirin-induced asthma may also be sensitive to benzoic acid derivatives, including tartrazines, which are used as coloring agents in many foods.

Metabisulfites

This food additive, used by restaurants for freshening lettuce, fruits, and potatoes (including potato chips), can induce severe asthma in susceptible individuals. Watch what you eat, and check the ingredient list when making purchases. Metabisulfites are also used in certain beers, wines, liquors, dried fruits, avocado dips, shrimp, and antiasthma medications, including Alupent, Isuprel, Bronkosol, and Metaprel multidose solutions. Alupent unit dose contains no sulfites.

Stress

It's important to learn to react appropriately to the problems of your life. You don't want to withdraw, afraid to face up when things are tough; yet if you overreact, you're left with mental and physical scars and exhaustion. Finding that middle ground means considering life's problems a challenge to be faced with vigor and a stout heart. The next time stress enters the picture and you are terrified or furious, ask yourself, "Could I settle for being scared and angry?" If so, could you instead be a little anxious and miffed? That's even better. Then ask yourself, "Did the whole thing really matter?" If it matters, accept some stress.

There are some situations you can't avoid, but try not to stress yourself about things that don't really matter.

Glaucoma and Cataracts

If you are taking steroid hormones, see your eye doctor twice a year for early detection and treatment of the possible side effects of glaucoma and cataracts. If you have glaucoma, take extra care not to spray ipratropium bromide (Atrovent) into your eyes when using the metered dose inhaler. You could precipitate an attack of glaucoma.

SHOULD YOU MOVE?

One of the questions we're asked most frequently is "I've read so much about air pollution. I'll move anywhere—just tell me where." Environment may definitely adversely affect your problem. There is, however, no exact magic spot. Based on what we've already told you, here's a five-point plan for thought.

1. Your present personal environment. If you are wheezing from your hairspray, moving to the mountains won't change a thing. So, first ensure that your personal habits are not contributing to your problems. You should not use any toiletries, cosmetics, or shampoos with scents, and your

clothes should be washed with nonscented products such as borax and baking soda (equal parts of each). Your clothes and bedclothes should emit no odors.

2. Your present home environment. Your home should be free of irritating chemical fumes such as bleach and ammonia. You must take every precaution to ensure your atmosphere is free of mold, dust, pollen, and dander. Naturally, there should be no smoke in your house. Your bedroom should not be near your garage. Adequate ventilation, air purification, and temperature and humidity control are very important, and—what's more appealing—doable!

3. Your neighborhood. Moving to a wonderful clean air spot may do you no good if you live next to a gasoline station or just under a busy highway or in the path of the winds from a nearby factory. If your neighbor burns wood and the smoke blows into your house or if a neighboring lawn is frequently sprayed with chemicals, you may have more pollution in your life than ever. You could move to the country only to find that the neighboring farmer's plowing stirs large amounts of molds and bacteria into the air.

4. Your present geographic location. Are you in a valley with smog settling around your property? Are you near factories and big-city traffic? Does the air pollution from a distant big-city rush hour arrive at your spot a few hours later? Is there an abundance of the very pollens and grasses to which you are sensitive?

5. A new geographic location. If you do decide to move, think what it will mean to uproot yourself; find out what your allergens are and ensure that they are not present in this new spot. In general, avoid big cities, industrialized areas, and valleys. Take an extended vacation at different times of the year in the area before you uproot yourself. Check not only the area but also the neighbors, the street, and the new home against the many things we discussed. Don't move to a new clean-air spot only to discover that the house has a moldy

basement. Consider whether moving to a nearby location, perhaps on a hilltop, would be less traumatic emotionally and just as effective. Check out any other triggering sources before you move. Try a dry climate.

There you have it—no easy answers but a way to proceed logically. Enjoy being a good detective.

Chapter 5

NUTRITION

JOIN THE DIET CRAZE

It seems as though everyone these days is worrying about diet—you should, too. Your nutritional concerns are very real and are related to more than looking good in a bathing suit. The kinds and quantity of food you consume may mean success or failure in your participation in an active or full life as described in this book. The average American diet is estimated to contain 37 percent fat, most of which is completely devoid of any essential vitamins or minerals and a great deal of which may contain harmful trans-fatty acids as well as other saturated fats that raise cholesterol. In addition, a large proportion of the rest of the diet frequently consists of refined and processed foods containing various preservatives and chemicals, also lacking in essential nutrients.

Recently we attended a special lecture by Donald R. Davis, Ph.D., director of the Roger J. Williams Nutrition Institute for Disease Prevention, Research, and Education, and a nutrition researcher at the University of Texas in Austin. Dr. Davis presented nutritional analyses of foods throughout the plant and animal kingdoms. He found that all whole foods (foods eaten as they grow) contain large numbers—that is, 25 to 35—of 42 known nutrients considered to be essential vitamins and minerals in relation to their calorie content. This was not true for what he called "dismembered foods," which contain few nutrients in relation to their calorie content. A whole food might be sweet corn. Corn oil is a dismembered food. Sweet corn contains large numbers of essential nutrients. Corn oil contains pesticide residues and few nutrients (see Fig. 5.1).

Dr. Davis measured the nutrients per calorie consumed and discovered that essentially all whole foods are well worth their calories; when we embellish whole foods with dismembered foods such as sugar and fat, the essential nutrients per calorie drop significantly. Let's go back to sweet corn. Eaten off the cob, it's healthy and nutritionally dense; eaten with butter all over it, there are many more calories and the nutrients per calorie decline. It's an important concept to keep in mind.

Look at the astounding difference between corn oil and whole corn in the number of essential vitamins and minerals, without which you cannot have a healthy body and a high level of energy. You are eating sufficient amounts of foods that are easy to prepare. But *what* do you eat? Is your diet predominantly junk food, food composed mainly of sugar and no other nutrients—smoked, salty, fatty, or fried foods such as salami, hot dogs, french fries, and greasy fried chicken? Do you eat mainly "empty" dismembered foods or predominantly whole foods? Now that you think about it, do you eat a lot of empty calories? You can't afford that and "live well." Here's why.

Recent investigations indicate that many patients with COPD are malnourished; even patients who have normal or excess weight may have below-normal muscle mass. Low muscle mass means poor strength and inability to be active. Studies have shown that individuals with COPD who have poor muscle mass also have weak respiratory muscles, with a markedly reduced ability to breathe deeply. It goes without saying that the ability to breathe deeply is an essential component of "living well." Furthermore, if your weight is normal, if your muscle mass is low, you have excess fat. An increase in fat weight means you must carry around unnecessary tissue that lends

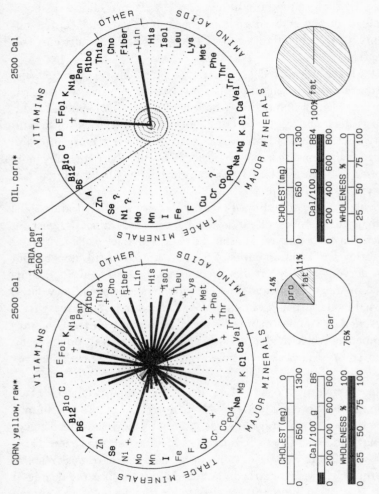

Diagram by NutriCircles Software © 1991

Figure 5.1 Nutritional Analyses of Raw Corn and Corn Oil

no strength to your body. You're already having enough trouble moving around; you don't need this added burden. Excess fat may be deposited in your coronary arteries as well as around your middle, resulting in heart disease as well as pulmonary disease. Lower-than-normal fat weight means you have inadequate protection if you cannot eat for a few days or weeks or if you are unexpectedly exposed to the cold.

And what about some of the other things you do or don't eat? Inadequate carbohydrate means limitation of energy, including energy supply to your respiratory muscles. Too much sodium intake means you'll be walking around with extra water weight, another added burden. Inadequate calcium intake may result in osteoporosis, a loss of bone tissue leading to painful and debilitating fractures most commonly in the back, hips, ribs, and wrists. A diet low in fiber may lead to poor bowel movements, with chronic constipation and rectal pain.

The work your body must do just to *breathe* is six to 10 times greater than that of a normal person (called increased *work of breathing*). If you want to have the energy and strength to live well, you can see how complicated the problem is. It can't be done with junk foods and empty calories.

You need to make some type of realistic assessment of whether you are over- or underweight, over- or underfat, or whether you may have high or low lean body mass. This is not easy and can only be approximated with the tests that are ordinarily available to you. You need to have a varied diet, buy the right foods, and cook them properly, all with a minimum expenditure of energy. That's going to take some study, but it can be done.

You will learn to formulate a sound diet, equip your kitchen, cook meals, and get your shopping done, all within the range of your physical capability. We will have special comments for those days when you don't feel well and your appetite is poor.

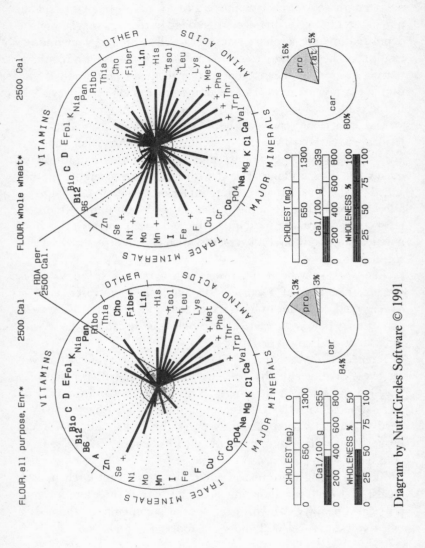

Figure 5.2   Nutritional Analyses and Comparison of White and Whole-wheat Flour

WHAT'S WHAT

Carbohydrates

Carbohydrates, eaten as sugar and starches, provide on-the-spot energy. There are two types: simple sugars such as table sugar, which if not used immediately are converted to fat, and complex carbohydrates such as those found in fruits, breads, and cereals. The latter are utilized slowly over a longer period, so the opportunities for immediate conversion to fat are fewer. A small amount of excess carbohydrate can be stored as a substance called glycogen (for emergencies), but the rest is converted to fat. It's important to have an adequate daily supply of complex carbohydrates.

Proteins

Proteins, composed of substances called amino acids and found in meat, fish, poultry, and some vegetables, are the building blocks of bone, blood, tendons, ligaments, muscles, and all the body cells. There are nine amino acids that the body cannot manufacture and therefore must be eaten daily. They are called essential amino acids. Animal proteins contain all the essential amino acids and therefore are called complete proteins. There's protein in vegetables, too, such as in soybeans, but vegetable proteins do not contain all the essential building blocks or amino acids and therefore are called incomplete proteins. Certain vegetables, such as rice and beans, "complement" each other and when eaten together result in the ingestion of complete protein. If you are missing one essential amino acid in your diet over a period of time, severe malnutrition will result. Excess proteins cannot be stored like carbohydrates and are converted to fat if they are not burned as energy.

Fats

Fats are oily substances found in meat, salad oils, and dairy products such as cream, whole milk, and cheese. Fat provides the largest store of potential energy in the body for most Americans. Once the body's small carbohydrate stores are used up, the rest of the energy must come from fat and protein. Therefore, the longer the energy requirement (i.e., exercise) continues, the more likely it is that the body's energy is coming from burned fat. Excess fats are metabolized by the liver and then carried into the bloodstream. All excessive food intake, including alcohol, results in the manufacture and deposit of fat.

Carbohydrates and proteins contain four calories per gram. Fats contain nine calories per gram. Three ounces equal 100 grams.

Fiber

Fiber, found mainly in certain vegetables, fruit, whole wheat, and bran cereals, is a nondigestible food element. Fiber is not absorbed. It adds bulk to bowel movements, making them softer and more easily passed by binding water and fats, including dietary cholesterol. Waste material leaves the body faster in a high–fiber diet. People who eat high–fiber diets generally have less constipation, and they may have lower cholesterol and possibly a lower incidence of cancer of the colon.

Minerals

Minerals are a part of every cell and are associated especially with the conversion of food to energy. *Sodium*, the principal content of table salt, is an essential ingredient in the chemical reactions that take place in the body fluids outside the cells. However, very little sodium, probably about two grams a day (one teaspoon or much less), is required by the body. A regular diet in which sodium is used in cooking but not added to the food upon eating usually contains four grams of sodium a day. Excess sodium may result in water retention, increased work for the heart, and high blood pressure. The latter contributes to heart disease and stroke. *Potassium* is an essential ingredient of chemical reactions that take place within the body's cells and is a food constituent found in all whole foods and most significantly in meat, bananas, oranges, prunes, and other vegetables and fruits. With normal kidneys there is no disorder from excess intake of potassium, but lack of potassium causes weakness, muscle cramps, and abnormal heart rhythm. *Calcium* is found most significantly in certain vegetables, cereal products, and particularly milk and cheese protein. It is the body's most abundant mineral and combines with the mineral phosphorus in the formation of bones and teeth. It is also important in the reactions that make muscles function. Your heart would not be able to pump without sodium, potassium, and calcium.

Vitamins

As their name describes, vitamins are minute amounts of food elements vital to life. They do not supply energy or contribute to body weight. They cannot be manufactured by the body, so they must be supplied in the diet, and they are absolutely essential for all body functions. Vitamins are widely distributed in all whole foods, including meats, fish, poultry, vegetables, and fruits, along with minerals. Without vitamins, the body could not make new tissue, fight infection, or produce energy.

Water

Water is a nonenergy-supplying liquid nutrient essential to life. It constitutes about 60 percent of our body weight and functions as the body's foremost transport medium for nutrients, gases, and waste products. Under normal circumstances two-and-a-half quarts of water a day are utilized, but that includes the liquid ingested in food. A person can live a long time without food (provided he or she has typical body muscle and fat) but only a few days without water.

Alcohol

Found in wine, beer, and liquor, alcohol is a food that supplies energy but has no vitamins, minerals, protein, fat, or carbohydrate. Whereas small amounts of about one ounce a day or less may in some instances lower the blood cholesterol, excess amounts may lead to deterioration of the liver and nervous system, including the brain.

Caffeine

Caffeine is a drug found in coffee, tea, cocoa, and many carbonated beverages. In low doses (e.g., the amount in one cup of coffee) caffeine may increase concentration; in higher doses it causes restlessness, nervousness, and insomnia and raises the pulse rate and possibly the blood pressure. When people consume a lot of caffeine, their heart rate goes up out of proportion to the amount of exercise. Therefore, they tire more easily and can do less.

Oils

Unfortunately, all oils are dismembered (nonwhole) foods that supply virtually no nutrients to accompany their exceptionally high calorie content. Even "unrefined" or "cold pressed" oils bear no nutritional resemblance to the whole foods from which they are derived, and their use should be restricted for the same major reason that table sugar should be restricted. We must have certain fats and vitamin E in our diet, however. The best sources of these are fatty whole foods such as nuts of all kinds, avocados, soybeans, olives, peanut butter (preferably the nonhydrogenated "old-fashioned" kind), and fish such as salmon, herring, and mackerel. For sparing use in cooking and salad dressings, we recommend cold pressed olive oil. Other recommended oils are nonhydrogenated safflower, sunflower, and canola oils. We avoid partially hydrogenated oils, which contain questionable *trans*-fatty acids, and most oils that are extracted with petrochemical solvents.

WHAT'S NEW

The Exercise-Fat Connection

Two separate groups of patients were put on identical reducing diets. One group entered into an exercise training program exactly as described in Chapter 6; the other group remained sedentary. The weight loss for both groups was identical. The group that remained sedentary lost 50 percent fat and 50 percent muscle mass; the group that dieted *and* exercised lost about 95 percent fat and 5 percent muscle mass. If you are a sedentary person who loses and gains weight and suffers from the "yo-yo syndrome," then when you are on the down "yo," you lose fat and muscle, and when you are on the up "yo," you replace muscle with fat. With each diet binge you will grow weaker and will have a lower muscle mass and a higher fat mass. *That's bad.*

The Vitamin-Cancer Connection

The National Research Council (NRC), a scientific advisory group to the federal government, has issued a report entitled "Diet, Nutrition and Cancer," urging us to eat more foods containing vitamins A and C, which may lower the risk of some cancers. Beta carotene is the safe and powerful precursor of vitamin A found in certain fruits and vegetables. Even heavy smokers reduce their risk of lung cancer by increasing their intake of these natural foods. In other studies heavy smokers who ate small amounts of beta carotene were four times as likely to have cancer as those heavy smokers who ate large amounts. Vitamin A seems to help the delicate cells lining the bronchial tree to reproduce and repair themselves in such a way that they are able to continue their normal functions. Without vitamin A the cells become dry and hard and show changes that resemble those caused by tumor-producing chemicals. Overdoses of vitamin A, on the other hand, can cause severe liver damage and injuries to the brain and nervous system. Therefore, increasing the intake of vitamin A by tablets is not recommended. When you eat vitamin A in foods or in its natural form, beta carotene, the body controls the rate of conversion and there are no toxic side effects. Try to eat a daily source of natural vitamin A, or beta carotene.

Vitamin C stops the formation of nitrosamines, a group of substances that cause cancer in animals. The National Research Council pointed out in studies that it reviewed that those population groups observed who ate fruits and vegetables containing vitamin C had lower rates of stomach and esophageal cancer. A daily source of vitamin C is important.

The NRC has made further interim suggestions as its research continues. Americans have been advised to avoid excessive alcohol intake, minimize eating smoked or salt-cured foods such as ham and pickled herring, lower fat intake, and include whole-grain or high-fiber cereals as part of their daily diet.

The Calcium Link

We used to think that osteoporosis, or weak, thin bones that tend to get small fractures, and periodontal disease, a disease of the gums that results in the teeth loosening and falling out, were diseases of older or middle-aged people. They are, but now we know that their beginnings are rooted in the young who have sedentary lives and who possibly have a poor calcium intake.

We used to think that milk was a children's food. It's no longer so. Adults need an ample intake of calcium throughout their lifetime, coupled with exercise, as the best means now known of lessening the risk of osteoporosis and periodontal disease. It's long been known that steroid hormones such as prednisone, at times necessary medications for people with COPD, can also cause the breakdown of bone and contribute to osteoporosis. Vigorous upright exercise, such as walking briskly, tends to stimulate new bone formation, and vigorous exercise actually reversed the bone loss and muscle loss found in our astronauts due to weightlessness. One final note: Smoking and excessive alcohol intake may also contribute to osteoporosis.

"Good" and "Bad" Cholesterol

Most people know there are two kinds of fat—saturated, as is found in fatty meats and cream and animal products, and unsaturated, as is found in vegetable oil. What's new is that all excess foods, including alcohol, are metabolized by the liver into fat and contribute to the formation of low-density lipoprotein, or LDL, and are then carried into the bloodstream. It's postulated that large quantities of LDL in the bloodstream injure the lining of blood vessels, especially in the coronary arteries, and that's how arteriosclerosis may begin. Unsaturated fats, unless they are eaten in excess, tend to lower the manufacture of LDL, or bad cholesterol, by the liver, and exercise tends to favor the manufacture of what's called high-density lipoprotein, or HDL, the good cholesterol, for HDL does not result in deposits in the coronary arteries. In fact, exercise can actually raise the ratio of HDL to LDL. It comes down to this: If you walk, walk, walk, and eat right, you might have more good cholesterol than bad. And good cholesterol is the kind worth having!

The Fiber-Cancer Connection

Populations that eat very high quantities of fibrous foods have extremely large stools and very low rates of cancer of the bowel. How can that be? Scientists are not sure, but they postulate that when bacteria "sit around" in the intestines they may create low-level cancer-producing compounds. By eating fiber along with fluids you may be fighting cancer as well as constipation.

Good and Not-so-good Starches

A high simple sugar load results in an outpouring of insulin from the pancreas. Insulin is quite efficient at getting sugar metabolized and deposited as fat if it's not burned quickly. It also tends to overshoot slightly, causing the blood sugar to drop, resulting in hunger. You eat a candy bar because you're hungry, but shortly after you're finished, you're hungrier than ever. This may set up a vicious cycle of overeating and a binge on sweets. Since starches, or as we described them, complex sugars, are metabolized more slowly, insulin levels tend not to rise rapidly. However, it's been discovered that all starchy foods are not alike, even when the starch is in a single food prepared in different ways (e.g., the wheat in pasta as opposed to that in bread), with some starches causing more of a blood sugar rise than others. We have divided starches into three groups based on low, medium, or high blood sugar responses. In the lowest, or most desirable, group are apples, oranges, milk, yogurt, dried legumes (beans, chick-peas, lentils, black-eyed peas), sweet potatoes, yams, spaghetti, bran, and oatmeal. In the middle group are raisins, bananas, beets, new potatoes, bread, shredded wheat, rice, and sweet corn. In the highest group are parsnips, carrots, instant potatoes, and cornflakes.

As regards simple sugars, here are some surprises. The blood sugar response to fructose (fruit sugar) is in the very lowest group, sucrose is in the middle, and honey is in the highest group, along with glucose and maltose.

To avoid a binge, choose foods from the lowest group. Also, if you are a binger, read the section on food allergies with great care. Hidden food allergy may be a cause of food addiction and overeating. We sometimes crave the very foods to which we are allergic. Try the elimination diet mentioned a little later on in this chapter. If you have any food problems at all, especially binging, try the multiple food elimination diet.

It's clear we think you shouldn't diet unless you're willing to exercise. You need the best muscle mass you can get. You don't want to be too thin or too fat. You don't want to carry around extra water and eat rich, salty foods that may increase the risk of hypertension and heart attack or smoked, cured foods that may increase the risk of cancer. You can't afford the consequences of empty calories. You want a diet high in fiber, foods containing calcium and vitamins A and C, and complex carbohydrates with adequate high-quality protein and not too much fat.

Nutrition

WEIGHT, FAT, AND MUSCLE

Locate your height and weight in Table 5.1. Are you too fat? Weight more than a little above the accepted normal range is considered to be unhealthy. Researchers have discovered that the distribution of fat is also important to health. Excess fat above the hips is correlated with fat deep in the abdomen, which is linked to diseases of the

TABLE 5.1

Suggested Weights for Adults

Height[a]	Weight in pounds[b]	
	19 to 34 Years	35 Years and Over
5'0"	97–128	108–138
5'1"	101–132	111–143
5'2"	104–137	115–148
5'3"	107–141	119–152
5'4"	111–146	122–157
5'5"	114–150	126–162
5'6"	118–155	130–167
5'7"	121–160	134–172
5'8"	125–164	138–178
5'9"	129–169	142–183
5'10"	132–174	146–188
5'11"	136–179	151–194
6'0"	140–184	155–199
6'1"	144–189	159–205
6'2"	148–195	164–210
6'3"	152–200	168–216
6'4"	156–205	173–222
6'5"	160–211	177–228
6'6"	164–216	182–234

[a] Without shoes.

[b] Without clothes. The higher weights in the ranges generally apply to men, who tend to have more muscle and bone; the lower weights more often apply to women, who have less muscle and bone.

Source: Derived from National Research Council, 1989.

circulatory system. This type of fat may also be linked to breast cancer in older women. Here's how to check your fat distribution.

1. Measure your girth at the narrowest part of your waist and at the widest point of your hips over the buttocks.
2. Divide the waist measure by the hip measure. A healthy ratio for women will be below 75 percent and for men, below 80 percent. A dangerous ratio for women is above 85 percent and for men above 95 percent.

Are you too thin? If your weight is more than a little below the normal range, you have cause for concern. Often patients with pulmonary disease lose weight no matter what they do. Try to eat as much as you can and to keep active. Don't get discouraged. More research needs to be done on your problem.

This book seeks to open up new worlds of choices and ranges of interests, but not when it comes to the food you eat. If you want to have a healthy body, you have to eat a healthy core of whole foods that are nutritionally dense, filled with vitamins and minerals as well as proteins, carbohydrates, and some fats.

THE HEALTHY CORE DIET

An easy way to analyze any diet is to divide it into basic food groups. We've done that here, but with our own special categories.

1. High-calcium contributors: including fat-free milk, yogurt, low-cholesterol cheese, frozen yogurt, canned sardines and salmon with their bones, and *broccoli*. Four or more portions equivalent to 1,000 milligrams or more of calcium per day.
2. Cancer-fighting foods containing vitamins A and C: including grapefruit (especially pink), oranges, strawberries, watermelon, cantaloupe, brussels sprouts, cauliflower, sweet peppers, spinach, tomatoes, carrots, sweet potatoes, and

broccoli. Three to five servings, supplying vitamin A (recommended dietary allowance, 5,000 units per day for men and 4,000 units for women) and vitamin C (recommended dieta ry allowance, 60 milligrams per day).

3. Energy elevators: including breads, cereals, pasta, rice, and beans. Three to four or more servings per day (125 grams of complex carbohydrate = minimum).

4. Muscle builders (proteins): including meats, fish, poultry, peanut butter, low-fat cottage cheese, and egg whites. Two or more portions a day to equal about one gram for every pound of your ideal body weight in kilograms (= body weight divided by 2.2). With increased stress, however, protein requirements also increase, as high as 1.5 to 2 grams for every pound of ideal body weight in kilograms.

5. Fiber foods: including bran, potato skins, carrots, brussels sprouts, cauliflower, bananas, cabbage, corn, oranges, raw apples, pears, dried apricots, high-fiber cereals, whole-grain, long-cooking cereals, and *broccoli*. No particular minimum daily requirement has been established. Try for 20 or more grams of fiber per day.

Some foods actually cross over several categories. For instance, low-fat milk provides high-quality protein as well as being dense in calcium. For clarity's sake, we have generally avoided listing foods under more than one category but rather in the area in which they make their most important contribution. Isn't broccoli a knockout? It's loaded with beta carotene and vitamin C, as well as calcium and fiber, and there's some vegetable protein and carbohydrate there, too.

How do you know your *exact* requirements for calories, carbohydrates, fats, and protein? That's difficult. Your doctor is in the best position to help. If you are very thin and quite short of breath all the time, it may be best to have a nutritionist make sophisticated estimates of your body composition and needs.

The Healthy Core Diet (see Table 5.2) is high in complex carbohydrates (40–55 percent of daily calories), has little or no simple sugar,

TABLE 5.2
Healthy Core Diet: 1,500 Calories

	Calories	Protein (gm)	Carbohydrate (gm)	Fiber (gm)	Cholesterol / Total Fat (gm)	Ca (mg)	A (units)	C (mg)	Sodium (mg)
Breakfast									
Bran cereal, 1 oz.	71	4.0	22	8.5	0 / 0.5	23	1,250	15.0	320
Skim milk, 1 cup	86	8.4	11.9	0	0 / 0.4	302	500	2.0	126
1/2 pink grapefruit, 4 in.	37	0.7	9.5	0.2	0 / 0	13	318	47.0	1
Bread, whole wheat, 1 slice	61	2.3	11.3	0.4	trace / 1.0	30	trace	trace	121
Coffee, 1 cup	4	0.2	1.6	0	0	6	0	0	8
Lunch									
Low-fat cheese, 2 oz.	144	30.6	1.6	0	32 / 9.0	366	332	0	264
Peanut butter, 2 tbsp.	190	9.2	5.0	0	0 / 16.4	10	0	0	6
Pita bread, small, whole wheat	106	4	20.6	0.3	trace / 0.6	31	0	trace	215
Carrot, 1 large	31	0.7	7.3	1.1	0 / 0.1	19	20,253	19	25
Pepper, lettuce, tomato, mixed	40	1.5	6.0	0.6	0 / 0	14	600	40	8
Apple, medium	81	0.3	21.1	2.8	0 / 0.5	10	74	8	1

	Calories	Protein (gm)	Carbohydrate (gm)	Fiber (gm)	Cholesterol (mg) / Total Fat (gm)	Ca (mg)	A (units)	C (mg)	Sodium (mg)
Dinner									
Poultry, white meat, without skin, 3½ oz.	157	29.9	0	0	69 / 3.2	19	0		64
Sweet potato, baked, 1 medium	118	2.0	27.7	2.1	0 / 0.1	40	24,877	23	12
Lettuce or salad	14	1.2	2.5	0.5	0 / 0	35	970	2	9
Homemade dressing (oil & vinegar), 1 tbsp.	72	0	0.4		0 / 8.0	1	7	0	7
Broccoli, 3 stalks	78	9.3	13.5	4.5	0 / 0.9	264	7,500	270	30
Orange, 3 in.	65	1.4	16.3	0.8	0 / 0.1	56	256	80	1
Snacks									
Popcorn, 2 cups popped, no fat or salt	46	1.6	9.2	0.3	0 / 0.6	2	0	2	0
Skim milk, 1 cup	86	8.4	11.9	0	0 / 0.4	302	500	2.0	126
TOTALS	1,504	126.3	186.1	17.6	101 / 36.3	1,279	49,937	245	1,314

Source for data: Bowes and Church's *Food Values of Portions Commonly Used*, 15th edition, revised by Jean A. T. Pennington, Ph.D., R.D. (New York: Harper and Row, 1989).

TABLE 5.3

Modifications of Healthy Core Diet to Varying Calorie Counts

Calories:	1,200	1,500	2,000	2,500	3,000
Breakfast					
Bran cereal, 1 oz.	X	X	X	X	X
Skim milk, 1 cup	X	X	X	X	X
1/2 Grapefruit (pink)	X	X	X	X	X
Bread, whole wheat, 1 slice	X	X			
Coffee, tea, etc.	X	X	X	X	X
Large roll, whole wheat			X	X	X
Raisins			1 tbsp.	2 tbsp.	3 tbsp.
Lunch					
Low-fat cheese	3 slices	3 slices	3 slices	3 slices	3 slices
Pita, small, whole wheat	X	X			
Carrot, 1 large	X	X	X	X	X
Peanut butter		1 tbsp.	2 tbsp.	3 tbsp.	3 tbsp.
Vegetables, raw	X	X	X	X	X
Apple	½. 2 in.	2 in.	X	4 in.	4 in.
Tea, cereal beverage	X	X	X	X	X
Large roll, whole wheat			X	X	X
Tuna			½ cup	½ cup	1 cup
Mayonnaise			1 tbsp.	1 tbsp.	3 tbsp.
Dinner					
Poultry, white meat	3½ oz.	3½ oz.	3½ oz.	3½ oz.	7 oz.
Sweet potato	½	1	1	1	1
Salad	X	X	X	X	X
Salad dressing	1 tbsp.	1 tbsp.	1 tbsp.	1 tbsp.	1 tbsp.
Salad oil				2 tbsp.	2 tbsp.
Broccoli, 3 stalks	X	X	X	X	X
Orange, 3 in.	X	X	X	X	X
Snacks					
Popcorn	1 cup	2 cups	2 cups	2 cups	2 cups
Skim milk, 1 cup	X	X	X	X	X
Fruit				1 large	2 large

TABLE 5.4
Fruits and Vegetables Containing Vitamins A and C

Food	Calories	Vitamin A (units)	Vitamin C (mg)
Fruits			
Apricots, dried, 10 halves	83	2,534	1
Cantaloupe, 1 cup	57	5,158	68
Grapefruit, pink, half	37	318	47
Orange, one medium	65	256	80
Papaya, 1 medium	117	6,122	118
Peach, 1 medium	37	465	6
Strawberries, raw whole, 1 cup	45	41	85
Watermelon, 1 cup	50	585	15
Vegetables			
Asparagus, 1 cup cuts, spears	44	1,492	38
Beans, snap, 1 cup	30	680	15
Broccoli, medium stalk	46	2,198	98
Brussels sprouts, 8	60	1,122	96
Cabbage, 1 cup	32	128	36
Carrots, 1 cup slices	70	38,302	4
Cauliflower, 1 cup pieces	30	18	68
Collards, 1 cup	27	8,436	38
Kale, 1 cup	42	9,620	54
Lettuce, looseleaf, 2 leaves	10	1,064	10
Peas, 1 cup	134	956	22
Peppers, sweet, 1 cup	24	528	152
Potatoes, 1, ½ lb., baked with skin	220	trace	52
Pumpkin, canned, 1 cup	82	53,816	10
Squash, winter, 1 cup baked & mashed	204	7,256	20
Sweet potatoes, 1 medium, baked	236	49,754	56
Tomatoes, raw, one	24	1,304	44
Turnip greens, 1 cup boiled	30	4,256	34

Source for data: Bowes and Church's *Food Values of Portions Commonly Used,* 15th edition, revised by Jean A. T. Pennington, Ph.D., R.D. (New York: Harper and Row, 1989).

TABLE 5.5
Sources of Calcium

Food	Calcium, (mg)	Calories
Skim milk, protein fortified, 1 cup	352	100
Skim milk, 1 cup	302	86
Whole milk, 1 cup	290	157
Sardines, canned in oil, 2 medium	92	50
Yogurt (skim milk), 1 cup fortified	452	127
Canned evaporated milk, 1/2 cup	329	169
Milk powder, dry non-fat, 1/4 cup	377	109
American cheese, 1 oz.	159	82
Creamed cottage cheese, 1 cup	126	217
Cottage cheese, low-fat, 1 cup	138	164
Canned salmon (with bones, 3 oz.)	203	130
Dandelion greens, raw, 1/2 cup chopped	52	13
Collard greens, boiled, 1/2 cup chopped	148	27
Tofu, 3½ oz.	128	72
Broccoli, 1/2 cup boiled	89	23
Spinach, 1/2 cup boiled	122	21
Green beans, 1/2 cup canned	18	13
Oysters, canned, 3 oz.	38	58
Brazil nuts, dried, 1 oz.	50	164
Almonds (dried), 1 oz. (24 nuts)	75	167
Whole-wheat bread, 1 slice	30	61
English walnuts, dried, 1 oz. (14 halves)	27	182

Source for data: Bowes & Church's *Food Values of Portions Commonly Used*, 15th edition, revised by Jean A. T. Pennington, Ph.D., R.D. (New York: Harper and Row, 1989).

is low in fat (25–30 percent of total daily calories) and cholesterol (less than 300 milligrams a day), has adequate protein for moderate stress (20–27 percent daily), and is high in fiber, low in alcohol (less than 60 milligrams a day or none), and high in calcium (1,000-plus milligrams a day), vitamins A (15,000 units-plus) and C (250 milligrams-plus). It also contains all other essential vitamins and minerals, according to the National Research Council's recommended dietary allowances.

Fifteen calories per pound of ideal body weight provides adequate

Table 5.6*

How to Add Calories

Bread, wheat, 1 slice—61
Popcorn, popped, no salt or fat, 1 cup—23
Low-fat 1% cottage cheese, ½ cup—113
Rice, 1 cup—223
Apple, 1 medium—81
Kidney beans, boiled, 1 cup—225
Bagel—163
Tuna, water-packed, ¼ cup—60
Peanut butter, 1 tbsp.—95
Vegetable oil, 1 tbsp.—124
Egg substitute, equivalent to 2 eggs—60
Sweet potato, 1 medium, baked—118

*Source for data: Bowes and Church's *Food Values of Portions Commonly Used*, 15th edition, revised by Jean A. T. Pennington, Ph.D., R.D. (New York: Harper and Row, 1989).

nutrition for those who are moderately active and undergoing no unusual stress. For those who are very thin, or in high-stress situations, 20 calories per pound of ideal body weight is suggested. Overweight men should follow a 1,500-calorie diet and women a 1,200-calorie diet. Therefore, we've adapted the Healthy Core Diet to calorie counts of 1,200, 1,500, 2,000, 2,500, and 3,000. Whatever variations you make, retain the principles of the Healthy Core Diet. Eat poultry or fish five or six times a week and lean red meat once or twice a week. Use the diet exchange charts that follow to help with your choices.

If you are not undermuscled or subject to increased stress, you may require less protein. Excessive protein intake results in the loss of calcium in the urine. Check with your doctor.

HEALTHY CORE SHOPPING LIST

We've given you a shopping list for the first week. The proportions are for one person. The meat, however, is a two-week supply. Does

TABLE 5.7
First Week Healthy Core Diet
Shopping List for One
(Two Weeks' Meat Supply)

Calories:	1,200	1,500	2,000	2,500	3,000
Produce					
Grapefruit (pink), 4	X	X	X	X	X
Oranges, 3 in., 7	X	X	X	X	X
Fruits, small—2 in., 7	X	X	X		
Fruits, large—4 in., 7				X	X
Tomatoes, 3	X	X	X	X	X
Lettuce, 1	X	X	X	X	X
Peppers, 4	X	X	X	X	X
Carrots, 7	X	X	X	X	X
Sweet potatoes, medium	3	5	5	5	5
Broccoli, 2 large bunches	X	X	X	X	X
Meat					
Chicken breasts, whole	3	3	3	3	6
Lean ground beef	½ lb.	½ lb.	½ lb.	½ lb.	1 lb.
Fish	½ lb.	½ lb.	½ lb.	½ lb.	1 lb.
Dairy					
Cottage cheese, 1% fat	X	X	X	X	X
Skim milk (1 gal.) or equiv. powder	X	X	X	X	X
Cheese (low-fat) 2 12-slice packages	X	X	X	X	X
Baked Goods					
Bread, whole wheat	X	X			
Pita (small, whole wheat), 7	X	X			
Large rolls or bagels, whole-wheat, 14			X	X	X
Other					
Oil (unsaturated)			X	X	X
Popcorn kernels	X	X	X	X	X
Bran cereal	X	X	X	X	X
Spices as needed	X	X	X	X	X
Raisins			X	X	X
Salad dressing, Italian type (not sugared)	X	X	X	X	X

Calories:	1,200	1,500	2,000	2,500	3,000
Canned Goods					
Stewed tomatoes	X	X	X	X	X
Low-sodium bouillon	X	X	X	X	X
Beverages					
Tea, cereal beverage, etc.	X	X	X	X	X
Frozen Foods					
2 weeks: main dishes	4	4	4	4	8
Broccoli (if fresh not available)					

Comments: If milk produces gas, bloating, or abdominal cramps, you may have lactose intolerance. The solution lies in adding LactAid, an enzyme that digests the lactose for you. If it is not available at your drugstore, call 1-800-257-8650, the LactAid Hot Line, LactAid Inc., Pleasantville, NJ.

We've suggested low-fat cottage cheese instead of butter or margarine. Please check the ingredients list of all cheeses. Some varieties contain synthetic food coloring, which may exacerbate asthmatic symptoms.

that sound peculiar? Here's our grand plan: Five nights each week, cook one more portion than you need and freeze immediately in a plastic heat-sealed boilable/freezable bag. Label it with a felt-tip pen. The second week you'll only have to boil the bag. We suggest you cook five nights a week. Two nights a week eat salad and high-quality, reduced-calorie frozen meals (this may not be advisable if you're on a very-low-sodium diet) or eat out (see Chapter 10). If you're on the 3,000-calorie diet, eat two frozen meals. Stick to the Healthy Core Diet as outlined. In a few weeks you can make your own adjustments. Comfort yourself by thinking of all the supermarket aisles you don't have to walk down anymore.

FOOD ALLERGIES

Food allergy may cause asthma. After all, foods contain chemicals, and substances in foods may precipitate a variety of symptoms, including stuffy nose, itching, tearing of the eyes, sore throat, water retention, headaches, hives, wheezing, and cough. There are two types of reaction to food. The first is usually easy to detect. You eat a food; you wheeze immediately. This is called an immediate reaction. Sometimes, though, you could eat a food and not wheeze for up to 24 hours. This is called a delayed reaction. If you eat foods to which you are sensitive every day, these foods may very well be the reason that you wheeze every day. The most common food allergens are milk, corn, eggs, and wheat. Other common offenders are yeast and molds, soy, peanuts, shellfish, and food coloring, especially yellow dye #5. Some other chemicals commonly found in foods—such as meta-bisulfites, monosodium glutamate, and aspartame—can cause similar symptoms. A simple, no-cost way to determine whether or not foods might be contributing to your asthma is to eliminate them for a period of at least 10 days, remembering that it is common to be allergic to more than one food.

Even though we recommend milk, some people think that milk increases mucus production. If, in fact, you believe that milk affects you adversely, eliminate it from your diet. Milk is contained in all dairy products. It is contained in cheeses, baked goods, butter, ice cream, yogurt, cottage cheese, and creamed foods.

Wheat is found in baked goods, crackers, many cereals, breaded foods, gravies, pastas, and whiskey.

Corn is found in some flours, vegetable oils, thickeners, corn syrup, and many packaged foods, such as cold cuts and sausage. If an ingredient list contains the word *starch*, it probably means corn-starch. Even many vitamin pills and other medications contain corn as a binder. The ingredient *syrup* usually means corn syrup. Sorbitol is made from corn. Dextrose, glucose, baking powder (usually made from cornstarch), many carbonated beverages, sweetened fruit juices, beer, gin, some soybean milk, and any beverage or food prepared in a waxed carton may contain corn products. Canned and frozen fruit with sweeteners, vegetables in waxed containers, suc-cotash, candied fruits, graham crackers, corn flakes, pancake mix, and other foods on which corn is sprinkled, such as pizza dough, contain corn. Fish may be packed in corn oil. If you have a corn allergy, you should also avoid hot dogs and luncheon meats, many ice creams, gelatin desserts, commercial spaghetti sauce, candies, brown sugar, cake mixes, corn oil, jams and jellies, dressings with corn oil, some peanut butter, some aspirin tablets, monosodium glutamate, and adhesives found on envelopes and stamps. Are you surprised at how pervasive corn products are?

Yeasts are found in such baked goods as bread, cheeses (including cottage cheese), alcohol, vinegar, pickled foods, smoked meat and fish, coffee, chocolate, mustard, malt drinks, ginger ale, root beer, black tea, wine, whiskey, rum, buttermilk, frozen and canned juices, dried fruits, mushrooms, fermented beverages (cider, beer), chili peppers, and tomato sauce. Many cereals are fortified with malt and with B vitamins that are yeast-derived. Most baked goods, sour cream, mayonnaise, soy sauce, sauerkraut, salad dressings, ketchup, horseradish, and pickles contain yeast, as may leftovers (e.g., fish and meat).

You might now be asking yourself, "What is it I can eat?" Good replacements for wheat bread are rice cookies and rice cakes. For those eliminating yeast, but not wheat, whole wheat matzos are a good choice. Oatmeal is an acceptable cereal and can be eaten without milk. Soy milk may be an acceptable substitute for milk. An egg replacer or arrowroot can be used in baking in lieu of eggs.

Another approach is to eliminate all the common allergens at once for a period of 10 days. In addition, eliminate all food coloring (in fact, you should probably not eat foods that contain food colorings, especially yellow dye #5, anyway). Clean vegetables thoroughly, because pesticides are other chemicals that can cause asthma. The multiple-food, low-allergen diet would be as follows: Eat only fresh or frozen foods, nothing packaged in a box. Soak vegetables thoroughly for one half hour and then scrub them well with a vegetable brush. Eat only vegetables, meat, fish other than shellfish, chicken, and nonwheat cereals such as oatmeal for 10 days. A sample menu would be as follows:

Breakfast: oatmeal with rice cakes, no milk.

Lunch and dinner: three vegetables with meat, fowl, or fish other than shellfish.

You will notice that this diet eliminates all the common allergens and also contains no fruits, nuts, or sugars. If after 10 days you feel better, add back one food in a plain, unadulterated form every three or four days. For instance, when adding back milk, don't do it by eating yogurt and drinking milk that is packaged in a waxed carton, since corn may have been used in the packaging.

In addition, some people feel much better if they don't eat any particular food more often than every four days. This is called a rotation diet (see Table 5.8).

In the following rotation diet, foods from the same family are not eaten more often than every four days. When you start this rotation diet, first cross out any foods to which you know you are sensitive. Next, put parentheses around foods you eat often and save them for later rotations. If you wish to make changes in the diet, do so by moving those foods with a two-sided arrow, because each is from a separate family. Sometimes wonderful things happen on a rotation diet—although you may have some temporary food cravings for the first few days, both food cravings and wheezing may diminish. Give a rotation diet at least a one-month trial.

If you find a significant difference in your asthma or if you are not sure, continue with the rotation diet another few rotations and then bring this information to your doctor.

In general, people with asthma and any hint of food sensitivity or chemical intolerance should learn to read ingredient lists. Ingredient lists should be simple, and all ingredients should be recognizable. An ingredient list that contains more chemicals than recognized foods should not be eaten. Foods containing food colorings are best eliminated. One last note: Foods can also exacerbate symptoms of sinus disease, and, as previously stated, exacerbations of sinus disease may worsen the symptoms of COPD.

TABLE 5.8

A Diversified Rotation Menu Plan

	Day 1	Day 2	Day 3	Day 4
Protein	Fish with fins cod, perch, halibut, salmon, tuna, mackerel, sole, anchovy, catfish, butterfish, flounder, snapper, bass, trout, herring, turbot, etc.	Red meat beef, veal, lamb, goat, pork, venison, buffalo, moose, etc. milk, cheeses, yogurt, butter, gelatin	Shellfish abalone, clam, crab, lobster, scallop, snail, shrimp, octopus, squid, other fish with fins not eaten on Day 1	Poultry and eggs chicken (egg), duck (egg), goose (egg), quail (egg), turkey (egg), pheasant, etc.
			frog legs ⟵⟶	*rabbit* ⟵⟶
	Legumes all beans and peas, lentils, soy, peanuts, alfalfa and bean sprouts	*amaranth* ⟵⟶	Grass family barley, corn, millet, oats, rye, rice, wheat, bamboo shoots, etc.	buckwheat
	sprouts	sprouts	sprouts	sprouts
Nuts and Seeds	*sesame* ⟵⟶ peanut, soy, walnut, pecan	*filbert* ⟵⟶ *pine* ⟵⟶ pumpkin seeds	*chestnuts* ⟵⟶ *macadamia* ⟵⟶ *Brazil* ⟵⟶ almond	cashew, pistachio, sunflower seed

	Day 1	Day 2	Day 3	Day 4
Oils and Fats	peanut, soy, walnut sesame ↔	olive → avocado ↔ butter, animal fat	corn, cottonseed, coconut, almond, apricot	sunflower, safflower, chicken, turkey, poultry fats
Grains and Flours	peanut, soy, and garbanzo flour, arrowroot ↔ kudzu root →	agar agar ↔ flax seed meal ↔	Xanthan gum ↔ grass family (grain) flours chestnut flour →	tapioca ↔ quinoa → buckwheat flour
Sweeteners	honey ↔ fig → raisins ↔	molasses ↔ whey, lactose	Palm family date, sago, coconut, corn syrup	maple syrup ↔ currants ↔
Vegetables	Carrot family carrot, celery, parsnip, parsley, dill, etc. Lily family asparagus, onion, garlic, leek, shallot, etc. Peas, string beans	Gourd family all squash, cucumbers, pumpkin, zucchini, etc. Beet family beets, spinach, swiss chard avocado ↔ olives → sweet potato ↔	Mustard family cabbage, bok choy, broccoli, brussels sprouts, cauliflower, kale, radish, greens, etc. bamboo shoots, corn okra chestnuts →	Composite family lettuce, endive, artichoke, dandelion greens, etc. Nightshade family potato, tomato, eggplant, pepper, etc. rhubarb yam, yucca ↔ mushroom ↔

	Day 1	Day 2	Day 3	Day 4
Fruits	Apple family apple, pear, quince, etc. Rose family boysen, black, raspberry, strawberry, loganberry, etc.	Heather family blueberry, cranberry, huckleberry, etc. all melons, cantaloupe	Prune family apricot, cherry, peach, plum, prune, etc.	Citrus family lemon, lime, orange, tangerine, etc. gooseberry
	papaya ⟷ *fig* ⟷ *grape, raisin* ⟷	*pomegranate* ⟷ *kiwi* ⟷	*guava* ⟷ *persimmon* ⟷ *pineapple* ⟷	*currant* ⟷ *mango* ⟷ *banana* ⟷
Bulk	*pectin*	*flax seed* ⟷	*chia seed* ⟷	*psyllium seed*

Source: Sally Rockwell, Diet Designs, Seattle

Chapter 6

EXERCISE

FINDING THE ATHLETE INSIDE YOU

P erhaps you haven't walked more than a block or two in years. You are a product of millions of years of roaming, hunting ancestors who survived by physical activity. Athleticism is as much a part of your inheritance as a human being as is your mental ability. All you have to do to let out the athlete buried inside of you is to claim that inheritance. Find the will and the courage to grasp what is rightfully yours. With rare exceptions, your performance can improve in a training program, just as any other athlete's performance improves. You can attain fitness based on your own individual needs and abilities.

But, you may be thinking, what *is* fitness, anyway? What can I *expect* from being fit? And why bother?

Being fit means that your body has sufficient flexibility, muscle strength, and heart and lung power to perform the tasks you need to do to "live well."

Here's what to expect:

- heart, lungs, and blood vessels that work better
- lower blood pressure
- possibly less chance of developing heart disease, and less

chance of pulmonary infections that develop in people who are sedentary
- less tension and stress
- better control over body fat
- fewer problems with deterioration of bones and joints
- a day-to-day feeling of well-being, physical as well as mental
- feeling happier
- feeling better about your body
- more energy at the end of the day
- energy and ability to do the things you'd given up—you thought—forever
- a natural high from exercise, instead of from cigarettes, alcohol, or drugs
- a better sex life

You might be thinking, "Can I really expect that?" Well, why not try and see for yourself? A great new world is about to open up for you as you experience the joy of moving your body once again. Here's exactly how to do it: step-by-step instructions to becoming an athlete.

CARDIOPULMONARY CONDITIONING

Cardiopulmonary conditioning results in the most efficient heart, lungs, and blood vessels possible for you. Each of us has a *maximum heart rate* (hereafter referred to as *MAX*). This is the upper limit of how fast our hearts can beat from doing vigorous activity. Predicted MAX is determined by age and not training. MAX is calculated by subtracting your age from the number 220. Therefore, a 55–year–old has a predicted MAX of 165 beats per minute. So, you might ask, if it's all predetermined, why bother training? After all, predicted MAX drops with age, and the greatest athlete cannot change it. But here's what *can* change: how fast and hard your heart will have to beat to do various tasks. If walking down the street makes your heart approach your MAX, you will be struggling for breath and can do no more. With the training we'll describe, however, you might be able to walk down five streets and still never approach MAX. *That's* what we're going to try to achieve. The kind of training that will result in your heart's beating slowly and evenly during exercises and tasks that you do all day will mean that you will have more energy and the ability to go longer and farther in your own daily activities. Your heart will not have to beat furiously to do a minor task. Can you imagine what a difference that will make in your life? What you will gain can be called *endurance.* If now you have to huff and puff and stop after climbing only a few stairs, or after walking only half a block, with training you might be able to do that with a very moderate amount of effort. Endurance can be the difference between barely accomplishing your activities of daily living and having enough energy at the end of the day to enjoy yourself, to socialize, to go to the movies, to go shopping and carry your own bundles, to drive your car, or to go for a walk with your mate or a friend. It can mean not sitting around all day doing only sedentary activities, and it can mean increased ability to have sex and enjoy it more. Because your heart and lungs will be stronger and more efficient, oxygen will be delivered throughout your body with less work. New and expanded blood vessels may form in exercised muscles, providing roadways to carry oxygen. Blood vessels may become more pliable and blood pressure may fall to more normal limits. Fatigue, that terrible enemy of the pulmonary patient, can *decrease!*

To attain cardiopulmonary conditioning, you need your doctor's permission, help, and guidance. When not contraindicated, exercise testing is a valuable tool to help assess your pulmonary function and to help in designing your exercise program. Here's how you can start to attain cardiopulmonary conditioning and begin a training program in an easy-to-follow step-by-step procedure.

TAKING AN EXERCISE TOLERANCE TEST
(STRESS TEST)

An exercise tolerance test is the observation and recording of an individual's cardiopulmonary responses during increasing levels of physical work. A stress test is usually done to rule out heart disease. In your case you also need a measurement of your lungs' ability to take up and utilize oxygen. In a stress test, with a doctor in the room, you walk on a treadmill or ride a special bicycle called an ergometer while your heart waves and rate are continuously monitored.

In addition, there are several ways in which your blood oxygen can be measured. You might wear a small, nonpainful clip on your ear containing a sensing device. This device will constantly read the amount of oxygen in your blood. This is called ear oximetry. A second method is to have your oxygen and other blood gases measured by drawing blood from an artery before, during, and immediately after the exercise test. A third method is to measure your body's actual uptake of oxygen by a mouthpiece attached to a small computer. This is called a metabolic measurement cart. We feel that it is important for the pulmonary patient to have this additional measurement during an exercise test.

You may have no visible signs of heart disease, but if your blood oxygen falls off instead of rising as it should as the energy and oxygen demands of the test increase, you might do better exercising with portable oxygen. In fact, your doctor may want to do two exercise tolerance tests, one with and one without oxygen, to see whether your endurance can increase with the use of oxygen, and this test may be repeated again at a later date to check on your improvement. The pulmonary laboratory at the nearest medical center may be the best place for you to take your exercise tolerance test. *Remember,* measurement of oxygen and blood gases is very important.

Here are some hints to help ease the stress of your stress test. Don't eat for at least two hours before being tested. The preceding meal should be a light one, low in fat. Eliminate all sources of caffeine, including coffee, tea, and caffeinated beverages such as colas, for at least 12 to 24 hours prior to the test. Unless otherwise advised, take all your medications as usual. Wear jogging shoes or sneakers (or the best walking shoes that you have); don't bring slippers! Bring gym shorts, Bermuda shorts, or a pair of loose-fitting light trousers or sweatpants. Women should wear a bra and a loose-fitting short-sleeved blouse that buttons in the front. Don't wear one-piece undergarments or panty hose. Men will have their chest shaved before the test in order to allow placement of the electrocardiogram electrodes.

Go through the test calmly and with a sense of adventure. There will be a doctor in the room with you. Insist on a trial walk on the treadmill before starting a treadmill test. If you feel light-headed, have chest pains, get anxious, and want to call the test off at any time, that's your option. Just say so.

You will start off by moving very slowly on the treadmill, and measurements will be taken constantly. The treadmill will not go faster or be elevated in any way until the doctor is assured that you are doing well and can handle a slightly harder task, and then the workload is increased very gently and gradually. Talk to the doctor giving you the test and get a feeling of confidence in him or her.

After the completion of the walking part of the test, you will lie down. Measurements will continue as your heart and lungs return to a resting state. It's a good idea to have someone go with you when you take the test in case you are exceptionally tired at the completion. Look at stress testing as an exciting experience; have courage and don't be afraid. This is the first step toward becoming an athlete!

THE EXERCISE PRESCRIPTION

The exercise tolerance test has told your doctor the capabilities of your heart, lungs, and muscles and whether you need portable oxygen during your training program. It also can inform your doctor of the safe heart rate range over which you can train. To produce cardiopulmonary efficiency, you must train at a rate as close as possible to 70 to 85 percent of your maximum heart rate (MAX). At first, you may not be able to achieve that and may have to begin at 60 percent. You should, however, work toward this goal, for such a heart rate range will produce maximal cardiopulmonary benefits and the kind of endurance and—yes—athleticism that we described. This heart rate range as prescribed by your doctor is called the *training sensitive zone* (hereafter referred to as *TSZ*). A typical TSZ for an average healthy 55-year-old would be as follows: MAX 220– 55 = 165 and 70 percent of 165 = 115; 85 percent of 165 = 140. Therefore, the TSZ for an average person 55 years of age is 115 to 140 beats per minute. Your training zone may be different because of the limitations of pulmonary disease. No matter. Unless your doctor disapproves of the TSZ concept for you, don't leave the office without this exercise heart range. This is the range that is safe for you.

You will use your TSZ once you get used to it, not only during exercise but during all your activities. You won't have to be afraid anymore. You will know that you are within a safe pulse range. You will use your TSZ when walking, having sex, going to the movies, shopping, fishing, climbing a hill. This is your safe heart rate zone. It can change, because people change. It can go up or down. But you need your TSZ as a guide to begin this program.

You also need the rest of the exercise prescription. How long should you keep your heart in the TSZ? How often? Should you walk or ride a stationary bicycle? Should you use supplemental oxygen? If so, how much? These are all important questions for you. Even if you haven't had a stress test, get exact answers. For most people, we suggest walking. Show your doctor the walk program (see page 125). Ask if you can use it, and ask the doctor to check the starting level that's appropriate for you. The most likely choice will be Level 1.

You now have your exercise prescription. Becoming an athlete is within your grasp. Let's get to work! Don't overdo, but don't be worried by a few minor aches. Get your doctor's support, and start working!

SUGGESTED TRAINING PROGRAM

If there is a group exercise program in your area, perhaps at the YMCA, perhaps designed for the cardiac patient and regulated by pulse and exercise time, try to get into it. You will be able to exercise under supervision. This will be helpful, especially at the beginning. Perhaps there is a cardiac rehabilitation program at your local hospital. The level at which you function might be different, but the principles are the same. See if you can entice the staff to let you into it. If you are really lucky, there might even be a pulmonary rehabilitation program. Once *you* get going, perhaps you can get a community pulmonary exercise program started!

The components in the pulmonary exercise program for cardiopulmonary conditioning are: stretching-flexibility warm-up, stretching-flexibility exercises, warm-up phase, TSZ time, cooldown phase, and post-cool-down flexibility and stretching.

Before we begin explaining these components of your training program in detail, here are a few exercise how-to's.

How to take your pulse: Place the tips of your fingers on the thumb side of your wrist. Having found your pulse, it is important to count accurately. You are going to count for only 10 seconds and multiply by six, and therefore accuracy is essential. If you are off by one beat, then your minute reading will be in error by six beats. You should take your pulse while moving, but if you can't, just try moving in place and take your pulse right away. Know your 10-second heart rate zone and practice. To get your 10-second pulse zone, divide the upper and lower limits of your TSZ by 6: TSZ of 115–140 = 10-second zone of 19–23. If you absolutely can't get your pulse at the wrist, buy an inexpensive stethoscope at a surgical supply store. Tape it to your chest under your left nipple, or wherever your heart sounds the loudest, put it in your ears when you are ready, and count your heartbeat.

The times to take your pulse are as follows:

1. Take a resting pulse in the morning before you get out of

bed. Your resting pulse should decrease as fitness improves. If your resting pulse drops from 80 to 70, this means there are 10 fewer beats per minute; there will be 600 fewer beats required per hour; in 24 hours, 14,400 beats are "saved"—a sign of the heart's increased efficiency.

2. Take the next pulse before you begin to exercise.
3. During exercise, take your pulse every two minutes. Once you can exercise continuously for 15 minutes, take it every five minutes.
4. Take your pulse again at the end of the cool-down period.

When you walk, keep your body erect or lean slightly forward, your shoulders relaxed and down. Let your arms swing naturally. An exaggerated arm swing is inefficient. Step right out, gazing straight ahead. Focus on an object about 30 feet away. Do not shuffle. Increase your stride length to increase efficiency. If you would like to walk faster, raise the arms to about waist height and bend at the elbows and make a gentle opposing swinging action of the arms as you swivel your hips slightly. This will increase your stride length and the speed at which you can move. Remember, most of us get places by walking, not jogging or running. Always try to go longer, not necessarily faster. Keep to the lower level of your TSZ as much as possible. Don't go above your TSZ and never go to MAX except under laboratory conditions.

The ideal temperature for exercising outdoors is between 40° and 60°F. The windchill factor on colder days must be taken into account. Rapid walking will cause a tenfold increase in heat production over that associated with the resting state. Therefore, you can dress quite lightly and just risk being a little cold at the start. On the other hand, do not go far afield on a cold day. The sun may disappear or the wind may come up, affecting the windchill factor and lowering the temperature drastically. (See the Windchill Chart in Chapter 4.) When you exercise, sweating is a natural product of a good workout. The body produces heat, as we just described. Sweating cools the body, but it can also freeze, leaving you feeling wet or damp and chilled on a freezing cold day. Therefore, when you are exercising in the winter, exercise in an area that is effectively in a circle with your home in the middle, so you can get back to your home quickly before hypothermia (excessive coolness of the body) occurs.

After exercise, get yourself into dry, warm clothing such as a turtleneck and a pair of slacks. Never take a hot shower or steam bath after exercising. Take only a lukewarm shower, and then it is best to wait 30 minutes before doing so. A hand-held shower with a vibrating head is inexpensive and will feel wonderful.

You can dress yourself in layers during the cool seasons. The first layer could be long polypropylene or wool blend underwear and socks to wick away sweat. Over that, wear a woolen sweater and pants. If you need additional layers over that, put on another sweater made of wool or a garment made of insulating material, such as down or fiberfill, and then a nylon-type wind-breaking outer layer. If possible, all the upper-body garments should be zipped or buttoned in such a way that they can be loosened easily when you are overheating. At night, wear reflective strip material on your clothing. Woolen mittens are warmer than gloves. Be sure to wear a hat down over your ears. For those people sensitive to cold air, put a scarf under both sides of your hat, over the nose, and under the eyes. Inexpensive cold-weather masks are available at your drugstore. Modify your own wardrobe generally to fit this category. Inexpensive sweatpants that have elasticized bottoms are very helpful as well as a zippered jacket with a hood. You might also consider an outdoor nylon running suit with a vented jacket.

When you exercise in warm weather, wear sunscreens and dress lightly in running shorts and a short-sleeved top. You're an athlete, so dress like one! Do not exercise outside if temperatures are above 85° or humidity above 70 percent. (See the Temperature and Humidity Chart in Chapter 4.) Once again, if you keep yourself in a circle around your home base, you can always "call it off" and go home and you will not find yourself overheated. Drink water any time you are thirsty. Don't worry about overdoing it: You can't. Water should be cool—not ice-cold.

You will need the same great shoe as any runner or jogger. Go to the best-stocked sporting store available. Don't worry if your physique is different from that of the other customers. Your purpose is the same. You're in the exercise crowd now. Check out the following:

1. Is the shoe extremely light?
2. Is there leather reinforcement on the sides of the shoe to prevent "foot drift"?
3. Is the tongue padded to prevent blistering from friction of the laces?
4. Is the toe box roomy enough to accommodate your toes so they can flex while standing, with no prominent stitchery in the toe box?
5. Does the shoe fit relatively snugly without being tight, with no feeling of discomfort from external pressures anywhere?
6. Is there a sole to provide support for your arches?
7. Is the outsole thick, yet soft enough to cushion your foot and to keep it from turning?
8. Is there a padded Achilles tendon protector?
9. Is there an ample collar, padded to reduce pressure and friction and hold your heel in place?

Here is the training regimen. Take it and adapt it to your own needs and abilities.

Stretching and Flexibility

These exercises stretch the muscles and tendons to increase the range of motion of the joints, thereby minimizing the number of injuries. Tight muscles may result in strains and cramps, and besides, having a supple, flexible body feels good.

Stretching routines are as important after exercises as they are before. After exercise, stretching will reduce the tightening effect that occurs as a result of vigorous movement of muscles.

Important points to remember while doing flexibility stretching exercises:

1. Stretch slowly and smoothly—*don't bounce*; bouncing can pull muscles.
2. Let the muscle stretch itself by attaining the position in which you feel a slight pulling sensation, and *hold* that position for 10–30 seconds.
3. Breathe easily during stretching; don't hold your breath.
4. Remember, the purpose is to stretch and obtain suppleness and *not* to strain yourself.
5. *Train—don't strain!*

Stretching-Flexibility Warm-ups

1. Sit comfortably in a chair and make a circle with both feet simultaneously, slowly and easily, for about 30 seconds.
2. Tap your feet gently for another 30 seconds, one after the other. Go slowly; you are just warming up.
3. While sitting, extend both arms out to the side and do arm circles, five circles forward and five backward to begin.
4. Repeat steps 1, 2, and 3 twice.

While doing the above, do not slouch. Sit up and keep the spine straight.

The Warm-up

To warm up, walk, gradually increasing the speed, to bring your pulse rate to just below your TSZ over a seven-minute period. Do not enter your TSZ. This allows your cardiopulmonary system and muscles to adjust *gradually* to increasing energy and oxygen requirements and prevents early burnout, pain, and exhaustion. *Do not skip the warm-up!* You may lengthen it, but do not shorten it.

Training-Sensitive-Zone Time

This is the most important component of your training regimen. During your TSZ time, you increase your effort and bring your heart rate into the prescribed range. It's increasing your TSZ duration that leads to endurance. Stretching-flexibility and warm-up are all appetizers. *This* is your main course! Your ultimate goal is to keep your pulse in the TSZ for 20 to 30 minutes three times a week (four times is even better!) on nonconsecutive days. It may take many weeks or months to accomplish this. Consider this a long-term, lifetime project. Increase your TSZ time very gradually. We have given you a suggested training table.

On alternate days do less strenuous activities. When exercising in your TSZ, exercise by pulse and time. Do *not* try to cover a preset distance. By this we mean: do not try to complete the same distance every training day. Factors such as wind, humidity, pollution, and pollen count change the amount of effort required. Sometimes you will have to walk slowly or your pulse will be too rapid.

Exercising by time and pulse allows for these changing conditions and gives you flexibility. You can vary your "fitness trail" from somewhat hilly terrain to a walk in the mall. In fact, your local mall is a great place to exercise in bad weather.

If your TSZ time is 15 minutes or more, take your pulse every five minutes. If your TSZ time is less than 15 minutes, take your pulse every three minutes.

Self-evaluation in the TSZ is important. In addition to pulse taking, learn to notice how you are feeling and how you are breathing. You should be breathing deeply, but not be "hungry" for air. You should be working hard, but exertion should not be severe. If you can't talk, you're overdoing. Test this even if you have to talk to yourself. Anxiety, nervousness, nausea, light-headedness, and chest pain are all signs that you should slow down. Do not stop abruptly unless you can't avoid it. (See "Cool-down" below.) When you finish exercising in your TSZ, you should feel happy, not tense, and you should be looking forward to your next "TSZ encounter."

If you absolutely need an additional aid to keep your pulse in your TSZ, you might want to look into the purchase or use of the Exersentry electronic heart rate monitor made by Respironics, Inc., available at athletic or surgical supply stores. This small sensing device attaches to the chest and reads out your heart rate constantly. The lower and upper limits of your TSZ are then dialed in.

If you go above your TSZ, a gentle alarm will sound and continue sounding until you have slowed down and your heart rate has fallen back to a safe range.

Cool-down

The purpose of the cool-down is to allow the heart, lungs, and muscles to recover gradually. It also gives a chance for the large pool of blood that is now in the extremities to be redistributed back to the central part of the body. In the cool-down you simply return to the warm-up walk rate. Cool down by walking for approximately five minutes. Remember to *keep moving* and do not stop! Blood pooling can cause fainting. At the completion of the cool-down, take your pulse. It should be below 120 or back to resting level. If not, decrease your TSZ time by going back one level on your training sheet.

Post-cool-down Stretching Flexibility

This relieves the increased contraction of muscles that occurs with strenuous exercise, decreases the number of postexercise aches and pains, and contributes further to overall suppleness and flexibility. Repeat *all* the stretching-flexibility exercises at this point.

If your physician doesn't wish to give you a TSZ, you can still follow all the previously described principles of exercise. Try to obtain at least an upper limit for your safe heart rate.

A Twelve-minute Test

Now that you understand the basics of a training program, why not take a 12-minute walk test and record the results? Simply put, this is the distance you can walk in 12 minutes—comfortably and with no strain. Pick a safe walkway, preferably around your house. You don't need to continue walking for the full 12 minutes. You may stop any time you want. In fact, be sure there are plenty of chairs and stop areas along your walkway. Just walk comfortably, and at the end of 12 minutes record the approximate distance. Here are examples: 550 yards; five times around the living room; one time the length of the mall. Record the results. You will want to repeat the 12-minute walk test regularly to check your progress. During the test, take your pulse now and again to make sure you're not out of a safe range. You may take the test with or without oxygen. Be sure to record that information. Don't overdo during this test. This is *not* a maximum stress test!

The Exercise Diary

Your progress may astound you. Each time you exercise, you should make an entry in your exercise diary (see Table 6.1). Please look carefully at it now as we explain each column. Take a large index card or other firm piece of paper that can fit comfortably in your pocket, and copy the columns onto it. At the top, write your TSZ and your 10-second TSZ. If these change, go to a new diary card. The first column, of course, is the date. The next column is your morning resting pulse. Take this *before* you get out of bed. Your pulse rate should eventually drop as your cardiopulmonary efficiency increases. You will find some variation in your pulse from day to day. Learn what is acceptable regarding variation in pulse for you and what may be your relapse rate (see Chapter 3). The next column is for recording your pulse just prior to any exercise activity, including stretching and flexibility. There are then three columns in which to record subsequent pulses during exercise. The next column is to

TABLE 6.1
Exercise Diary

Training Sensitive Zone _____
10-second TSZ _____

Date	A.M. Resting Pulse	Pre-Exer. Pulse	Exer. Pulse (1)	Exer. Pulse (2)	Exer. Pulse (3)	Post-Exer. Pulse (minutes) 3 5	Duration (total exercise time)	Time at Training Zone	Comments

record your pulse at three and five minutes after exercise is completed. Next, record your total duration time of exercise and then your TSZ time. You will want to see those figures going up. Remember, even an increase of 30 seconds in TSZ time could be a triumph. The last column is for comments, such as "easy day" or "easily winded today." Be sure to record any of the danger signals already discussed, should they occur.

You should show the diary to your doctor regularly, and, in fact, if you don't see your doctor very often, ask if you might mail your results in to him or her. If you are sending the original cards, remember to ask that the doctor return them to you after checking to see that there are no untoward signs or symptoms being recorded by you. Solicit your doctor's cooperation here; you need the help and guidance that a professional can provide.

Walk Program

Do *not* progress to the next level until you have successfully completed a level at least six times. After two weeks on this program, you can tell all your friends that you "work out" regularly!

Starter Level

	Warm-up	Training-Target TSZ in Minutes	Cool-down	Total Time
Level 1	Walk slowly 7 min.	Then walk briskly 3 min.	Then walk slowly 5 min.	15 min.

You may increase your TSZ time by 1 min. instead of 2 (or 30 sec. instead of 1 min.!)

	Warm-up	Training-Target TSZ in Minutes	Cool-down	Total Time
Level 2	Walk slowly 7 min.	Walk briskly 5 min.	Walk slowly 5 min.	17 min.

	Warm-up	Training-Target TSZ in Minutes	Cool-down	Total Time
		Intermediate Level		
Level 3	Walk slowly 7 min.	Walk briskly 7 min.	Walk slowly 5 min.	19 min.
Level 4	Walk slowly 7 min.	Walk briskly 9 min.	Walk slowly 5 min.	21 min.

Bronze Level

	Warm-up	Training-Target TSZ in Minutes	Cool-down	Total Time
Level 5	Walk slowly 7 min.	Walk briskly 11 min.	Walk slowly 5 min.	23 min.
Level 6	Walk slowly 7 min.	Walk briskly 13 min.	Walk slowly 5 min.	25 min.
Level 7	Walk slowly 7 min.	Walk briskly 15 min.	Walk slowly 5 min.	27 min.
Level 8	Walk slowly 7 min.	Walk briskly 17 min.	Walk slowly 5 min.	29 min.

Award yourself the Bronze Medal upon completion of the above!

Silver Level

	Warm-up	Training-Target TSZ in Minutes	Cool-down	Total Time
Level 9	Walk slowly 5 min.	Walk briskly 23 min.	Walk slowly 5 min.	33 min.
Level 10	Walk slowly 5 min.	Walk briskly 26 min.	Walk slowly 5 min.	36 min.
Level 11	Walk slowly 5 min.	Walk briskly 28 min.	Walk slowly 5 min.	38 min.

Award yourself the Silver Medal upon completion of the above!

Gold Level

	Warm-up	Training-Target TSZ in Minutes	Cool-down	Total Time
Level 12	Walk slowly 5 min.	Walk briskly 30 min.	Walk slowly 5 min.	40 min.

Give yourself the Gold!

If you can't go outdoors, go to your local mall. At home, move your arms and legs to music, or walk around your living room. Ride a stationary bicycle or jump rope *without* a rope by a loping action with one foot in front of the other. Always follow your training schedule. Always use the same format of stretching, warm-up time, TSZ time, and cool-down. And, last but not least, get yourself one of those inexpensive, sporty black plastic LCD watches with a stopwatch feature. And how about a personal radio or cassette player?

Bodybuilding and Weight Training

Yes! You can do it! You want to have good general upper and lower body strength. You want a good strong back, and for that you need strong abdominal muscles. You want to be able to open up a jar that's stuck, and to carry a package. Not only do you want cardiopulmonary conditioning, you also want to attain good total body strength and flexibility. The good athlete is an all-around person. To "live well" with COPD, you must be restricted as little as possible from enjoying the ordinary activities of daily living that are available to you. You're not going to become a professional weight lifter, but weight training—that is, lifting light weights—can make an enormous difference in your everyday life.

A good time to do weight training is directly after completing the cardiopulmonary training program for the day. Your muscles will be supple and still ready for action, and you will have a glorious feeling following your walk or after riding your bicycle. Begin with one-pound weights. Try one-pound cans of food as the simplest way to start weight lifting. When you have determined that one-pound weights feel extremely light to you, switch to three-pound weights, which are easily purchased. Try six repetitions to begin with for each of the following exercises and call this one set. Try to build up the number of repetitions to 12. Eventually you can build up the number of sets. Set reasonable goals. Back off if your muscles become sore—it's not necessary. If there is a burning sensation in your muscles, they are exercising vigorously. Once you feel the burn, that's enough of that exercise for the day.

Sit back in the chair in which you did your stretching warm-ups. Ideally, it should have no arms. Try to do each of the following exercises six times to start.

HALF A HEAD ROLL. Gently roll the head from side to side. Roll the head to the right, then back to the left. Rolling the head in both directions is one repetition.

SHOULDER ROLL. Rotate the shoulders gently forward six times and gently backward six times.

SMALL FORWARD ARM ROW. With the arms extended, rotate the arms six times in a small circle forward.

LARGE FORWARD ARM ROW. With the arms extended, rotate the arms six times in a large circle forward.

LARGE BACKWARD ARM ROLL. Rotate the arms six times using a backward motion with the arms held extended.

OPEN SHOULDER FLEXIBILITY. Put the right hand behind the head and try to grasp your fingers with the left hand behind the back. Now switch off and put the left hand behind the back and try to grasp the fingers of the right hand. This exercise can be done three times instead of six. It keeps the shoulder joints open. Women need open shoulders to do such basic tasks as fastening their bra. Men need it to pull up their pants.

FORWARD LIFT WITH WEIGHTS. Pick up a one-pound weight in each hand. Proper breathing technique is now essential. Inhale *prior* to lifting the weight. Exhale *as the weight is being lifted*. Lift the weights to shoulder height in front of you. Slowly bring your arms back to your sides.

SIDEWARD LIFT WITH WEIGHTS. Take a breath. As you are exhaling, slowly bring the arms sideward to shoulder level and then back down slowly.

BACKWARD LIFT. Bring your arms gently backward at no more than a 30° angle behind your body and return slowly. Use the same proper breathing techniques.

FORWARD ROW. Simulate a rowing action. Do this slowly and remember to use the proper breathing techniques.

BICEPS CURLS. Start with arms at your sides, then contract the elbows and bring the weights to your shoulders.

Now put your weights aside.

ABDOMINAL MUSCLE CONTRACTIONS. Sit comfortably in a chair. Contract your abdominal muscles. Bring your belly in.

PC CONTRACTION. *PC* stands for "pubococcygeal muscle." This is the muscle that contracts during sexual activity. Better development will heighten sexual sensation and control. This part of your body should be as well conditioned as the rest of you. Contract the muscle by making the same motion as you would to stop the flow of urine.

KNEE TO CHEST. Bring your knee to your chest, clasp your hands around them. Keep your back straight and your foot pointed. Try to touch your knee to your chest for about two seconds.

ANKLE FLEX. Rest heels on ground. Flex the feet slowly forward and backward.

ANKLE CIRCLES. Make slow circles to right and then to left. You may rest your heels gently on the ground.

Respiratory Muscle Training

Sit still and increase your respiratory muscle power! This is a new exercise concept. You can sit still, use the device we are about to describe, and increase your respiratory-muscle endurance. Just as all your other muscles have come into disuse because you are sedentary, so the muscles that control the vital movement of your lungs as you breathe have become weak from disuse and lack of exercise. As the settings on the inspiratory muscle trainer increase, the air hole diameter decreases, thus "exercising" your inspiratory muscles by making them work harder to inspire the same amount of air.

We recommend that your physician consider your using the P-flex inspiratory muscle trainer (a prescription is necessary). This is a small, plastic whistlelike device made by the HealthScan Company (908 Compton Avenue, Cedar Grove, NJ 07009-1292; phone 1-800-962-1266). It is very inexpensive. It's also convenient and practical for use at home. Enclosed in the trainer's package are complete instructions for an exercise program for your inspiratory muscles. In a recent study with a group of patients who used the trainer and a group who used a sham device, there was marked improvement in maximum work rate and respiratory muscle endurance in the group that used the trainer. The patients who used the sham device showed no improvement. All you do is sit quietly breathing through your P-flex and your respiratory muscles will grow stronger. A nose clip will ensure that all your air comes in through the trainer. You can perform this part of your exercise program while watching TV or reading.

You need your doctor's permission, cooperation, and advice. Read the brochure enclosed in the inspiratory muscle trainer *carefully*. Begin with 15 minutes daily, but try to achieve 30 minutes a day.

When you use the muscle trainer, your respiratory rate and pulse *should not go up*. They should either *remain the same or go down*. If your respiratory rate or pulse is rising, you are using too high a setting.

You may want to follow this procedure, used in studies with the respiratory muscle trainer, to determine whether it is safe for you to go to a higher setting:

1. Use setting number 1 until you can breathe comfortably for 30 minutes and your respiratory rate and pulse are not rising. Do this for a *minimum* of one week. Note your respiratory rate and pulse while breathing on number 1.
2. Increase the respiratory rate setting to number 2. Breathe for 10–15 minutes. Are you breathing comfortably? Is your respiratory rate and pulse *the same or lower*? If so, report this to your doctor and ask for permission to use the second setting.
3. Use the second setting for a *minimum* of one week until you are breathing comfortably for 30 minutes. Note your respiratory rate and pulse while on that setting.
4. Increase the setting to number 3. Over a 10-minute period of time, note your respiratory rate and pulse. If they are *the same or going down*, and if you feel comfortable, notify your doctor and ask for permission to increase the setting by one number.
5. Continue the use of the trainer in this manner with your doctor's permission until you reach the highest number tolerable for you. Continue to use that setting indefinitely, working your way slowly up to 30 minutes a day.
6. When you move up to a higher setting, you may be able to breathe comfortably, but only for five to 10 minutes daily. Therefore, at that higher setting, gradually increase your time back up to 30 minutes.
7. If you are ill and unable to use the trainer for some period of time, go back at least one setting.
8. Be sure to note the care and washing instructions in the pamphlet.

Another device for respiratory muscle training is called the Threshold®. The Threshold is a device that contains an air flow valve on one end, an internal pressure regulator controlled by spring tension, and a mouthpiece at the other end. The tension must be set by your physician after he or she measures your maximal inspiratory force. Maximal inspiratory force is simple to measure but does require a special device. A physician usually sets the tension at approximately 30 percent of the maximal inspiratory force. The training principles are the same, with special caution to avoid overbreathing and soreness of the chest wall. Both devices are manufactured by HealthScan.

We have come to the end of this chapter on exercise. If you've come along with us, you've learned a great deal. Ideally you've been through a stress test and obtained a TSZ. In certain cases, your doctor may not think a stress test is appropriate but may fix a TSZ for you based on his or her knowledge of you as a patient. You've taken a 12-minute walk to sample your progress. You've had the experience of going to an athletic store and buying jogging shoes and weights. You're beginning to do things that the rest of the world is doing. When you open up a magazine, you'll understand what is meant by warm-ups, cool-downs, and TSZ, or, as it's sometimes called, exercise heart range. You should buy runners' magazines and read them—why not? Buy other books on walking and cardiovascular fitness, because cardiovascular fitness treats more than the heart: It treats the whole person. You should also continue to expand your training in calisthenics. Do simple exercises that will not hurt your back or joints. Continue to lift light weights, perhaps increasing to five pounds in time. Watch your strength and endurance improve. This is your ultimate goal. You cannot become a competitive athlete, but you can become an all-around stronger person and be able to live a full day filled with a wide range of activities that include taking care of yourself, exercising, eating right, relaxing, enjoying recreational activities, and having fulfilling sex.

Keep reading about exercise; keep trying. Remember, this is a lifelong program. Think about it in terms of months and years, not days or weeks. You will notice improvement. A small improvement is a lot. Don't get discouraged. Ask questions, and seek advice when you need it. Don't let anything deter you from keeping up your physical activity. Keep in mind the adage "Use it or lose it!" And remember that "success breeds success."

Chapter 7

EMOTIONS

The other chapters in this book have dealt with the physical you: anatomy, physiology, nutrition, medicines, and mechanical aids. Now we're going to talk about the psychological you: your attitudes, knowledge, emotions, and the way you behave toward others and yourself, a subject no less complicated. The physical and the emotional are irrevocably intertwined. If you don't feel well physically, it's hard to keep your spirits up. Likewise, if you're "mentally down" all the time, your physical self will also be depressed. Therefore, it's important to do some soul-searching as you read through this chapter if you don't feel happy and contented most of the time. Let's start with a brief quiz.

LEARNING ABOUT YOURSELF

1. I feel afraid a lot of the time.   Yes _____ No _____
2. Experiencing emotions, even trying to enjoy myself, makes me too short of breath, so I keep my feelings inside.   Yes _____ No _____
3. I have no one to comfort me.   Yes _____ No _____
4. I have no one to set me straight when I go wrong.   Yes _____ No _____

133

5. I get very short of breath when I get
   angry.   Yes _____ No _____
6. I avoid contact with others.   Yes _____ No _____
7. Activities outside the home don't
   interest me.   Yes _____ No _____
8. I feel worthless and dissatisfied
   with everything.   Yes _____ No _____
9. I often look back at what I've lost.   Yes _____ No _____
10. Nothing can change my situation.   Yes _____ No _____

This quiz reveals pertinent information about you. Before you read our explanation, do some thinking about why you answered the way you did. Make your own analysis first.

Would you say, after taking this quiz, that your situation might be described as living in a psychosocial prison? If this expression sums it up, then together we have to figure out how to get you out, make a "prison break."

Let's discuss the significance of the answers you gave in the quiz. A "yes" answer to any of the questions means that you have a problem you must deal with.

1. A "yes" answer denotes excessive fearfulness or anxiety. We all feel afraid some of the time, but most of the time is far too much. Don't settle for it—life can be much better than that. You deserve *not* to feel afraid most of the time.
2. A "yes" answer here means you are in what Dr. D. L. Dudley, professor of psychiatry at the University of Washington, has called an emotional straitjacket, an inability to express your emotions because you are afraid they will give you physical symptoms you can't handle, such as shortness of breath and fatigue. You can't allow this either. You have to be able to cry when you must and laugh when you can.
3. Number 3 indicates social isolation, having no one who intimately cares for you and lacking a "comforter" in life.

We feel that an intimate involvement with another is essential. (We'll tell you why shortly.)

4. A "yes" denotes social isolation again, not having the kind of intimate involvement in which you have not only a comforter but also a "concerned confronter" in life.

5. "Yes" means you're in the emotional straitjacket.

6. "Yes" means social isolation, but of another kind: lack of involvement as what we call a citizen of the world.

7. Another description of social isolation. If you answered "yes" to 3, 4, 6, and 7, you are alone on all counts. Being alone for most people can be too difficult, too impossible, too undesirable, too sad. You owe it to yourself to correct the situation.

8. A "yes" answer denotes excessive sadness or depression, a very painful feeling. You deserve better.

9. A "yes" answer denotes depression or sadness as in question 8, coupled with a grief reaction over loss of vigor— looking backward instead of forward.

10. "Yes" means you feel that nothing, even after reading all the chapters in this book, can change your situation. Tell your doctor.

Did you get anything out of this quiz? Are these your problems? Let's add them up: (1) anxiety, (2) social isolation, (3) depression, and (4) the emotional straitjacket. These add up to the psychosocial prison we mentioned earlier.

INTERPRETING WHAT YOU'VE LEARNED

The human spirit is amazingly resourceful and resilient. Your first obligation is to be for yourself. You must practice enlightened self-interest. You have to care about yourself and take care of yourself. Caring about yourself means eating the proper food, knowing your medications, protecting yourself from illness, and exercising regularly. It means looking out for yourself, making sure that you do things that will make you happy and content. That's what enlightened self-interest is all about. If you don't care about yourself, who will? If you want respect and dignity, you have to quietly inspire that by the way you carry yourself in life. If you act heroically, you'll be treated that way. If you're infantile and dependent on other people for everything, people will look at you in that light. You have to think of yourself as unique and precious and begin to focus on all the things that *you* can do for *yourself*.

But you cannot be a whole person if you are centered *only* on your own needs; nor can you expect someone else to spend his or her life centered on your needs. Give and take are necessary parts of living and loving well. You have to give to get. You must involve yourself with other people in two separate ways. The first is to become as intimately involved as possible with a single other person in a caring relationship. The kind of involvement we're talking about requires communication, reasoning, caring, and concern. These are human qualities that you possess. Make use of them. If your every thought is centered on your own needs, you will have nothing left over for someone else, and that someone else is essential. If you have made even some parts of this book part of yourself—if you know how to eat right, exercise, take care of yourself, and if you can touch someone in any conceivably meaningful way—you definitely have something to offer to another person. You can have a genuine give-and-take relationship. If you don't have one now, find one. If you do have one, work to improve it.

The second way to involve yourself with others is as a citizen of the world—for that is what you are. You must become involved with problems and issues beyond your immediate concerns. Work may meet this need. If not, seek activities that ensure your place as a citizen of the world. Are you wondering what we're talking about? You are a resident of a neighborhood, a town or city, and a state. Are there problems there? Can you help? This is your country. Can you lend a hand to a local government project? You are part of the human race with all its problems.

Can you help the environmentalists?

Can you help neighborhood children who can't read?

Can you help others break the smoking habit?

Can you call the nearest chapter of the American Lung Association and become involved? (The national office is at 1740 Broadway, New York, NY 10019.)

Can you call your doctor and local community center and start a pulmonary rehabilitation program?

Can you help an organization fight poverty, disease, and starvation on the other side of the world?

Start now. Don't give up anymore. Don't waste time grieving over the past. Start now to change things—today, this minute.

We're now going to give you proposed solutions. They are not the only solutions. Add your own, but you must come up with solutions to the problems the quiz may have disclosed. If you cannot, you must be sure to convey this to your physician.

ACTING ON YOUR DISCOVERIES: A FOUR-POINT PROGRAM

1. Start with exercise. Knowing your training sensitive zone, a safe pulse rate for you, is a valuable tool. You'll know what a healthy amount of shortness of breath feels like. You'll begin to know automatically what your body can tolerate with ease or moderate discomfort and what's too much for you. Utilize this perception of how you're doing and how hard you are working or breathing when interacting with others, shopping, having sex, laughing, getting angry, or even feeling sad or blue. Knowing you can handle the emotion and the situation will provide an instant comfort. To know your training zone, however, you have to read the chapter on

exercise carefully, go to a physician, obtain an exercise prescription, and really follow an exercise training regimen.

2. Learn all you can about your disease. Understanding your medications, knowing how to manipulate some of them with permission from your doctor, and doing your own physical self-evaluation will give back to you control over yourself. You won't be living in a fearful world, not knowing from day to day whether you will be healthy or sick. Relapses usually don't happen in a moment. They begin in a subtle way over a period of a few days. Previously, during that time, you might not have known that you were getting sick. You might not have known whether to call your doctor. We hope that by this point in the book you do know how to recognize the beginnings of a relapse, or at least you know how to work toward this goal. Think what that can mean to you. You will not be helpless. To do this, however, you have to study, take notes, keep diaries. You have to look at yourself and give yourself time and attention each day that you may not have been used to doing before this. Your anxiety will drop when you understand your illness and how to handle it.

3. Try to get involved with a single other person and with the world as we've just described. It's time to look forward and say "I won't give up" instead of grieving over what is past and gone. Can you still enjoy the sunshine and the seasons, laugh, reason, love, get angry, want someone, need someone? If so, you can find someone. You have something to offer. Someone also needs you. Involve yourself in community activities. Give to others who are less fortunate than you are. Join social or religious organizations. Volunteer your time and talents. Do you still think you have nothing to offer to the world? Take this test: Are you reading this book? If so, could you volunteer your time to read it to somebody who is blind? If you don't take that first step toward meeting and involving yourself with others, both intimately and in the broader sense as we have described, no one will take it for

you. If you do take that first step, we doubt you'll ever be sorry or want to go back to a restricted atmosphere of social isolation.

4. You've had three do's—now here's a don't. Don't give way to despair. We know you have lost a lot, but you have not lost as much as some people in this world. You have probably already had more than many millions will ever have. You can look forward. You are worthwhile. You may need help, particularly when the going gets rough and you're trying to exercise, learn about yourself, and meet new people; it all seems like an awful lot. What's wrong with getting help? Who can help? Your physician! Getting needed help is well worth your time and effort. Your alternative is to sit alone and sad, feeling sorry for yourself. In a sense, that could be easier. That's right—to give way to despair, and sit smoking and eating junk food may be easier than facing life, finding something to be happy about and to laugh about, and finding someone to care about. Give this a lot of thought. There's much at stake. Replace anxiety and despair with action.

Chapter 8

SEX

Have you given up sex because you thought you could no longer perform? But why? You need less energy to have sex than to climb up a flight of stairs slowly. Caring about sex is as legitimate a concern for you as caring about any other physical function in your life. Just as your capacity to exercise can be improved by a regular program, so your sexual functioning can get better and better if you want it to and if you admit that you care about it. Think it over.

You and your partner must commit yourselves to the idea that you can have sex regularly. You should plan your sexual activity, just as you plan any other important part of your lives. Don't expect it to be spontaneous. Pick a time of day when you're both fresh. If you must unexpectedly put off the act, pick an alternate time. Both of you must be committed to the idea that sexual relations can improve your overall well-being. Living and loving go hand in hand. Don't make sex the last item on your list of activities for the day. Plan a special time and place that's right for both of you.

MANAGING COUGHING AND SHORTNESS OF BREATH

Sex takes preparation for the person with COPD. Pick a time of day when your chest is clear and your sputum volume is down. Use your bronchodilator and do postural drainage if necessary. If you use supplemental oxygen, you might want to turn it up about a liter with your doctor's permission. If during sex you become short of breath or have bronchospasm, don't be coy about it. Tell your partner frankly. You might want to call it off for a few moments. Put your head down and do postural drainage again. Don't get overly anxious and you'll succeed. You also must be frank. Don't expect your partner to know that at this moment your chest is constricting or that the kiss is too long and you can't breathe. Say so, and continue enjoying yourself as soon as you can.

A TECHNIQUE FOR WOMEN WITH COPD

Position is extremely important. Prop yourself up against the head of the bed with pillows or, if necessary, sit in a chair. Your lover must bring the part of his body to be stimulated to you. You must indicate to him what he is to do. For instance, gently guide his mouth toward yours. You are capable of licking with the tongue while breathing through your mouth. Take one section of the body at a time so your partner isn't required to move constantly. Your lover can sit or kneel next to you, facing you. Give quick kisses, flicks of the tongue, and delicate touches over each area of the body you want to stimulate. Use your imagination. Guide his body to the right position.

As you are stroking, kissing, and licking other parts of the body, begin to manually touch the head of the penis and gently stroke your hand over the testicles. If they are up high and tight, your lover is highly stimulated and an ejaculation may soon occur. If you wish to prevent this, decrease the amount of stimulation that you are giving. Hold your hand still or hold the testicles lightly. You can also gently put your fingers around the top of the testicles and pull them down.

This will decrease excitement. If the penis is not fully erect or if you wish to increase stimulation, put the thumbs and forefingers of both hands around the penis and stroke away from the middle, squeezing lightly as you do that. Don't squeeze too hard, or you will decrease erection. As you are stimulating your lover, ask him where he would like to be touched. How hard? How fast? Remember, at this point you are giving him pleasure. Both of you should concentrate on that.

Oral sex is not out as a possibility for you. Have your lover stand beside the bed and bring his penis to your mouth as you sit comfortably. Breathe through your mouth and stroke with your tongue and use manual stimulation at the same time. Remember, the head of the penis is the most sensitive, the shaft the next sensitive, and lastly the scrotum. Keep checking the testicular elevation and gauge the degree of excitement by that and the firmness of the erection. Continue to stroke and caress and lick the penis until the erection is hard and firm. There is no rush! It may take a long time, but don't get anxious.

When you both mutually agree, either by word or gesture, that it is time for ejaculation to take place, you may have to stroke in a very firm manner for which you may not have the strength. Let your lover put his hand over yours and let your hand go limp. Let him set the pace and force of your strokes. Ejaculation will soon occur.

Another good position for you is with your lover lying on his back with his head toward the foot of the bed and his penis within hand's reach. Sit propped up comfortably. If you wish to complete intercourse by having the penis in the vagina, try the woman-on-top position or gently slip off the bed, putting your knees on the floor and supporting your chest on the bed. Your lover can then enter from the rear. You can also turn on your back, put your knees up, and use the traditional position of the man being on top. He should take special care, however, to support his weight on his elbows and knees.

Take your time; don't be afraid to use oral sex; avoid the maneuvers that require you to hold your breath for a long time; be happy and adventuresome about your task! Both partners, at this point, should concentrate on giving the male his orgasm.

Although we described bringing the male to orgasm first, we actually advise that the woman receive attention first. Assume your most comfortable position, as described in the previous section. Your lover can be kneeling or reclining beside you or sitting next to you. Try to assume a position in which both your clitoris and vagina are reachable for manual stimulation. Sitting up with knees flexed gently is fine. If you can lower yourself onto pillows in a semivertical position or sit on pillows on a chair, this should provide adequate entry to your genitals. Let your lover know by the way your body moves how stimulated you are. You should not be afraid to correct him immediately if his stroke is too fast or is painful. Let him know gently what is right for you. Both of you should concentrate on giving you pleasure. You might want to put your hand over his and gently guide him to stroke your clitoris until your level of arousal reaches its climax. Also, your lover can insert his finger into your vagina and locate your G spot to give you additional pleasure. (The G spot is a small round firm area inside the vaginal opening on the anterior wall.) You may prefer simultaneous stimulation of the clitoris and the G spot, or alternating stimulation of these areas. If you wish to have your partner put his penis into your vagina, assume one of the positions described above.

There is no reason why the male cannot be brought close to ejaculation and the female then be brought close to orgasm and positions changed to allow the penis to be inserted into the vagina if that is what you both wish. However, it may be difficult and not always best to achieve simultaneous orgasm. We recommend that the male partner bring you through orgasm if possible and then insert the penis into the vagina; you could at the minimum have additional pleasurable sensations from this. Although you may want to use the penis in the vagina, remember it's not necessary. Each of you can have a satisfying and pleasurable experience without actual intercourse in the traditional sense.

A TECHNIQUE FOR MEN WITH COPD

Position is extremely important for the male with COPD and is the key to success. Prop yourself up against the back of the bed or sit in an armless chair. Just as with the female, it is important for you to guide your partner's body toward you. Read the section on the female. The same principles apply. You can give short kisses and use your tongue and still breathe with an open mouth. Don't rush your partner. There's plenty of time. Use her stimulated appearance and the joy you are giving her to stimulate yourself while you are giving her pleasure. When it comes time for more intense stimulation, a good position for the woman to assume is on her back with her head toward the foot of the bed, her knees flexed, her genital organs facing you. If she wants, her clitoris can be stroked easily and effectively, and your finger can be inserted into her vagina to stimulate her G spot. Watch the movement of her body. If she moves toward you, she is finding the sensations pleasurable and her arousal is increasing. If she moves away, back off. The clitoris is extremely delicate. Let her put her hands over yours and show you her magic spots and indicate to you the pace and the force with which she wants to be stroked.

To practice oral intercourse, you could kneel on the floor facing your partner. She can lie on her back on the bed with her genitals in front of your mouth. You will have plenty of air to breathe in this position. Remember to watch her body. If she is lifting her pelvis toward you and is lying comfortably and relaxed, she is enjoying herself. If she pulls away, you are making her uncomfortable. Ask what you can do. Is this too fast? Am I too firm? Remember, at this point you are both concentrating on her pleasure. Anything she indicates to you is the right way. To bring a woman to orgasm through clitoral stimulation, usually no extra firmness or particular strength is required. This can be done with the tongue or with the fingers. If, however, you are having trouble achieving the ultimate goal, your partner should put her hand over yours. Your hand should go limp and she should direct the pace and firmness of the stroke until orgasm is achieved.

To have an orgasm, stay in a position that feels comfortable. Your partner has free access to your body whether you are sitting in a chair or propped up in bed. Be relaxed and unafraid, and enjoy yourself. Indicate any movements that are not pleasurable. Correct these movements immediately. Don't be afraid to communicate! Do it freely, gently, and firmly. Read the principles in the previous section: They apply to you as well. If you are having trouble achieving ejaculation, you can guide your partner's hand or her mouth. She may be kneeling in front of you, or she may be on the floor in front of you as you sit in a chair or on the edge of the bed. Any way you are comfortable is acceptable. If you wish to enter her vagina with your penis, here are some recommended positions: Your partner can lower her vagina onto your penis while you sit. If you like, you can stand while your partner leans over a bed or table and you can thus make a rear approach. This position requires more energy expenditure. Remember once again, you don't need to have intercourse in the traditional sense to have wonderful sexual experiences. You can have the ultimate orgasm by manual or oral stimulation. You just have to be willing and open-minded enough to do it.

Covering every possibility is beyond the scope of one chapter. However, you can use the principles you've learned here and experiment for yourself. If you want, find books that graphically demonstrate sexual positions. Accept what you like; reject the rest. Find ways to stimulate each other at the same time and/or concentrate on ways for the both of you to concentrate on one partner at the same time. Don't forget communication! Leave any bitter or angry remarks out of the bedroom scene. If you have any real criticisms, save them for a time well after sex is over. The postcoital period is a time for further talk and romance, not for corrections or criticisms. Consider developing your sexuality a lifelong task. Work hard at it and the rewards will be great.

Chapter 9

CONSERVATION OF ENERGY, RELAXATION EXERCISES, AND PANIC TRAINING

Here are five top-priority activities we want you to concentrate your energies on:

1. eating right
2. working out regularly
3. getting as much sexual stimulation and satisfaction as you need
4. participating as a member of your own health care team
5. keeping your mind alert and stimulated

These areas require your urgent daily attention and commitment. In all other activities you want to conserve energy and do things as quickly and as efficiently as possible. You want to have enough stamina left over for the top-priority items. You want to eat a great diet, but you want to expend as little time and energy as possible cooking and shopping. You want to dress well and have clean, nice-looking clothes, but you don't want to spend hours hand-washing delicate materials. You want your house sparkling and dust-free, but with no time to cook and certainly no time to scrub clothes, you definitely don't want to spend a great deal of time and energy doing housework. That's what this chapter is all about: conserving time and energy. Look at our five top-priority items, and we hope you'll notice that these are the activities essential to a great life for anyone. Look at someone you admire, let's say an executive in a top company. If that person doesn't have the time to highlight these activities, we don't think he or she is "living well." Now that you've got the general idea, let's get down to specifics.

CONSERVATION OF ENERGY (COE) FOR PERSONAL HYGIENE

Take good care of your teeth. Infected and broken teeth lead to poor nutrition because of inability to chew properly and comfortably and multiplication of germs, which in turn can infect your lungs.

This is as good a place as any to tell you how to make our special invention—a bib-style holder. Take a chain designed to keep you from losing your eyeglasses and attach metal electrical clips to each end. Sling the chain around your neck and attach to it any appropriate length of paper toweling. You can use your special bib when practicing COE in the bathroom, and it will be equally handy for keeping your clothes clean while eating. We'll mention it again in the section on COE for housekeeping.

Obtain a rechargeable electric toothbrush (soft bristles) and a rechargeable electric shaver. Set up a personal hygiene center consisting of a comfortable chair, a table with mirror, round toothpicks, dental floss, disposable cups, a shaver, and necessary combs, brushes; and makeup. At the sink have paper cups, a toothbrush, and toothpaste. Sit comfortably at your personal hygiene center and shave first. Next brush your teeth, angling the brush up for the upper teeth so that the ends of the brush gently massage the gum line and the base of your teeth. Angle the brush down for the bottom teeth. If your inner jaw is narrow in the center, you can hold the brush vertically. The major problem with teeth is the presence of plaque, a gritty substance you can feel with your tongue at the base of your teeth near the gum. Plaque control is essential if you want to retain the teeth that you have and prevent gum disease. Most teeth from middle age on are lost from gum disease and not from cavities. As you hold the brush over each section of your teeth, count slowly to 10. Finish by brushing the chewing surfaces. You are sitting comfortably—take your time. You need a full three minutes.

When you have finished brushing, it's time to use dental floss to clean the loose triangles of gum tissue between teeth. Wind 18 inches of the floss mostly around the middle finger of one hand and the rest around the middle finger of the other, leaving a few inches in between. Use your thumbs and forefingers to guide the floss gently between the teeth. When the floss reaches the tip of the triangular gum flap, curve the floss in a C shape against the tooth. Move the floss five or six times up and down along the side of the tooth gently, going under the gum line until you feel resistance. Without removing the floss, curve around the base of the adjoining tooth and floss that one, too. Turning your middle fingers brings you fresh floss. Take another three minutes. Take care not to injure your gums when either brushing or flossing—gums are delicate. Lastly, slide your tongue over the brushed areas.

Once you've finished at your hygiene center, return to the sink, empty any cups you've used, and rinse your mouth. You might like to use a dental irrigator also. Using the lowest setting, aim the jet tip between your teeth to remove any final particles, using a constant side-to-side motion. It's also convenient to use around bridgework. You should practice oral hygiene at least twice a day and preferably after each meal. You can floss in bed in the evening if that's more appealing.

Conserve energy by having a chair or stool to sit on in the shower. Exchange your old shower head for a hand-held shower that can be switched to a variety of delightful sprays. It will not only be easier to clean yourself without getting your hair wet or water in your ears, but you will also be able to use the shower head to rinse off the walls of the shower and the bathtub. And besides, a vibrating massage is a luxury you'll appreciate after a brisk exercise session. We recommend that after you shower you use standard-size towels rather than heavy bath towels that may be luxurious but fill with water and are difficult to launder.

Don't rush your bowel movements. Once eating is over, a gastrocolic reflex occurs. This means that the large bowel gets stimulated by food in the stomach. Therefore, after meals might be an easier time for defecation. The occasional use (no more than once or twice a week) of simple glycerin suppositories available at any supermarket or drugstore may help you avoid straining and decrease the work of breathing during the act.

Do as many of your personal hygiene tasks as you can while wearing your pajamas. If you get a little toothpaste on your pajamas, it's not nearly as difficult to live with as getting the same stain on other clothes.

A special note: Now might be a good time to take a renewed interest in your appearance. We highly recommend a snappy new haircut, one that's attractive without requiring much maintenance or frequent visits to the hairdresser. Women may want to try using some makeup that will look great and not take much time or energy from the morning's routine. (Hypoallergenic cosmetics are readily available if needed.) A few simple changes can make both men and women look better and *feel* better—and you're worth it.

COE IN THE KITCHEN

The kitchen is not a good place to get your exercise. In fact, contrary to popular opinion, the kitchen is a good place to take it easy. You don't want to use up a good deal of your precious energy making meals and then be too tired to eat them. If you have too many dishes, ingredients, or cooking utensils, if you get overheated or overtired, you simply won't cook. You will be tempted to eat junk foods. You also won't have enough energy left over for the important things described in this book. Unless cooking is the love of your life, read this chapter carefully and learn how to cook with a minimum of effort. Tasty food, however, is one of the true joys of life, so the aim of this section will be to show you how to make tempting and nutritious meals. The foods we have mentioned in Chapter 5 provide a good diet with little or no preparation. Don't worry about getting bored with the food. You're free of the drudgery of complicated cooking and extensive cleanup. Set your mind to using a minimum of mixing and measuring tools.

If you need oxygen, bring it into the kitchen. If necessary, obtain 50 feet of tubing. You may need that anyway to walk around your house comfortably during the day. You do not, however, want to have oxygen in your nose when using an open flame. Do not use a gas stove while using oxygen—it's just too risky. Luckily, however, you really don't need any stove, and you certainly should not be bothered with an oven. Ovens change the humidity in the room; they require bending and lifting of heavy, hot pans. The well-equipped kitchen for the pulmonary patient has a toaster oven with a pop-out shelf, an electric nonstick frying pan, an electric can opener, a blender, and a second electric frying pan with a rack in it for steaming or a nonstick electric wok to use as a steamer. If you can, buy a microwave oven and an electric warming tray.

Put your electric frying pan next to the sink in such a manner that you can lift the handle, leaving the front part of the frying pan on the counter, and dump residue right into the sink. Never put away your electric frying pan, blender, toaster oven, electric can opener, or any other piece of equipment that you find useful.

Get out your favorite spices and leave them out where they can be easily reached. If you want to use salt, put one level teaspoon at a time in a small, clear glass shaker. You will want to know how much—that is, how little—you are using. Leave flour out in a small canister or shaker container.

Have several rolls of paper towels placed at strategic spots in the kitchen. Have small wastepaper baskets lined with disposable plastic bags also placed in important spots around the kitchen. You must be able to dispose of paper towels, napkins, bones, and other garbage directly at your feet. We're aiming for a minimum number of steps.

A nontoxic, nonfume-emitting liquid multipurpose glass, appliance, and cabinet cleaner should also be in evidence. (See Chapter 4.)

Obtain a heat-sealer, boilable and freezable cooking bags, and labels. Cook an extra portion each night and seal it in a bag. If you do this for one week, the following week you'll only have to boil water and drop in a bag to make your main dish.

Get breakfast, lunch, and dinner ready all at the same time. We recommend preparing three meals just before dinner. Dirtying the kitchen and cleaning it up once in 24 hours is all that's necessary. You will be cooking dinner for that day and breakfast and lunch for the next day.

Begin by getting your main meal cooking. *Now* try the *three-tray system*—one tray for each meal. Here are some suggestions for breakfast and lunch.

Tray 1 contents (breakfast):

1 paper cup filled with skim milk
1 paper cup filled with bran cereal or other equivalent
   high-fiber cereal
1 paper cupcake holder filled with low-fat cottage cheese
   (your "butter")
Roll or slice of whole wheat bread
½ grapefruit
Napkin, grapefruit spoon, teaspoon, cereal spoon, knife

Tray 2 contents (lunch):

Pita sandwich with low-cholesterol low-fat cheese, 1
   tablespoon peanut butter (if allowed), and lettuce
Carrot
Cucumber
Sweet pepper
Tomato
Apple
Knife, spoon, napkin

Cover all items appropriately and place the trays in the refrigerator. If one tray is smaller, you can place it on top of the other and carry both in one easy trip (and it will take less space in the refrigerator).

On the counter have two disposable cups containing a tea bag or instant-drink powder. The above menu is for the 1,500-calorie Healthy Core Diet. Consult Chapter 5 for other appropriate variations.

In the morning take tray 1 from the refrigerator. Stop off at an electric coffee pot that was turned on by an inexpensive timer and is now filled with hot water. Add the water to the appropriate cup and take tray 1 to the table. You will have one trip to the table going and only one trip coming back. Throw the disposable plates and cups out in a convenient basket on your way back to the kitchen. Use the same system with trays 2 and 3 for lunch and dinner.

During week 1 make dinner five nights for double the number of people who eat it. If you're one, for instance, cook for two. Seal one portion in the boilable cooking pouch and freeze. Week 2—just boil the bag and steam your vegetables. Label the bags. (Be careful not to buy bags that are bigger than you need.)

On the day you shop, do not cook. That's a good time to eat out or consume a high-quality prepackaged dinner. Try to limit yourself to buying foods with 10 grams of fat or less per serving as listed under the nutritional analysis on the label. Eat out or use prepared foods one other night per week, but keep the sodium content of this meal in mind.

When you cook dinner at night, limit the number of utensils you use to three. Use one electric frying pan, and another as a steamer. A wok can be used for stir-frying *and* steaming. Remove any excess grease or oil from your pans by using a wad of paper toweling. Virtually eliminate all chopping, mincing, and cutting.

Learn to look at recipes critically and change items that increase work; adapt recipes to your own use. For instance, for sliced onions, use frozen chopped onions or onion powder; for minced garlic, use garlic powder; for fresh peeled, seeded tomatoes, use canned stewed tomatoes; for potatoes, use canned boiled potatoes.

You can also utilize a powdered egg substitute. This is cholesterol-free and can be used in place of eggs in many recipes.

Make special arrangements right now for those days on which you don't feel well. You should have on hand at least a one-week supply of powdered, high-calorie foods (try drugstores), whose packages state that they contain 100 percent of the recommended daily allowance of protein, vitamins, and minerals. Even though some of these are sweet, you may not be able to eat when you don't feel well, and in this way you'd be able to keep your nutrition up.

You should puree meat, soup, and vegetables in a blender and pack them in boilable-freezable bags or other freezing containers, label them, and put them in the freezer. If you can eat only liquids, at least they will have a familiar taste and be as nutritious as regular foods. Have powdered milk and canned milk on hand, as well as vacuum-sealed bags of dried fruits and nuts.

When cooking, use no measuring spoons or cups. Substitute the following for measuring equipment. You already know how much a cup is: the amount of water you pour in when you make yourself a cup of tea or coffee. If you're not sure, take the pans you are cooking in, such as your electric frying pan, and pour one cup of water in there now and see what the level is. That will be a cup every time. Think about things as a shake, a long pour (which is about three seconds), or a short pour (which is to tip the bottle and flip it back again). A couple of heaping tablespoons is a small handful. If you're not sure, measure it once.

Protect your clothing in the kitchen and while eating: You don't want a lot of wash. Use the bib we described in the personal hygiene section. Roll out a longer length of paper (or clip on a towel or cloth napkin). You have an instant, disposable apron. Use caution with a paper bib near the stove. (By the way, you should take the same little gadget with you to restaurants and use the restaurant napkin. Ask for an extra napkin for your lap. Recently we went all over New York in very good restaurants and used this little gadget. People didn't even care, and some asked us where they could buy one.)

Don't use anything but paper towels in the kitchen. Buy a brand

153

that is safe for both cooking and cleaning and is made with natural fiber.

In all of your cooking, think: How can I use the minimum number of dishes and make the least mess to clean up? How can I take the minimum amount of steps? How can I minimize lifting, twisting, bending, chopping, and cutting? How can I make an entire dinner using only one or two pots and perhaps a spoon and fork? You'll find that combining COE in the kitchen with the Healthy Core Diet is easy to do.

COE FOR HOUSECLEANING

COE for housecleaning means having a lightweight electric broom, a rechargeable electric hand-held vacuum, a lamb's-wool duster with an 18- to 24-inch handle, a lightweight carpet sweeper, a nontoxic all-purpose liquid appliance and cabinet cleaner in a plastic spray bottle, a hospital magnetic-type dust mop (as large as is practical), and a long paper towel bib. You may need a bucket to hold all your equipment.

In the bathroom, keep paper towels and appropriate cleaners right out in the open.

Wipe off the sink and faucets with the cleaner immediately after using the bathroom. Likewise, wipe down the shower quickly with a squeegee mop. Use a toilet brush once a day. Use unscented liquid soap in the bathroom, bathtub, and shower to prevent soap buildup in the soap dish.

Your real enemy is dust. Wear a mask to protect yourself when you stir up dust. Armed with your lamb's-wool duster for high places, damp dust cloth, electric broom, lightweight carpet sweeper, and hand-held vacuum, you can prevail.

Make sure there are mats outside your front door for removing dust and other debris from shoes.

A foam squeeze mop should be adequate for doing kitchen floors.

For spills and stains, saturate the stain with a nontoxic liquid cleaner and wait. Let the cleaner do your work for you.

Your bed is a critical place. You want it comfortable, but you don't want to spend a lot of energy fixing it up. We call this our hypoallergenic conservation-of-energy bed. Put cotton barrier covers over the box spring and mattress, and put a fitted sheet over the box spring. Leave the fitted sheet on the box spring indefinitely. Next put an all-cotton mattress pad on the mattress, and over that a fitted sheet, a top sheet, and an all-cotton duvet filled with all-cotton blankets. The last item serves as both a bedspread and a blanket. You will be perfectly warm and comfortable in all weather.

When arising in the morning, grasp the top sheet and duvet and with one tug pull them up under the pillow, pat, and your bed is made. An alternate way to make your bed is to leave the duvet and sheet at the bottom of the bed folded over. When you get into bed you only have to pull the bedclothes up.

To change the sheets, put a chair or bench near the foot of the bed. Lay the comforter and blanket back on it. Change the fitted bottom sheet on a different time schedule from the top sheet so you'll only have one sheet and a pillowcase to wash at one time. The first and third weeks of the month you might want to change the bottom sheet and the second and fourth weeks of the month the top sheet. Use the occasion of changing the bedclothing to make extra sure that dust is not accumulating under the bed.

COE FOR SHOPPING

Map out the supermarket according to your Healthy Core shopping list. Go blithely past the huge varieties of foods. You don't require any variation to know you are eating well. For staple items, which include toilet paper, bathroom tissues, napkins, paper towels, foam plates, and cups, we suggest bulk buying. Look in the Yellow Pages and find a dealer who will deliver a half or whole case of these items. If you have a storage problem, you'll have to work around this idea. We bet there's a closet somewhere in your house stuffed with clothes you never use. Get a family member or friend to go with you a few times a year to buy other staple items such as soap, toothpaste, soap powder, and cleaning solution. Make a list of any items that you know do not spoil and that you can buy in bulk in advance. This will make your weekly shopping load much lighter.

Buy frozen foods, particularly vegetables, in large bags in which vegetable pieces are each frozen singly. You can take out as many pieces as you want at a time. Boxes of frozen vegetables are handy if you are cooking for more than one person but may be less convenient to use for a single portion.

Find a grocer who will cut meat the way you want it cut, with a minimum of bone in a small enough portion, and who possibly can deliver. It will be worth the extra money. If not, make friends with the butcher in your supermarket. He or she can be very accommodating.

Do most of your clothes shopping by using catalogs. Think about wearing a cotton jumpsuit. This will be lightweight and washable, and can be worn almost anywhere; with a one-piece item you're dressed and ready to go. You could have one jumpsuit that you don't wash very often and use for housecleaning and other chores. Don't buy any clothes that are not colorfast (including socks), and don't buy any clothes that can't go in both the washer and the dryer. All washing instructions should be the same on your clothes, something like "Wash Warm and Tumble Dry Medium."

Use the Yellow Pages. Phone ahead. Don't go to a store unless you know you have a good chance of finding the item you want. Get as many items delivered as you can. Bank by mail whenever possible. Use a bank close to your supermarket or grocery store. Consider keeping a month's worth of "cash" in traveler's checks.

COE FOR WASHING CLOTHES

COE for washing clothes means buying the right kind of clothes that we've just told you about. Now here's how to make it even simpler. Obtain two to six mesh laundry bags. As you use your underwear, put T-shirts or bras in one, shorts or panties in another, and socks in a third (or if you're not that fussy, put all the dirty underwear in one bag). When the bag or bags are moderately full, drop the entire bag filled with soiled laundry into the washing machine. When washing is completed, take the bag out and put it in the dryer. When drying is completed, do not empty your clothes out of the bag. Hang the bag or bags on pegs and take out your clothing as you need it. Don't worry if your underwear is wrinkled: it's a small price to pay to free yourself from so much drudgery. Just think—a minimum of effort at the washer-dryer. Wash everything at the same temperature, for example, warm wash and wear or cold rinse. Dry everything at medium. If you happen to be washing only towels, you might want to go to a hot drying cycle. Wash towels and sheets together, shirts, slacks, and underwear together.

COE FOR DAILY ACTIVITIES

General COE for daily chores means not bending at the waist. Bring any items to your midsection, putting your center of gravity there for lifting, using both arms if possible. Bend from the knees gently. Pull an item along the floor or counter rather than lift it. Wherever possible, sit down while you do your chores. Make work centers for yourself: Store all equipment for a task in a central place and leave it there.

COE for keeping current may mean not buying a daily newspaper (possibly a bother to get and a lot of waste to get rid of) but rather using the TV or radio to keep up with daily news. You can subscribe instead to a weekly news magazine.

Let timers work for you: for instance, a timer on the TV set so you can fall asleep without getting up, a timer to turn your lights on in the morning and off in the evening. Inexpensive timers are available for your thermostat, and other timers can be attached to room heaters to make sure that a room is warm and comfortable before you enter it and then cools down after you customarily leave it. You can save on fuel bills and yet keep your home at a comfortable, stable temperature as you move from room to room in the winter. Air conditioners may also be regulated by timers.

Your daily chores may require you to climb stairs. If so, figure out the fewest number of daily trips you can make. Plan your day and your week. Make a list of necessary tasks, applying the principles demonstrated in this chapter to other activities of daily living that we may not have covered.

Incidentally, here's an easy way to walk up the stairs: breathe in standing still, walk up about three stairs while breathing out, using pursed-lip breathing if comfortable. Stop a moment, breathe in, and then continue. Your stop may be long or so momentary that no one notices it, but if you need COE walking up the stairs, try this method.

COE FOR MEDICATIONS

COE for medications means opening your bottles just once a week yet never missing a pill! Obtain one to four different-colored, divided, one-week-size medication dispensers (one for each time of the day you take medications). Label the dispensers for the appropriate times. Not only are you now all set for a week, but you'll also be able to know if you forgot to take any of your pills.

RELAXATION EXERCISES AND PANIC TRAINING

We all know what provokes anxiety and fearful feelings. What we don't know how to do is turn them off. That's what we're going to show you in this section. These techniques, called relaxation exercises and panic training, should be practiced every day. Relaxation involves the mental as well as the physical. Be completely carefree while practicing the exercises. If any worrisome thoughts occur, let them float away.

Let's get started with relaxation training:

1. Sit in a comfortable position in a quiet room. You want to be awake and refreshed after these exercises, not asleep, so don't lie down.

2. Systematically tense and relax the muscle groups to be described. In each case feel the tension and the disagreeableness that go with it, and then enjoy the relaxation, light feeling, and return of blood flow into the muscle.
3. At the end of all the relaxation exercises, if any part of your body is still tense, do those exercises again.
4. In each case, while contracting or tensing the muscle, slowly count "one one-thousand, two one-thousand, three one-thousand" to yourself and then relax for a similar or slightly longer count.

Here are the specific maneuvers:

Make a fist with the right hand. Count—relax. (Remember, study the tightness, the tension; squeeze the muscles to the count of "one one-thousand, two one-thousand, three one-thousand," and then note the feeling of lightness, relaxation, and blood flowing back into the muscles.)

Make a fist with the left hand. Count—relax.

Bend the arm at the elbow, feeling the tension in the upper arm. Right arm first, then left arm. Count—relax.

Grasp the left shoulder with the right hand and pull, feeling the tension in the right lower arm. Count—relax.

Grasp the right shoulder with the left hand, feeling the tension in the left lower arm. Count—relax.

With the feet flat on the floor, push the toes away, feeling tension across the top of the feet. Count—relax.

Curl your toes upward, producing tension in the front of the shin. Count—relax.

Squeeze the buttocks together and feel tension across the back of them. Count—relax.

Push the abdomen out as you breathe in, as though you were filling it with air. Count—relax.

Arch the back forward and put your shoulders back, producing tension in the lower back. Count—relax.

Contract your abdominal muscles. Count—relax.

Bite down with your teeth, clenching the jaw, and then allow the mouth to fall slightly open. Count—relax.

Put your tongue to the roof of the mouth, feeling tightness in the tongue and on the top of the mouth. Count—relax.

Wrinkle the forehead and the nose, feeling tightness across the face. Count—relax.

Grimace, pulling the lips back and feeling tightness across the mouth. Count—relax.

Now feel as though you are floating on a cloud, and think of your own secret word that means "calm" to you. Repeat it in your mind. Feel as though you are being supported by the cloud. Count backward from five to one slowly.

Are you relaxed? Did you answer "no"? If so, have you had the right mental attitude toward these exercises? Remember, in many cases it can be easier to be tense and fractious than calm and happy. Your job is to work on the latter.

Don't expect to break bad habits overnight. Practicing COE and relaxation techniques in all of the multivaried activities of daily living may sound simple when you read it. Don't get discouraged when you try to incorporate them into your daily routine and find out that it takes a lot of discipline. Keep working at it. Each time you find a system or idea that works, grasp it, make it your own, and integrate it into your personality and routine as soon as you can. Take one idea or half a dozen ideas, whatever you can work with comfortably; then go on to improve yourself with practice.

Before you know it, with each task you have to do, your mind will begin applying COE techniques.

Keep practicing relaxation exercises. Give them the few moments a day they deserve.

Panic training is for those times when relaxation exercises aren't sufficient: those times when you find yourself breathing fast with rising fear you can't control. Rapid, shallow, uncontrolled breathing is very ineffectual, as you well know by now; it will merely drop the pressure in the bronchial tree and cause airway collapse. Begin panic training today. If possible, sit down at a table and rest your shoulders and your head quietly on the table top. Support your feet by having them rest gently on the floor. Push the chair slightly back from the table so you are sitting up and leaning slightly forward with your shoulders on the table. This will expand the rib cage. Use the secret word you invented for relaxation training that means "relax" or "be calm." Tell yourself, "———— down." That means relax, let go, stop grabbing at the air. Allow more time to breathe in. You might want to hold your breath at the end of inspiration as you count "one one-thousand, two one-thousand," and then allow more time to breathe out. Try to let your belly wall balloon out as you breathe in to allow more room for the diaphragm to drop. Purse your lips gently on expiration. Practice slow, even breathing; this will keep up the air pressure in the bronchial tree. It will allow more time for the oxygen to cross over that delicate alveolar membrane into the bloodstream before you breathe out. Transfer the same feeling of relaxation of body from relaxation exercises to relaxation of breathing. If you exercise and know your training sensitive zone, otherwise known as a safe pulse range, you will have less of a reason to panic. You will know what is a safe pulse range for you, and you will learn that one of the most important things to learn from an exercise program is how to pace yourself. Long before panic, if you think that you're beginning to grab at the air, check your pulse. The pulse is a very sensitive indicator of the status of the cardiopulmonary system. If your pulse is over your safe range, slow down before panic sets in. If you are not near a table, then try sitting and using the same respiratory maneuvers.

161

Practice relaxation exercises once a day and panic training once a day, and use both techniques in tight situations—relaxation when you're tense, and panic training when short of breath. With practice you'll become quite an expert. You'll be able to save the situation and avoid unnecessary distress.

You should control your emotions; they shouldn't control you. Remember, with conservation of energy, relaxation, and panic training, you are using as little energy as possible on necessary but unimportant tasks in order to have all the energy and joie de vivre necessary for the important things in life.

Chapter 10

LEISURE, WORK, AND TRAVEL

BEING ACTIVE

How can you be as active as possible? Force yourself to get started. Doing nothing is easy. It's also boring, depressing, and degrading to the human spirit. Doing something is harder. It's also invigorating, uplifting, inspiring, and ennobling to the human spirit. Keep going. Use rest periods, relaxation exercises, panic training, and your training sensitive zone as aids, *but keep moving*. Risk a little. After you've pushed yourself to do something, ask yourself if it was worth it. And if it was, push yourself some more. If it wasn't, change the activity.

Force yourself to do the things you find worthwhile. When you think you've had it, try this: Get in your most comfortable position for 10 minutes. Can you change your mind and go ahead? You might be wondering, What has pushing myself got to do with a chapter on leisure anyway? We're not talking about driving yourself when you're short of breath, but rather about those times when you feel like sitting around and vegetating. Recreation is a necessary part of *every* day, and having fun does take effort. We want you to understand and think about the kinds of recreation that are available to you and at the same time make sense for you.

ENERGY COSTS

One MET (metabolic equivalent) is the energy expenditure at rest, or, more simply explained, the amount of oxygen required while sitting quietly. Normally, it is 3.5 milliliters of oxygen per kilogram of body weight. That is to say, the heavier you are, the more oxygen you need both at rest and with exercise. You may burn more than 3.5 milliliters of oxygen per kilogram of body weight per minute at rest because your work of breathing may be increased. Nevertheless, for our purposes we will say that one MET will be considered baseline energy expenditure at rest for you. There are many worthwhile activities that require virtually no energy expenditure above one MET. We define these as activities for hand and mind. Energy expenditure increases as activity increases. Running burns approximately 10 METs, and this is the average maximum number of METs that a vigorous person can expend. Activities with energy expenditures higher than one MET will be grouped as recreation for hands, mind, and body and will be given numbers from 2 to 10, representing the relative need for oxygen above the resting level—for example, 10 METs is 10 times the resting oxygen requirement. You can't take these values as absolutes. An expert tennis player may require fewer METs to play than a novice. It's helpful, however, to think about activities in terms of their energy cost to you as being at or above your resting level.

Recreation for hands and mind includes knitting, crocheting, needlepoint, embroidery (acceptable activities for men as well as women in this day and age), reading,* assembling electronic kits, rug hooking, macramé, and similar activities. Think how nice it is to give someone a present you've made. It says, "I'm back in this world." And what about making something for yourself? Other one-to-two-MET activities include playing cards, chess, and checkers.

---

*Reading, strictly speaking, doesn't involve the hands, but it is a great one-MET activity.

Since we separate therapeutic exercise from recreation, vigorous activities are not required. Engage in as many recreational endeavors as please you and at levels of physical activity that are comfortable and appropriate. Recreation means fun—do whatever gives you the feeling of having it. Remember—it's *right* to have fun every day.

Now what about a personal computer? For a small expenditure, you can open up a whole new world: learn to program, keep track of your diet, daily physical examination, budget, and finances. For a little more you can connect by phone to computers around the country and communicate with other computer operators.

Have you ever thought of drawing, perhaps just with charcoal, or with watercolors or acrylics?

Keep yourself busy with projects. Have something to take up with your hands *every day*.

Activities for hands, mind, and body include swimming if you know how (if you use oxygen, get your long tubing and leave the tank on the side of the pool). Take up golf, for two to three METs with a power cart, or three to four pulling the bag. Light shoveling and gardening take five to six METs. Don't forget to go to movies, shows, concerts, national historic sites, and museums. As a point of reference, splitting wood is about six to seven METs; jogging, seven to eight METs; moderate basketball, seven to eight METs.

We consider sex a recreation (an orgasm is four METs).

Eating out is an important and pleasurable activity. Set the MET count yourself, depending upon how dressed up you get and how difficult it is to get to the restaurant. If you need oxygen, put it over your shoulder or pull it behind you without feeling self-conscious. If you feel like it, take the little bib chain we described in the preceding chapter and ask for an extra napkin. Put one on your lap and attach one to the chain. Just be sure you sit in a no-smoking section. Try not to overeat. Restaurants usually serve about twice as much food as you ordinarily require for a meal. Eat half and ask for the rest in a "doggie bag"; it'll be one less meal to cook.

Here's how to stay on your Healthy Core Diet and still enjoy yourself while eating out:

First course: Light soup such as vegetable or French onion without the cheese or croutons.

Second course: Salad—dressing on the side. Pick dressing closest to Italian and spoon on two to three teaspoons.

Main course: Broiled or baked fish, minimal crumbs and butter on lean poultry or meat; baked potato, sour cream on the side, use one teaspoon sour cream; vegetables—skip if oily.

Dessert: Fresh fruit, frozen yogurt.

WORK TO YOUR HEART'S CONTENT

What is a section on work doing in a chapter on leisure? Work seems to have more in common with fun than with any other activity in this book. It requires an active mind, possibly an active body, involves you as a citizen of the world, is elevating to the human spirit, and adds to self-esteem and efficiency. If you already have a job, try hard to keep it. You may have to sacrifice some time for recreation or limit recreation to hands-and-mind forms for a short time each evening. If you work in a service-type profession, such as in a hospital or in a professional office, that may be sufficient involvement with others and may supplant that activity altogether. If you no longer have a job, what about trying to start a new career? How about a telephone answering service, mail order sales, secretarial or typing services? Could you learn to bake one item, such as a pie, and contract for its sale to several restaurants? You don't necessarily need to do much of the physical activity of baking and delivering yourself once you make the contacts and sell the idea. Or try the federal government. Your "handicap" may actually get you a job. Is there a service you could perform for a neighbor, even if it is only for an hour a day? Remember, people who do any kind of a job well are always treated with dignity. You can't work? Don't be bothered by that. Remember, the benefits (mental and physical stimulation and satisfaction) of leisure activities are identical to those of work. With either work or leisure you ought to learn how to network. Here's what networking is and how it works.

NETWORKING

Let's say that you decide that photography would provide satisfying leisure or occupational activity. It's not just enough to take pictures. You could also join a photo club. Once you've met other members and made friends, this is a good time to plan a hike or a walk or a field trip to take more pictures. Now make a set of slides to show at club meetings. Finally, can you volunteer to teach photography? Learn to network with all your recreational activities if it's possible; particularly involve that one significant other as much as you can.

So now you know that networking is a technique in which you utilize activities to meet other people, expand your horizons, begin new activities, and so greatly enrich your life.

TRAVEL

Travel should be considered when you have long periods of stability and you have an excellent understanding of your disease and self-care. Your physician can provide you with the names of other physicians from various reference books such as the American College of Chest Physicians Membership Directory. If you use oxygen, ask your local supplier to call ahead and make arrangements for an adequate supply at your destination. Take more than enough medication and copies of your medical history with you. Avoid places that are so remote that there is no way to get any help if you need it. Railroad and bus lines allow you to utilize your own oxygen. A driving trip in your own car or van offers you maximum flexibility.

Here's some additional information you may need if flying. The air pressure in a plane at 30,000 feet is similar to that on earth at 6,000 feet above sea level. You may therefore need oxygen to fly, although you don't need it on the ground. Your physician can decide.

Should you need oxygen, you must notify the airline at least 48 hours before your flight. No personal oxygen can be carried on any U.S. airline; some foreign carriers do allow it. Any portable tanks must be emptied and stored as luggage. Should you have a stopover and need oxygen on the ground, you must make additional arrangements. Once again, check with your supplier.

Only nebulizers with leakproof (gel-cell) batteries can be used aboard planes.

Request the no-smoking section and an aisle seat near the rest rooms. Move your legs around frequently during long flights. The humidity in the airplane cabin is only 10 to 12 percent, so drink plenty of fluids. Unless you have other special requirements, order diabetic meals; they are calorie-controlled, low in fat and sugar, and usually have fresh fruit for dessert.

Lastly, think carefully about your needs at your destination. You might need a wheelchair in addition to oxygen.

Utilize the same principles of energy conservation and expenditure that we've been discussing throughout this entire book.

If your medical condition is extremely stable, you might consider the grand adventure of a cruise. Be on the lookout for one of the cruise groups specially designed for people with pulmonary disease. Recently, we cruised to Alaska and noted the following: The ship goes along the inland passage, and without leaving a protected, glassed-in deck one gets a constant panorama. When it's not raining, the humidity is low and the temperature a delightful high 60s to low 70s. The pollen count at sea is zero. It's not really necessary to do more than walk around the towns and not really necessary to leave the ship to enjoy the trip thoroughly. There was a physician, a nurse, and oxygen on board, but if you require constant oxygen, you must make your own arrangements, making sure that oxygen would be available if you should need a refill or that you take a sufficient supply aboard. There is a national distributor network for liquid oxygen. You should look to your supplier anytime you want to travel. Your supplier should be able to provide you with additional portable containers and central tanks as necessary for this or any other trip.

We made such a call to our supplier. We found that if an empty central tank could be flown to Vancouver, the usual departure point, there was a dealer able to provide a full tank. You should know exactly how long your tank will last at the liter flows you use. It's possible that for a trip such as the Alaskan one you might need two central tanks. You must discuss your situation directly with the passenger liaison officer. When we interviewed that officer on the ship, she was very open to having people with COPD aboard, as were the physician and nurse.

Difficulties may arise because a hospital is not immediately available. On the other hand, you are not too far from land at any one time. The incline of the gangplank, depending upon the water level, may be steep, but it is also short. You will really have to watch your diet and let them know in advance about such things as skim milk. You can bring your own low-cholesterol cheese slices aboard along with other special foods and keep them in a small foam chest filled with ice, which is automatically supplied to the rooms several times a day (you supply the chest).

On this particular cruise there were three professors aboard discussing the oceanography, geology, and history of the area. There was also a full library and a librarian. The cruise itself was relaxed. You would not require more than one or two dress-up outfits. Otherwise, a windbreaker, a plastic poncho, a sweater, and the usual shirts and slacks would be adequate. Don't forget your jogging shoes and a copy of your medical history, including a list of your medications.

You also need either to be near an elevator or to be able to climb stairs. Once again, a talk with the passenger liaison officer will put you in a cabin that you as an educated pulmonary patient know will fill your most pressing needs.

You may want to pay an additional fee for one or more of the many side trips that are offered. In general, we don't recommend long trips on buses. There is no place to stretch, the carbon monoxide level may rise, and the sites visited may be remote. Be content to take city tours and walk through the streets. You need easy access to the ship. Another option is to rent a car with other travelers.

If you love scenery, nature, whales, eagles, mountains, fjords, glaciers, and clean air and you understand that there could be bad weather, possibly somewhat rough seas, and some remoteness from a hospital, the adventure of a cruise up the Alaskan inland passage can provide the thrill of a lifetime.

Be sure to consult with your doctor before making any plans.

AGENDA FOR LIVING WELL

Below is a sample agenda for a nonworking day. If you work, you obviously must make adjustments in this schedule. You may have to forgo involvement with the world and consider that work fulfills this obligation. You will have to do your exercise walk either in the morning before work or right after. If you work, certain other duties might be delegated to others, such as cooking and housecleaning. Your requirements for exercise, recreation, eating right, taking care of yourself, however, do not change. A word about involvement with another person. We did not discuss this separately because that involvement should be woven as much as possible into the fabric of your entire day. Try to involve the closest other person in many of your activities, and vice versa.

7:00–7:30 A.M.	out of bed, morning treatment while listening to the news
7:30–8:00 A.M.	breakfast
8:00–8:15 A.M.	physical exam and record results
8:15–8:45 A.M.	housework
8:45–9:15 A.M.	relaxation exercises
9:15–10:00 A.M.	dress, shave, shower—don't forget plaque control
10:00–11:00 A.M.	exercise walk, followed by weight lifting
11:00–11:30 A.M.	change clothes and recover
11:30–12:15 P.M.	recreation
12:15–12:45 P.M.	noon treatment while listening to a book on tape

12:45–1:30 P.M.	noon meal and cleanup, plaque control (optional)
1:30–3:45 P.M.	involvement with the world
3:45–4:15 P.M.	rest followed by panic training
4:15–4:45 P.M.	late-day treatment while listening to a book on tape
4:45–5:45 P.M.	prepare breakfast, lunch, supper
5:45–7:00 P.M.	dinner and once-a-day kitchen cleanup, plaque control (optional)
7:00–9:00 P.M.	evening activities—include cleaning respiratory therapy equipment, using inspiratory muscle trainer
9:00–9:30 P.M.	evening treatment while listening to a book on tape
9:30 P.M.	personal hygiene—don't forget plaque control—and ready for bed

171

Chapter 11

HOSPITAL STAYS—
IGNORANCE ISN'T BLISS

A hospital's a place where you can depend on someone for every conceivable need at any conceivable time. There's a difference, however, between total, blind dependency on others and trusting capable professionals you know can help you. Lack of knowledge fosters fear, and fear may lead to unnecessary suspicions, poor cooperation, and often panic. You can become a hazard to yourself. *Believe us, ignorance isn't bliss.* When you are hospitalized, no matter how sick you are, you *must* continue to be a member of your own health care team. To that end, we want to tell you about the professionals and procedures you may encounter when hospitalized.

NURSES

Nurses are in charge of seeing that the floor runs properly and that the orders of the physician are implemented. Nurses also administer direct care to patients. An important function of nurses that you may not know about is to make clinical decisions as to changes in your condition. They are your guardians and will spend much more time with you during the day than the physician. It is the nurse's responsibility to note changes and to call the physician, and that responsibility is important and not a little awesome. It behooves you,

172

then, to communicate freely with your nurse. Don't "save" things for your doctor. It is a common practice for the doctor to come to the floor and check with the nurse first and review your chart. If the nurse knows your symptoms, she will tell them to the doctor, who can think about your problem while walking to your room.

RESPIRATORY THERAPISTS

Respiratory therapists are highly trained members of your health care team, specializing in the use of equipment and techniques necessary for the treatment of respiratory disease. This includes equipment used to administer bronchodilators deep into the bronchial tree and the performance of chest physical therapy. They may assist you not only with treatments for bronchodilation but also with postural drainage, chest percussion, vibration, and cupping, if ordered by your physician. You may be familiar with these techniques from your own home pulmonary toilette regimen. (If you don't have to practice postural drainage at home and you are asked to do it now, you should be familiar with the use of gravity to facilitate drainage. At times, your head and shoulders may be put in a position lower than the rest of your body. This may be necessary because the exacerbation of your COPD has resulted in excessive mucus production.) Respiratory therapists understand pulmonary disease; they are also in a position to note changes in your condition and report them. Communicate freely with your respiratory therapist, who, along with the nurse and the physician, is a partner in your health care.

CONSULTANTS

A consultant is a physician who your doctor feels knows more about some aspects of your problem than he or she does. A good doctor knows when to ask for help; no doctor can know everything. If your doctor asks for a consultant, think more of him or her and not less. Consultants may see you and just write their suggestions on a separate sheet of paper, or they may become active members of the treatment team on your case. Either way is acceptable. Just make sure that a take-charge person is running the show and that somebody is coordinating the suggestions of your consultant or consultants, since in some cases several consultants may be involved.

Communicating with Your Consultant

Give the consultant a history that he or she can comprehend, so your problem can be understood immediately. The doctor is starting the search for the reason that you've had to be admitted. This is called the *chief complaint* and is the beginning of your history. Ninety-five percent of all diagnoses are made by history as opposed to physical examination. Here are all the parts of a proper history. You should know them and practice being able to express yourself. There are minor variations among physicians, naturally, but essentially this is the manner in which a physician investigates your problem.

THE CHIEF COMPLAINT. This brief statement describes the events that resulted in your hospitalization. For instance:

Doctor: What brought you to the hospital?
You: For four days my cough has been getting worse and worse in spite of taking antibiotics and adding steam and postural drainage.

At this point the doctor may want a brief description of other relevant facts about you, including your age, marital status, occupation or previous occupation, the names of any other diseases you have, and the length of time you have had pulmonary disease. When the doctor "writes up" your case, the first sentence may read as follows: "This is a fifty-five-year-old, married, retired truck driver with mild diabetes who has had pulmonary disease for eight years and enters the hospital now with chief complaint of four days of increasing shortness of breath and uncontrolled cough in spite of intensification of pulmonary toilette and the addition of antibiotics

174

to his regimen." This opening sentence, ending with the chief complaint, sets the stage for the description of the rest of your history.

HISTORY OF THE PRESENT ILLNESS. In this section you tell your story in detail. Look how much the doctor already knows about you, including a knowledge of your home situation, whether you have a helpmate in life or not, your occupational exposure, how long you've been sick, and what symptoms were uncontrollable. Your doctor may now say, "Well, how did this all start?" You should begin your story by describing this relapse rather than your entire pulmonary history. On the other hand, you want to give the doctor an indication of how you feel when things are going well, so you might begin by telling your story something like this:

You: I felt the way I usually do. I bring up about two tablespoons of sputum each morning, and I'm quite active. Then I noticed that my sputum began to increase in volume. I phoned my doctor, and he told me to take my on-hand antibiotics and to increase my updraft nebulizer treatments to every four hours from four times a day. Nevertheless, my sputum volume continued to go up, and my sputum became thick and turned a greenish yellow, and I felt as though I couldn't get it up out of my chest. My breathing became difficult, and I had a constricting feeling in my chest.

Doctor: Then what happened?

You: Nothing helped. So my doctor suggested that I be admitted to the hospital.

Doctor: What has happened here in the hospital?

You: My sputum volume still seems to be high, and the color is off. I'm constantly wheezing and have a constricting feeling in my chest, and I feel exhausted and anxious, as though I'm not getting enough air. This morning I had such a violent coughing spell that I became terrified.

In this part of the history you give the consultant the facts concerning what has happened from the onset of this relapse until the time the consultant has seen you. Respond to the doctor's questions directly and succinctly. There may be many other ancillary questions regarding your current medications, home regimen, functional capacity, and so on.

Once you are done telling the doctor all the relevant details of this portion of your present illness, he or she may want to know the rest of your pulmonary history. This is also considered part of the present illness but is usually discussed at this point, after the acute phase of your problem is covered.

Doctor: When did you first begin to notice you had a pulmonary problem?

You: About five years ago, after smoking for 15 years, I noticed that I became short-winded with exertion.

At this point the consultant may want a summary of how much difficulty you have had with your pulmonary disease and may ask about previous hospitalizations, their relative dates, and the reasons for admission. If you cannot memorize these, you should have them written down.

OTHER RELEVANT MEDICAL HISTORY (PAST MEDICAL HISTORY). In this section of the history you will be asked to discuss all other diseases that you have, such as diabetes, high blood pressure, and heart disease. Your consultant will ask you directly. Have the information at your fingertips. He or she does not need to know the exact year or date but does need to know the relative year, the medications that you take, and their exact dosages. You know the names of all of your medications and treatments, and the doses that you use. You should explain to the doctor how you manipulate medications if you've been given permission to do so and how you are usually affected by a change of medications. For instance, if increasing your prednisone (steroid hormone) alleviates your wheezing and short-

176

ness of breath within a few hours, your consultant would like to know it, and if increasing your theophylline preparation by one tablet a day produces nausea, the doctor would like to know that, too.

Other important parts of the history that your consultant may or may not ask you include your family history, about your mother, father, siblings, and children. The doctor may want to know what diseases they have had and whether they are living or dead, and, if deceased, at what age they died. He or she might also ask about your work history (occupational history); social history, including use of alcohol and cigarettes; allergies to medicines and other substances; or any unusual exposures to inhaled chemicals, fumes, or particles.

REVIEW OF SYSTEMS. The last section of a history is called the review of systems, and if it's relevant for you, the doctor may ask you questions about every other "system" in your body, such as Do you have any trouble with your head, eyes, ears, nose, or throat? Do you have any nausea, vomiting, diarrhea, or constipation?

You might want to practice writing out your history. Here's an outline to use as a guide.

Opening sentence: Age, sex, race, occupation, marital status.

Chief complaint: What's happening.

History of the present illness: Recent events; details of the entire course of your pulmonary problem; medications: names, dosages, times taken, their effects; other hospitalizations.

Past medical history: Other major illnesses, any surgery or medication. Previous hospitalizations: why, where, what dates. Immunizations.

Family history: Mother, father, siblings, children. (Living, dead, their diseases and allergies.) Include significant diseases in other family members.

177

Occupational history: Include former and present jobs, especially those involving chemicals, fumes, dust, and so on.

Social history: Hobbies; smoking; alcohol; activities; exercise, and usual functional capacity; education.

Allergies and adverse reactions: Include known allergies and also "bad seasons" of the year when wheezing or cough is intensified. Describe any adverse reactions to medications, places, animals, food, chemicals, and so forth.

Review of systems: Other medical problems or symptoms not already mentioned.

You can ask your own physician to review your history to ensure that it's clear and accurate. Always keep a copy with you. It might also be important for you to have copies of final summaries of previous hospitalizations.

HOW TO EVALUATE YOUR CONSULTANT

You might think we're going to say that a good consultant is one who spends a great deal of time in the room talking to you. Not necessarily so. A good consultant is probably a popular one, and may have a fast, quick mind and be able to synthesize facts rapidly. On the other hand, a slow and steady mind may be equally effective. So you can't judge a consultant by how many minutes the consultant spends with you.

Your doctor has put your pertinent history on the chart and the consultant may indicate to you a familiarity with the facts, but he or she should spend time talking to you and checking out the pertinent facts, looking for those clues that may have been overlooked or have suffered from underemphasis. When you're speaking to the consultant, that person should listen attentively, especially when your responses are clearly organized and relevant to your present problem.

A good consultant does at least those parts of the physical examination that are pertinent to your problem, such as listening to your chest, asking you to cough, and checking your leg and neck veins. When you ask a sensible question, he or she shouldn't hesitate to give you an answer you can understand. If you don't understand something told to you, ask again. A good consultant has a clear picture in mind of the problems involved in COPD and should be able to give you an answer you can understand. A good consultant might also tell you that he or she doesn't yet know what's wrong with you. Always admire the physician who admits he or she doesn't know. You're in trouble when the doctor doesn't do something about it.

BRONCHOSCOPY

Almost all bronchoscopies are now done with a fiberoptic instrument rather than a rigid steel one. The fiberoptic bronchoscope contains thousands of glass fibers that carry light and images. The instrument has a flexible tip that is controlled by the physician and can bend to a considerable angle both forward and backward. It provides a direct look inside the bronchial tree without requiring surgery. There is a special channel to the bronchoscope for suctioning secretions and instilling medications, including local anesthetics. Tiny brushes and biopsy forceps can be passed through the channel to obtain specimens from suspicious areas. The fiberoptic scope can find out why you coughed up blood or why your pneumonia won't "clear up." If thick secretions are stubbornly plugging your bronchial tree, small amounts of mucus-thinning agents can be instilled followed by suctioning, resulting in an unobstructed airway.

Most of the time you'll be wide awake during the procedure. Only a mild sedative is necessary. The discomforts are minor—the possible gains major. Don't be afraid.

179

INTUBATION, VENTILATION, AND TRACHEOTOMY

Sometimes the going gets rough and your doctor might feel that he or she is "losing control over the airway." That means the doctor believes that you may not be getting enough oxygen in and carbon dioxide out to sustain life adequately. The situation usually occurs when there is a large volume of secretions plugging the bronchial tree, and no amount of postural drainage, suctioning, antibiotics, or other measures has helped. Usually you have become exhausted because the work of breathing against this large resistance is so great. If that happens, your treatment may include one or all of the following: *intubation, ventilation,* and *tracheotomy.*

The bad news is that it is frightening and uncomfortable, and you can't talk when intubated. The good news is that you will be safe, feel more relaxed, can communicate by writing, and can put yourself in other people's hands with confidence.

For intubation, a semirigid, soft plastic tube—an endotracheal tube—is inserted either through the nose or mouth down through your voice box (larynx) into the upper part of the trachea. For one method of intubation, the doctor will stand behind you, lifting the base of your tongue out of the way so that he or she can see the larynx to insert the tube. The doctor needs to use a metal instrument, called a laryngoscope, to see the larynx. Another technique requires the tube to be inserted down through the nose. Once the tube is inserted into the trachea, a soft balloon is inflated to fix the tube in place and permit air to be ventilated into and out of the lung without a leak around the tube and also so the contents of your stomach cannot get into your lungs and choke you. When this happens, no air can vibrate your vocal cords, so you cannot talk. At first, the tube may feel very uncomfortable and may make you cough. Substances that will suppress the cough can now be put down the tube, and you will soon adjust to it. Intubation provides a clear channel to suction secretions out and, once having accomplished this, to get that miracle substance, oxygen, in.

Once you are intubated, a ventilator is usually necessary. This machine assumes the work of breathing and is attached by simple connectors to the endotracheal tube. Once on the ventilator, you should feel relaxed, as though the strain is off. Let the therapist or nurse know if you are not getting enough air in or out. Remember, this situation is uncomfortable, but you are now safe. Try not to panic and fight the machine. The ventilator is a machine that is tried and true and extremely reliable, and you have an excellent chance of survival with no loss of function. A clipboard with a pencil and paper will allow you to communicate with the staff.

If you require mechanical ventilation for a more prolonged time, a tracheotomy may be necessary. Fortunately, this is an uncommon requirement. In this procedure a small hole is actually made through the neck in the trachea and an airway (or tracheotomy tube) is inserted into that hole. This airway functions in the same way an endotracheal tube does to allow for suction of secretions and connection to a ventilator if necessary. It allows you to eat. A tracheotomy may also be done when intubation is impossible for any reason or when there is an obstruction that has to be bypassed.

If you have to be intubated or have a tracheotomy and be put on a ventilator, your job is to be calm, let people around you know that you are in contact, and inform them when you do not feel the flow of air is proper. You must also keep yourself oriented. If a clock is in view, look at it. Know what day it is. Wear your glasses. Try to move your legs in bed at least every hour. If possible, ask your doctor to prescribe bedside physical therapy. Ask to sit in a chair. You may be able to walk a few steps with a therapist using what is called a manual ventilator. This soft, squeezable bag can be attached to the endotracheal tube or tracheotomy tube to assist your breathing while walking.

Once your secretions are cleared out and infection and exhaustion are over, you will soon be "weaned" from the ventilator. This is usually done gradually by removing the ventilator and attaching the endotracheal tube to a tube delivering oxygen. Sometimes the dials on the ventilator are set so that in effect you are breathing on your own. There are many procedures for weaning, but rest assured that as soon as possible the medical team taking care of you will gradually remove the support mechanisms. Once the endotracheal tube is removed, your voice might be hoarse, but you'll be able to speak immediately. The same is true for the tracheotomy tube. The hole it leaves will close over naturally, leaving an inconsequential scar.

We hope that understanding these procedures and knowing that they are safe and effective, with few side effects, will help to keep your spirits up if you should have to go through this difficult and trying time. Remember, you can make it; don't let despair defeat you.

HOME VENTILATION

What happens, however, if you cannot be weaned from the ventilator and the only way that you can survive is with ventilator assistance? Is this a horrible prospect, or can you still "live well"? The answer is that you can live well if you want to, and here's how. First of all, expect that a trained, multidisciplinary team will be in charge of your discharge planning. You will need people at home to help, and they will work with this team, which may consist of your doctor, a respiratory therapist, a nurse specialist, a social worker, probably a physical therapist, and an occupational therapist. You and your family must be knowledgeable about at least the following: suctioning, changing tracheotomy tubes, range-of-motion exercises, troubleshooting the ventilator, checking the ventilator, cleaning equipment, chest physical therapy, changing of ventilator circuits, emergency troubleshooting, and tracheotomy care. You should receive written individual instructions on all of these topics.

The portable home mechanical ventilator is usually small, lightweight, quiet, fits on the back of a wheelchair, and runs both from wall current and battery current. With modifications, such as the insertion of a Passy-Muir valve into the ventilator tubing, you will be able to speak again. Here is a list of most of the items that will be required at the time of discharge:

1. two ventilators, one portable without water humidification and one bedside ventilator with a water humidification circuit
2. Thermavent 600 (functions as an artificial nose) for the portable ventilator when there is no water humidification
3. wheelchair
4. two deep discharge batteries: one to function as the battery you are using and one as a backup in case the first fails; a battery charger
5. portable suction machine
6. bedside suction machine
7. normal saline
   a. individual bullets for instilling and suctioning
   b. 1,000-ml bottles
8. sterile water in 1,000-ml bottles
9. suction catheters that match the specific size you were discharged with
10. cotton swabs
11. hydrogen peroxide
12. spare tracheotomy tubes, both the same size you were discharged with and one size smaller in case some swelling occurs and the original size cannot be inserted
13. tracheotomy tape
14. Velcro tracheotomy tube holders
15. stethoscope
16. clean gloves
17. sterile gloves
18. complete ventilator circuit, including air filters
19. water-soluble lubricant
20. oxygen tank with oxygen tubing
21. manual ventilation device for temporary use when needed

Additionally, depending upon the ability of your family to care for you, there may be a requirement for twelve-hour nursing care at night, while you are sleeping.

What else can you expect? You can expect not only to go home but that once you are home you can have a great deal of mobility and retain a good deal of your own independence and feelings of self-esteem. Try to be as independent as possible. Try to do your own self-care, such as brushing your teeth. Try to still reach out to others; remember, there are still others probably worse off than you. As for enjoying yourself, remember that the ventilator can go anywhere a wheelchair can go. Lastly, you might ask, "How do I get exercise?" Use a stationary bicycle and low-level weights, following the same guidelines we discussed in the chapter on exercise. You may come home weak after a long, hard hospitalization, and it will be up to you to be forward-looking and try as hard as you can to get stronger and to increase your own independence. Above all, don't give way to despair. Please remember, if you want to find a way to live well, you will.

GETTING OUT OF BED TO GET WELL

You may have a vision of yourself relaxing in the hospital lying in bed being cared for by nurses. Forget it. The hospital is no place to sit around in bed. If you really want to get sick, if you really want to get pneumonia if you don't already have it, or if you want your pneumonia to get worse instead of better, you'll lie in bed thinking that's the way to get well. You must be as active in the hospital as your doctor will allow. If you usually walk with oxygen, insist on a small portable tank so that you can take walks. If you need help to walk and nobody comes to take you on a regular basis, ask your doctor to write it as an order so that you'll be walked on a schedule, let's say four times a day, just as you'd be given a medication. Ask for a physical therapist to help you if necessary. Just one day in bed produces significant weakening of muscles. You don't want to lose all that you've gained in terms of fitness and training. Get someone to bring your weights and get your jogging shoes out, and, as much as you can, be active.

Landing in the hospital is not the most pleasant of experiences.

However, you are there to get well, and your chances of survival are much greater in the hospital when your doctor believes that you belong there. Cooperate, keep your spirits up, keep active, and try to get out as soon as you can. Understanding who's who and what's what should help you feel more comfortable with the hospital environment.

WHAT TO TAKE TO THE HOSPITAL IN AN EMERGENCY

Problem: You feel terrible, but you have enough energy to gather a few things to take to the hospital. Essential items are (1) walking shoes and socks, (2) eyeglasses, and (3) a copy of your history.

The hospital has plenty of items for personal hygiene such as toothbrushes, combs, and razor blades; books and magazines are readily available. You need your glasses to keep oriented and to see well. A copy of your history will help your health care team, as we've described. The indispensable items are your walking shoes and socks (yes, the very same ones you use in your exercise program). They'll help you to be active again as soon as you can and show the staff you have that fighting spirit.

Appendix

Plan for the Significant Other

HOW TO GET THAT SPECIAL PERSON OUT OF AN EMOTIONAL STRAITJACKET, OR NEVER LET HIM OR HER GET THERE IN THE FIRST PLACE

COPD affects many more people than just the victim; it affects the whole family. A cardiac patient frequently suffers an acute event such as a heart attack and then can pick up his or her life and sometimes feel better than ever before. Victims of chronic pulmonary disease, however, suffer long years of disability, joblessness, loss of income, depression, repeated hospitalizations, and loss of normal activities that give life meaning, such as recreation, sex, and work. When this happens, you, the important other, suffer also. Working together, however, you can accept this disease as a challenge instead of going down in defeat. You may find that not only do you help your loved one to live well, but you also improve your own sense of health and well-being at the same time.

COPD is a disease characterized by secretions blocking the airways and actual destruction of the lung tissue itself coupled with frequent infections and spasm of the bronchial tree muscles. Because of this, the sufferer must expend extra effort to breathe, even at rest.

This leads to easy fatigability. The COPD victim begins to give up a little and "take it easy." When that happens, the sufferer loses even more, giving up friends, fun, and work, and struggles with loss of self-esteem while dealing with repeated relapses and what can be a bewildering array of medications and repeated hospitalizations. The end result is high levels of fearfulness and anxiety coupled with feelings of depression and isolation. When there is unwillingness to express any emotion, happiness or sadness or even fear, when the physical work of laughing or crying is too much, that is an emotional straitjacket. How can you be a vital partner in getting your significant other out of this state or prevent this sorry state of affairs to begin with? Here is a five-point plan:

1. *Start with control of the environment.* Carefully read the all-important chapter on self-protection. Know the air quality and pollen count. Be cognizant of high-traffic times. Check the humidity. Be careful about cosmetics and soaps. Make sure that the bedroom and bathroom are a refuge of clean, non-polluted air. Eliminate all cleaning agents that contain respiratory irritants and use only nontoxic fume-emitting chemicals in the house. For new construction, use only nontoxic building material, and try as much as possible to stick to 100-percent cotton clothing from which the sizing has been washed. Use baking soda, borax, and kosher soap, vinegar, and lemon juice in cleaning. Take care to clean the house thoroughly of all animal dander and house dust. Naturally, no smoking is allowed.

2. *Exercise together.* The ability to walk for 10 minutes opens up a whole world. It means being able to go out to movies, into a mall, to take care of oneself, to buy something in a store. Athletic accomplishment provides a very natural high. Enter a walking program and light-weight-lifting program together, with your doctor's help. Take your planned exercise walks, plus as many other walks together as you can fit into your daily schedule. Keep an exercise diary together. When you are

walking, be cognizant of how the other is feeling so that neither has to be afraid. If a person cannot say four words without taking a breath, he or she may be overdoing it. Note that neither of you should feel fearful or light-headed, or have chest pains. At the end of the exercise walk, you should both feel that it has been a job well done, with a certain sense of having worked, but also being exhilarated. Neither of you should be so exhausted that you have to lie down for several hours and recover. If you can't walk outside because the humidity, air quality, temperature, or pollen prohibits it, walk in malls or around your living room. Or you could put on some music and do a walk-dance together, always touching, holding hands, looking at each other, and talking. Communicate while exercising. When you lift weights—a nylon stocking with a pound of beans in it with a knot on one end makes a wonderful weight—look at each other. Read the chapter on exercise in this book thoroughly, and discuss the program with your doctor.

3. *Make yourselves members of the health care team.* Remember, you are in this together. Learn all about chronic obstructive pulmonary disease. Learn all about medications, uses, doses, and side effects, and if you, the significant other, also have diseases and need to take medicine, the COPD patient should learn about your medical regimen also. For every drug a person takes, he or she should know the minor side effects—those that should be nonfrightening—and the major side effects—those that require calling the doctor immediately. If you know this about every drug you take, you won't have to be afraid. The daily physical examination or self-assessment (described in Chapter 3) is extremely important. Why don't you do that together and discuss the findings? If you know how your significant other "stacks up" on a good day and what the usual variation of the symptoms are, once again you will feel much more at home with this problem, not made fearful by minor variations or the feeling that you might wait too long to call the

doctor when you need help. Remember, you are in this to-gether; this is the challenge.

4. *Get back to sex.* It is very important that you both say that you care about sex. If it has been a long time since you have even touched each other, start with hug therapy—a hug four times a day. Begin talking about sex, thinking about it, and reading about it. Be inventive, open-minded, and flexible. Don't forget to use what you've learned in exercise about safe pulse ranges. If you are having sexual activity and you are worried that you are overdoing and you know the safe pulse range, you can check in a moment, and both of you can be involved. Holding each other closely and intimately, doing those very private things with each other is a beautiful experience, and you should not miss out on it.

5. *Make sure nutrition is adequate.* Remember, the COPD patient cannot afford to carry around extra water weight or fat weight, and if possible the patient should avoid becoming extremely thin or undermuscled. It is very important to eat a nutri-tionally dense (packed with vitamins and minerals) diet. Keep in mind the principles of the Healthy Core Diet, and use those principles to eat a wide variety of well-washed whole foods with as few pesticides and chemical additives as possible. These include:

(a) high calcium contributors, such as dairy foods—four or more portions per day equaling 1,000 mg calcium

(b) cancer-fighting foods containing vitamins A and C, such as broccoli, sweet potatoes, and carrots—three to five serv-ings, supplying 5,000 units of vitamin A and at least 60 mg vitamin C

(c) energy elevators: breads, pastas, and macaroni—three to four servings per day, at least 125 grams

(d) muscle builders (protein): meat, fish, poultry—50 to 100 grams

(e) fiber foods, such as bran and potato foods—no particular minimum daily requirement, but about 20 grams per day

So we say to you, "Don't just do what's easy; do what's right." Study and learn all about this disease together. Make it a joint project. You can both feel like the whole, precious people that you are and take control of your lives. Even though COPD is not curable, you can both participate in arresting this disease or stabilizing it. Try this five-point program, this new way toward freedom and living well with asthma, bronchitis, and emphysema.

GLOSSARY

AIR SACS. Delicate sacs at the end of each terminal bronchiole covered with blood vessels, also called *alveoli*.

AIR TRAPPING. Air caught behind collapsed bronchial branches during expiration (exhalation).

AIRWAY COLLAPSE. The actual collapse or closure of branches of the bronchial tree due to weakening of the bronchial walls secondary to disease.

ALPHA-1-ANTITRYPSIN. The natural enzyme that inactivates trypsin and keeps it from destroying lung tissue.

ALVEOLAR MACROPHAGE. A special cell in the lung that engulfs bacteria and foreign material and produces enzymes.

ALVEOLI. Synonym for air sacs.

ASTHMA. An obstructive disease of the lung that is characterized by inflammation (invasion by PMNs, especially eosinophils) and wheezing, which may be reversible.

ASTHMATIC BRONCHITIS. The coexistence of wheezing and chronic bronchitis.

BARREL CHEST. The shape of the chest in some patients with COPD, caused by air trapping that leads to overinflated lungs.

BLEBS AND BULLAE (sinkholes). Large holes in the lung due to rupture or destruction of the air sacs (alveoli).

BRONCHI. Branches of the bronchial tree.

BRONCHIAL TREE. The ductwork of the respiratory system (bronchi and bronchioles) that branches like a tree; the terminal branches lead to the alveoli.

BRONCHIOLES. The smallest branches of the bronchial tree; these eventually lead into alveoli or air sacs.

BRONCHOSPASM. Intermittent narrowing of the bronchial tree because of spasm of the muscles in the bronchial wall.

CARBON DIOXIDE. The gaseous waste product released by the cells that passes into the blood stream and then into the air sacs and must exit by way of the bronchial tree.

CHRONIC ASTHMA. A chronic obstructive pulmonary disease that is characterized by bronchospasm and is not completely reversible.

CHRONIC BRONCHITIS. A chronic obstructive pulmonary disease characterized by cough, sputum, chronic infection, and obstruction to the bronchial tree.

CHRONIC OBSTRUCTIVE PULMONARY DISEASE. A group of diseases characterized by obstruction and destruction of the bronchial tree and/or the alveoli, usually referring to chronic bronchitis, emphysema, and chronic asthma.

CILIA. Tiny hairlike structures of cells lining the bronchial tree that act as a defense mechanism by moving mucus and inhaled particles toward the mouth.

DIFFUSION. The movement of oxygen or carbon dioxide across the delicate membrane of the air sac (alveolus).

ELASTIC RECOIL. The ability of the lung to "snap back" at the end of inspiration.

EMPHYSEMA. A chronic obstructive pulmonary disease characterized by destruction of the alveoli, leading to enlarged air spaces, decreased elastic recoil, air trapping, and overinflation of the lungs.

EXPIRATION. Breathing out.

FEV_1 (forced expiratory volume at one second). The amount of air forceably expired in one second during a test of vital capacity.

GASTROESOPHAGEAL REFLUX. The regurgitation of sour stomach contents into the esophagus, causing heartburn and possibly exacerbating chronic asthma.

MUCUS. A gelatinous product secreted by special cells within the bronchial tree; it traps bacteria and foreign particles.

OXYGEN. The most important component of air, necessary for bodily functions.

PERFUSION. The passage of blood through the lungs (and other body organs).

PHARYNX. The back of the throat.

POLYMORPHONUCLEAR LEUKOCYTES (PMNs). White blood cells—special cells that fight infection, engulf bacteria and irritants, and secrete enzymes.

RELAPSE. Getting sick again after feeling well.

SINUSITIS. An inflammation of the walled cavities contained in the skull that may be a contributing factor in chronic asthma.

TRACHEA. The main trunk of the bronchial tree.

TRYPSIN. A natural enzyme that destroys invaders and may also destroy lung tissue.

VENTILATION. The passage of air into and out of the lungs.

VENTILATION PERFUSION INEQUALITY (MISMATCHED MATES). The most common cause of low blood oxygen. It occurs when the blood circulating in the alveoli cannot pick up oxygen because of mucus plugs obstructing the flow of air in and out of the alveoli or when oxygen cannot enter the bloodstream because of destruction of the blood vessels, although there is no obstruction to airflow.

VITAL CAPACITY. The maximum expiration after your deepest inspiration.

WHEEZING. The sound made by air moving through partially obstructed air passages.

BIBLIOGRAPHY

HELPFUL PUBLICATIONS FOR REFERENCE AND READING

Aslett, Don. *Is There Life After Housework?* Cincinnati: Writer's Digest Books, 1981.

Bower, John. *The Healthy House.* New York: Carol Publishing Group, 1989.

Dadd, Debra Lynn. *Nontoxic, Natural, and Earthwise.* Los Angeles: Jeremy P. Tarcher, Inc., 1990 (distributed by St. Martin's Press, New York).

Godish, Thad. *Indoor Air Pollution Control.* Chelsea, MI: Lewis Publishers, 1989.

Haas, Francis, and Haas, Sheila Sperber. *The Chronic Bronchitis and Emphysema Handbook.* New York: Wiley, 1990.

Petty, Thomas L., and Nett, Louise M. *Enjoying Life with Emphysema.* Philadelphia: Lea & Febiger, 1987.

Rousseau, David; Rea, W. J.; and Enright, Jean. *Your Home, Your Health, and Well-Being.* Berkeley, CA: Ten Speed Press, 1989.

Rudoff, Carol. *Asthma Resources Directory.* Menlo Park, CA: Allergy Publications, 1989.

U.S. Department of Agriculture/U.S. Department of Health and Human Services. *Dietary Guidelines for Americans*, 3rd ed., 1990.

U.S. Environmental Protection Agency/U.S. Consumer Product Safety Commission. *The Inside Story: A Guide to Indoor Air Quality.* 1988.

Young, Stuart H., with Susan A. Shulman and Martin D. Shulman. *The Asthma Handbook.* New York: Bantam, 1989.

SELECTED REFERENCES

General

American Thoracic Society. "Guidelines for the Approach to the Patient with Severe Hereditary Alpha-1-Antitrypsin Deficiency." *American Review of Respiratory Disease* 140 (1989): 1494–97.

Christopher, Kent L.; Spofford, Bryan T.; Petrun, Mark D.; McCarty, Dawn C.; Goodman, John R.; and Petty, Thomas L. "A Program for Transtracheal Oxygen Delivery: Assessment of Safety and Efficacy." *Annals of Internal Medicine* 107 (December 1987): 802–808.

Dolovitch, M.; Ruffin, R.; Corr, D.; and Newhouse, M.T. "Clinical Evaluation of a Simple Demand Inhalation MDI Aerosol Delivery Device." *Chest* 84 (July 1983): 36–41.

Dosnan, James A., and Cockcroft, Donald W., guest ed. "Obstructive Lung Disease." *Medical Clinics of North America* 74, no. 3 (May 1990).

Findley, Larry J.; Whelan, Donna M.; and Moser, Kenneth M. "Long-Term Oxygen Therapy in COPD." *Chest* 83 (April 1983): 671–74.

"The Green Way to Green a Yard." *Consumer Reports* 56, no. 6 (June 1991): 407–24.

Heimlich, Henry J., and Carr, Gerson C. "Transtracheal Catheter Technique for Pulmonary Rehabilitation." *Annals of Otology, Rhinology and Laryngology* 94 (1985): 502–504.

Heimlich, Henry J., and Uhley, Milton H. "The Heimlich Maneuver." *Clinical Symposia* 31, no. 3 (1979): 3–32.

Hodgkin, John E.; Zorn, F. G.; and Connors, G. L., eds. *Pulmonary Rehabilitation: Guidelines to Success.* Boston: Butterworth, 1984.

Johnson, Lloyd P., and Cary, Jeffery M. "The Implanted Intratracheal Oxygen Catheter." *Surgery, Gynecology & Obstetrics* 165 (July 1987): 75–76.

Newhouse, Michael T. "Proper Use of Metered-Dose Inhalers." *BronkoScope* 2, no. 2 (July 1983): 6–7.

Nocturnal Oxygen Therapy Trial Group. "Continuous or Nocturnal Oxygen Therapy in Hypoxemic Chronic Obstructive Lung Disease: A Clinical Trial." *Annals of Internal Medicine* 93 (September 1980): 391–98.

O'Hollaren, Mark T., and Bardana, Emil J., Jr. "Chronic Rhinitis: A Practical Approach to the Work-Up." *Journal of Respiratory Disease* 11, no. 5 (May 1990): 443–54.

Petty, Thomas L. "Home Oxygen—A Revolution in the Care of Advanced COPD." *Medical Clinics of North America* 74, no. 3 (May 1990): 715–729.

————, guest ed. "Diagnosis and Treatment of Chronic Obstructive Pulmonary Disease." *Chest* 97, no. 2 (February 1990): supplement.

Sahn, Steven A.; Nett, Louise M.; and Petty, Thomas L. "Ten Year Follow-up of a Comprehensive Rehabilitation Program for Severe COPD." *Chest* 77 (February 1980): supplement, 311–14.

Samet, Jonathan. "Environmental Controls and Lung Disease: Report of the American Thoracic Society Workshop on Environmental Controls and Lung Disease." *American Review of Respiratory Disease* 142 (1990): 915–39.

Sheppard, Dean. "Adverse Pulmonary Effects of Air Pollution." *Immunology and Allergic Practice* (February 1984): 25–35.

Tiep, Brian L.; Christopher, Kent L.; Spofford, Bryan T.; Goodman, John R.; Worley, Patricia D.; and Macy, Siobhan L. "Pulsed Nasal and Transtracheal Oxygen Delivery." *Chest* 97, no. 2 (February 1990): 364–68.

Yager, Jean A.; Ellman, Herman; and Dulfano, Mauricio J. "Human Ciliary Beat Frequency at Three Levels of the Tracheobronchial Tree." *American Review of Respiratory Disease* 121 (1980): 661–65.

Asthma

American College of Gastroenterology. "Gastroesophageal Reflux Disease." *GI Focus* (Spring 1990).

Barnes, Peter J. "A New Approach to the Treatment of Asthma." *New England Journal of Medicine* 321, no. 22 (November 30, 1989): 1517–27.

Cockcroft, Donald W. "A Stepwise Approach to the Outpatient Management of Asthma." *Modern Medicine* 58 (May 1990): 50–60.

Dolovich, J., and Hargreave, F. "The Asthma Syndrome: Inciters, Inducers, and Host Characteristics." *Thorax* 36 (1981): 641–44.

Dulfano, M. J., and Luk, C. K. "Sputum and Ciliary Inhibition in Asthma." *Thorax* 37 (1982): 646–51.

Habenicht, Herald A.; Preuss, Lawrence; and Lovell, Robert G. "Sensitivity to Ingested Metabisulfites: Cause of Bronchiospasm and Urticaria." *Immunology and Allergy Practice* (August 1983): 25–27.

Herrera, Alma M., and DeShazo, Richard D. "Sinusitis: Its Association with Asthma." *Postgraduate Medicine* 87 (April 1990): 153–164.

Juniper, Elizabeth H.; Kline, Patricia A.; Vanzieleghem, Michael A.; Ramsdale, E. Helen; O'Byrne, Paul M.; and Hargreave, Frederick E. "Effect of Long-Term Treatment with an Inhaled Corticosteroid (Budesonide) on Airway Hyperresponsiveness and Clinical Asthma in Nonsteroid-Dependent Asthmatics." *American Review of Respiratory Disease* 4 (1990): 832–36.

Kerrebijn, K. F. "Triggers of Airway Inflammation." *European Journal of Respiratory Disease* 69, Supplement 147 (1986): 98–104.

Klingelhofer, Edwin L., and Gershwin, M. Eric. "Asthma Self-Management Programs: Premises, Not Promises." *Journal of Asthma* 25, no. 2 (1988): 89–101.

Lam, Stephen, and Chan-Yeung, Moira. "Occupational Asthma: Natural History, Evaluation and Management." *Occupational Medicine* 2, no. 2 (April–June 1987): 373–81.

Mayo, Paul H.; Richman, Julieta; and Harris, H. William. "Results of a Program to Reduce Admissions for Adult Asthma." *Annals of Internal Medicine* 112 (June 1, 1990): 864–71.

Merchant, James A., guest ed. "Environmental and Occupational Asthma." *Chest* 98, no. 5 (November 1990): supplement.

Nelson, Harold S. "Is Gastrointestinal Reflux Worsening Your Patient's Asthma?" *Journal of Respiratory Diseases* 11, no. 9 (September 1990): 827–44.

Piyamahunt, Arkapol; Bernstein, David I.; and Bernstein, I. Leonard. "Is Your Patient's Asthma Caused by Occupational Exposure?" *Journal of Respiratory Diseases* 11, no. 8 (August 1990): 672–88.

Shim, Chang, and Williams, M. Henry, Jr. "Effect of Odors in Asthma." *American Journal of Medicine* 80 (January 1986): 18–21.

Sporik, Richard; Holgate, Stephen T.; Platts-Mills, Thomas A. E.; and Cogswell, Jeremy J. "Exposure to House-Dust Mite Allergen and the Development of Asthma in Childhood." *New England Journal of Medicine* 323, no. 8 (August 23, 1990): 502–507.

Home Ventilation

Giovannoni, Rita. "Chronic Ventilator Care: From Hospital to Home." *Respiratory Therapy* (July/August 1984): 29–33.

Make, Barry; Gilmartin, Mary; Brody, Jerome S.; and Snider, Gordon L. "Rehabilitation of Ventilator-Dependent Subjects with Lung Diseases: The Concept and Initial Experience." *Chest* 86, no. 3 (September 1984): 358–365.

COPD and Smoking

AACP Subcommittee on Smoking in the Physician's Workshop (Edward R. Munnell, Chairman). "The Management of Smoking in the Physician's 'Workshop.'" *Chest* 82 (September 1982): 359–61.

Bode, Frederick R. "Axioms on Smoking and the Respiratory Tract." *Hospital Medicine* (November 1978): 35–55.

Crofton, John; Campbell, I. A.; Cole, P. V.; Friend, J. A. R.; Oldham, P. D.; Springett, V. H.; Berry, G.; and Raw, Martin. "Comparison of Four Methods of Smoking Withdrawal in Patients with Smoking Related Diseases." *British Medical Journal* 286 (February 19, 1983): 595–97.

Doyle, Nancy C. "Even at Work, Second-Hand Smoke Can Affect Your Lungs." *American Lung Association Bulletin*, 66 (June 1980): 5–7.

Hunninghake, G.; Gadek, J.; and Crystal, R. "Smoke Attracts Polymorphonuclear Leukocytes to Lung." *Chest* 77 (February 1980): supplement, 273.

Janerich, Dwight T.; Thompson, W. Douglas; Varela, Luis R.; Greenwald, Peter; Chorost, Sherry; Tucci, Cathy; Zaman, Muhammad B.; Melamed, Myron R.; Kiely, Maureen; and McKneally, Martin F. "Lung Cancer and Exposure to Tobacco Smoke in the Household." *New England Journal of Medicine* 323, no. 10 (September 6, 1990): 632–36.

Luoto, Joanne. "Reducing the Health Consequences of Smoking: A Progress Report." *Public Health Reports* 98 (January/February 1983): 34–39.

National Cancer Institute. *Calling It Quits: The Latest Advice on How to Give up Cigarettes.* U.S. Department of Health, Education, and Welfare Publication No. (NIH) 79-1824. Washington, DC: U.S. Government Printing Office.

———. *Clearing the Air: A Guide to Quitting Smoking.* Washington, DC: U.S. Department of Health, Education, and Welfare Publication No. (NIH) 78-1647, 1988.

———. *Helping Smokers Quit: A Guide for Physicians.* U.S. Department of Health, Education, and Welfare Publication No. (NIH) 78-1825. Washington, DC: U.S. Printing Office.

Nett, Louise M. "The Physician's Role in Smoking Cessation: A Present and Future Agenda." *Chest* 97, no. 2 (February 1990): supplement, 28S–32S.

Repace, James L., and Lowrey, Alfred H. "Indoor Air Pollution, Tobacco Smoke, and Public Health." *Science* 208 (May 2, 1980): 464–72.

White, James R., and Froeb, Herman F. "Small-Airways Dysfunction in Nonsmokers Chronically Exposed to Tobacco Smoke." *New England Journal of Medicine* 302 (March 27, 1980): 720–23.

Diet and Nutrition

American Lung Association. "Juggle Your Diet to Include Carotene." *American Lung Association Bulletin* 69 (May/June 1983): 13–15.

Arora, Narinder S., and Rochester, Dudley F. "Respiratory Muscle Strength and Maximal Voluntary Ventilation in Undernourished Patients." *American Review of Respiratory Disease* 126 (July 1982): 5–8.

Bantle, John P.; Laine, Dawn C.; Castle, Gay W.; Thomas, J. William; Hoogwerf, Byron J.; and Goetz, Frederick C. "Postprandial Glucose and Insulin Responses to Meals Containing Different Carbohydrates in Normal and Diabetic Subjects." *New England Journal of Medicine* 309 (July 7, 1983): 7–12.

Bowes and Church's Food Values of Portions Commonly Used, 15th ed., revised by Jean A. T. Pennington, Ph.D., R.D. (New York: Harper and Row, 1989).

Brown, Stephen E., and Light, Richard W. "When COPD Patients Are Malnourished." *Journal of Respiratory Diseases* (May 1983): 36–50.

Bunker, Mary Louise, and McWilliams, Margaret. "Caffeine Content of Common Beverages." *Journal of the American Dietetic Association* 74 (January 1979): 28–32.

Driver, Albert G.; McAlevy, Merle T.; and Smith, Jack L. "Nutritional Assessment of Patients with Chronic Obstructive Pulmonary Disease and Acute Respiratory Failure." *Chest* 82 (November 1982): 568–71.

Evans, Marguerite, and Dwyer, Johanna. "Diet, Nutrition and Cancer: A Summary." *Cancer Institute Bulletin* 3 (Spring 1983): 2–3.

Goldin, Barry, and Gorbach, Sherwood. "The Relationship Between Diet and Breast and Colon Cancer." *Cancer Institute Bulletin* 3 (Spring 1983): 3–4.

Katch, Frank I., and McArdle, William D. *Nutrition, Weight Control, and Exercise,* 3rd ed. Philadelphia: Lea & Febiger, 1988.

Kuo, Peter T. "Hyperlipoproteinemia and Atherosclerosis: Dietary Intervention." *American Journal of Medicine* 74 (May 23, 1983): 15–18.

Mayer, Jean. Introduction. *Cancer Institute Bulletin* 3 (Spring, 1983): 1–2.

McCauley, Kathleen, and Weaver, Terri E. "Cardiac and Pulmonary Diseases: Nutritional Implications." *Nursing Clinics of North America* 18 (March 1983): 86–96.

Openbrier, Diana R.; Irwin, Margaret M.; Rogers, Robert M.; Gottlieb, Gary P.; Dauber, James H.; Van Thiel, David H.; and Pennock, Bernard E. "Nutritional Status and Lung Function in Patients with Emphysema and Chronic Bronchitis." *Chest* 83 (January 1983): 17–22.

Power, Lawrence. "Diet and Blood Cholesterol: The Important Role of Specific Fibers." *Physician & Patient,* May 1983: 46–52.

Selivanov, Val; Sheldon, George F.; and Fantini, Gary. "Nutrition's Role in Averting Respiratory Failure." *Journal of Respiratory Diseases* (September 1983): 29–32.

Whittaker, J. S., et al. "The Effects of Refeeding on Peripheral and Respiratory Muscle Function in Malnourished Chronic Obstructive Pulmonary Disease Patients." *American Review of Respiratory Disease* 142, no. 2 (August 1990): 283–88.

Exercise

Cheong, Tuck H.; Magder, Sheldon; Shapiro, Stanley; Martin, James G.; and Levy, Robert D. "Cardiac Arrhythmias During Exercise in Severe Chronic Obstructive Pulmonary Disease." *Chest* 97, no. 4 (April 1990): 793–97.

Cockroft, A. E.; Saunders, M. J.; and Berry, G. "Randomised Controlled Trial of Rehabilitation in Chronic Respiratory Disability." *Thorax* 36 (1981): 200–203.

Jones, Norman L. "Exercise Testing in Pulmonary Evaluation: Rationale, Methods and the Normal Respiratory Response to Exercise." *Medical Intelligence* 293 (September 11, 1975): 541–44.

Lake, Fiona R.; Henderson, Kathryn; Briffa, Tom; Openshaw, Janet; and Musk, A. William. "Upper-Limb and Lower-Limb Exercise Training in Patients with Chronic Airflow Obstruction." *Chest* 97, no. 5 (May 1990): 1077–82.

McArdle, William D.; Katch, Frank I.; and Katch, Victor L. *Exercise Physiology: Energy, Nutrition, and Human Performance*, 3rd ed. Philadelphia: Lea & Febiger, 1991.

Ries, Andrew L.; Ellis, Birgitta; and Hawkins, Randy W. "Upper Extremity Exercise Training in Chronic Obstructive Pulmonary Disease." *Chest* 93, no. 4 (April 1990): 688–92.

Shayevitz, Myra B., and Shayevitz, Berton R. "Athletic Training in Chronic Obstructive Pulmonary Disease." *Clinics in Sports Medicine* 5, no. 3 (July 1986): 471–91.

Sicilian, Leonard. "Mechanisms and Management of Exercise-Induced Asthma." *Practical Cardiology* 9 (August 1983): 143–52.

Sinclair, D. G. M., and Ingram, C. G. "Controlled Trial of Supervised Exercise Training in Chronic Bronchitis." *British Medical Journal* (February 23, 1980): 519–21.

Sonne, Leonard J., and Davis, James A. "Increased Exercise Performance in Patients with Severe COPD Following Inspiratory Resistive Training." *Chest* 81 (April 1982): 436–39.

Stein, David A.; Bradley, Bernard L.; and Miller, Warren C.

"Mechanisms of Oxygen Effects on Exercise in Patients with Chronic Obstructive Pulmonary Disease." *Chest* 81 (January 1982): 6–10.

Psyche

Dudley, Donald L.; Glaser, Edward M.; Jorgenson, Betty N.; and Logan, Daniel L. "Psychosocial Concomitants to Rehabilitation in Chronic Obstructive Pulmonary Disease." Part 1: "Psychosocial and Psychological Considerations." *Chest* 77 (March 1980): 413–20.

Dudley, Donald L. "Psychosocial Concomitants to Rehabilitation in Chronic Obstructive Pulmonary Disease." Part 2: "Psychosocial Treatment." *Chest* 77 (April 1980): 544–51.

McSweeney, A. John; Heaton, Robert K.; Grant, Igor; Cugell, David; Solliday, Norman; and Timms, Richard. "Chronic Obstructive Pulmonary Disease: Socioemotional Adjustment and Life Quality." *Chest* 77 (February 1980): supplement, 309–11.

Sex

Baucom, Donald H., and Hoffman, Jeffrey A. "Common Mistakes Spouses Make in Communicating." *Medical Aspects of Human Sexuality* 17 (November 1983): 203–19.

Brauer, Alan P., and Brauer, Donna. *How You and Your Lover Can Give Each Other Hours of Extended Sexual Orgasm.* New York: Warner, 1983.

Kaplan, Helen S. "Sexual Relationships in Middle-Age." *Physician & Patient* 2, no. 10 (October 1983): 11–20.

Kieran, James, with Nan Pheatt. "No End to Love." *American Lung Association Bulletin* 67 (December 1981): 10–13.

Korenman, Stanley G.; Viosca, Sharon P.; Kaiser, Fran E.; Mooradian, Arshag D.; and Morley, John E. "Use of a Vacuum Tumescence Device in the Management of Impotence." *Journal of the American Geriatrics Society* 38, no. 3 (1990): 217–20.

Kravetz, Howard M. "Sex and COPD: Counseling that Allays Patients' Anxieties." *Consultant* (July 1982).

————. "Sexual Counseling for the COPD Patient." *Clinical Challenge in Cardiopulmonary Medicine* 4, no. 1 (June 1982): 1–5.

————; Garland, Anne M.; Harner, Dave; and Harner, Carol. *A Visit with Helen: A Summary for the Patient.* Slide-tape presentation for patient education, Pulmonary Foundation, 1011 Ruth Street, Prescott, AZ 86301.

————; Weiss, Lillie; and Meadows, Rosalyn. *A Visit with Harry: A Summary for the Patient.* Slide-tape presentation for patient education, Pulmonary Foundation, 1011 Ruth Street, Prescott, AZ 86301.

Mooradian, Arshag, and Greiff, Vicki. "Sexuality in Older Women." *Archives of Internal Medicine* 150, no. 5 (May 1990): 1033–38.

Noehren, Theodore H. "Editorial Comment." *Clinical Challenge in Cardiopulmonary Medicine* 4 (June 1982): 5–6.

COE

Carney, Robert M. "Clinical Applications of Relaxation Training." *Hospital Practice* (July 1983): 83–94.

Recreation

Copolillo, Henry P. "The Value of Recreation." *Physician & Patient* 1 (September 1982): 66–68.

Dillard, Thomas A., et al. "Hypoxemia During Air Travel in Patients with Chronic Obstructive Pulmonary Disease." *Annals of Internal Medicine* 111, no. 5 (September 1989): 362–67.

Gong, Henry, Jr. "Editorial: Advising Patients with Pulmonary Disease on Air Travel." *Annals of Internal Medicine* 111, no. 5 (September 1989): 349–51.

Woodridge, William E. "Medical Complications of Air Travel." *Postgraduate Medicine* 87, no. 7 (May 15, 1990): 75–77.

INDEX

DREAMS

from the

MONSTER FACTORY

A TALE OF PRISON, REDEMPTION AND
ONE WOMAN'S FIGHT TO RESTORE JUSTICE TO ALL

Sunny Schwartz

with David Boodell

SCRIBNER
New York   London   Toronto   Sydney

SCRIBNER
A Division of Simon & Schuster, Inc.
1230 Avenue of the Americas
New York, NY 10020

Some of the names and identifying characteristics of people
in this book have been changed and some characters are composites.
All changes were made to protect the identities of those involved.

Copyright © 2009 by Sunny Schwartz and David Boodell

First Scribner hardcover edition January 2009

SCRIBNER and design are registered trademarks of
The Gale Group, Inc. used under license by Simon & Schuster, Inc.,
the publisher of this work.

For information about special discounts for bulk purchases,
please contact Simon & Schuster Special Sales at
1-800-456-6798 or business@simonandschuster.com.

Designed by Kyoko Watanabe
Text set in Aldine 401

Manufactured in the United States of America

1   3   5   7   9   10   8   6   4   2

Library of Congress Control Number: 2008020441

ISBN-13: 978-1-4165-6981-7
ISBN-10: 1-4165-6981-2

For Frieda, Lauren, Ella and the Chicago Cubs

The future belongs to those who believe in the beauty of their dreams.

—ELEANOR ROOSEVELT

You don't need to wait for a roof to collapse on your head to fix something.

—FRIEDA SCHWARTZ, MY MOTHER

DREAMS
from the
MONSTER FACTORY

PROLOGUE

I don't think my truant officer ever knew where I went. I'd ditch class and ride the El to Chicago's north side, jump off at Belmont and plant myself in the Wrigley Field bleachers. I'd soak up the squawk of the beer man, the steam coming from the bins of the Vienna Beef hot dog vendors, the gentle slapping sound of a ball dropping into a mitt in the outfield and the emerald green expanse of the diamond. Wrigley was my sanctuary when I was a gawky teenager stumbling through adolescence. Even if school gave me palpitations and my family drove me nuts, I still had the ballpark and the dream that bound all of us fans together: the dream that this year the Cubs would go all the way.

I was raised on the south side and by rights should have pledged allegiance to the White Sox, but my heart has always been with the underdogs and so it was the Cubs for me. Later, when I moved to San Francisco, I gave myself with equal passion to the Giants, who have validated my devotion by failing to win the big one year after year. I am like this in the rest of my life, too: I root for underdogs.

I work in the jails of San Francisco County, and my clients are thieves and wife beaters, gangbangers and murderers—underdogs, every one of them. They have hurt their victims, their families and their communities and are now paying the price, abandoned to society's scrap heap. There are lots of names for this scrap heap: the big house, the slammer, the joint, lockup. I think the best name is monster factory. In these factories, men exist in cells on long tiers, where they have nothing to do. They sleep in their bunks, play dominoes and cards, watch the *Jerry Springer* show on TV and scheme. They scheme about how to steal someone's lunch, how to pull one over on the DA, how to score black market cigarettes for five bucks a smoke and how to get even with whoever crossed them. They make shanks out of mops, pens and metal shards broken off their bunks. These are places where the strongest thugs are allowed to terrorize the weakest. In most of our nation's jails and prisons, violence in the form of beatings, racial threats and rapes is normal. The most predictable product of this system is rage, which builds and builds in each prisoner until he is set free—and about 90 percent are set free someday, released back into our communities.

It's no news flash to say that traditional criminal justice is in chaos. One out of every hundred adults in the United States is behind bars. This is the highest incarceration rate in the world. Recidivism rates—which are difficult to track since no one keeps comprehensive statistics—hover somewhere around 70 percent, despite state budgets for corrections that have been climbing for years now. "There is no other business in the world," one coporate attorney told me, "that gets an increase in their budget when they have a seventy percent failure rate."

I was trained as an attorney, and always thought I'd spend my life as a defense attorney, but have instead worked on what I call "true defense." True defense is working for the good of all: the victims of crime *and* the perpetrators as well as the community. It has been my life's work to fight the monster factories, to reject the presumption people make that nothing can ever change. It hasn't been a simple fight. The question I get most often is "Why should I care?" I've found there is no more persuasive way to answer this question than by taking people to see the monsters. I first show people the traditional jail. Then I take them to the jails I've helped set up. I take them to RSVP (Resolve to Stop the Violence Program), the program I'm most proud of, where we work with violent men to make them less violent. I tell people about the evaluation of our program, done by psychiatrist James Gilligan, who directed the Center for the Study of Violence at Harvard Medical School and now works at NYU. He is one of the country's leading experts on violence. His study showed an 80 percent drop in violent recidivism for inmates who had spent more than four months in our program. I take people to see the charter high school (the first charter school for incarcerated adults in this country) and the college classes, and show them what a jail can be like in a place where there are high standards, and where the presumption exists that despicable men and women can change for the better and rejoin the human race. One venture capitalist I took around with me came away thunderstruck. "Sunny," he exclaimed, "those programs for violent men. They could help me! They could help any man." The stories I tell in this book will take you on the same journey, to see both the worst the system has to offer, and the best.

Everyone has a stake in this, Republican or Democrat, liberal or conservative; this isn't a partisan issue, it is a human one. What do we do with the people who get out of jail and come back to our communities? I know that we can actually use the prisons to make us safer and our communities better. I know it because I've seen it happen. I've seen men who have committed horrible crimes defy all predictions, take responsibility for their lives and begin to make amends. Every time that happens, for me, it's like the Cubs have won the World Series. If RSVP stops just one person from committing a murder, that's an entire community of family and friends saved from devastation. Now imagine if across the country, every jail and prison challenged criminals to stop their violence, to stop using drugs, to get a job, to become responsible citizens, to become, as one friend described it, "taxpayers instead of tax drainers." If that happened, we wouldn't just change the prisons and jails; we would remake the face of American society. That's the dream I've had. That's what has sustained me in the monster factory.

CHAPTER 1

1980

Jails are about doors. You wait for them to open. You wait for them to close. There is nothing subtle about a jail door. It rumbles and clangs like a death knell. You don't open them yourself. Others decide whether you come in or go out.

I was waiting at Post 5, outside Mainline, the processing center for anyone arrested in San Francisco County. I was shoving my ID up to a window so that the annoyed-looking deputy sheriff could flip the switch and let me in. I was beginning to grow angry at how long the deputy was taking when an electrical buzzing shriek cut through my thoughts and the door shuddered open.

A wave of noise crashed over me, quickly followed by a rancid smell of ammonia and body odor. I stepped out onto the tier. Mainline was like a zoo, except uglier than any zoo I'd ever been to. Huge cages framed the long corridor in front of me, which stretched out the length of a football field. Every cage was filled with men wearing jail-issue orange—orange pants, orange T-shirts, orange sweatshirts, orange flip-flops or canvas shoes. A few prisoners wandered the corridor. They were workers with special privileges, allowed to be out of the tanks when going to or from their jobs. Half the cages were open dormitories filled with bunk beds; the other half were lined with two-man cells. The echoing of angry voices was deafening. There was nothing to absorb or interrupt the noise. Shouts and shrieks banged off bulletproof glass, steel bars and cinder blocks. There were probably four hundred prisoners in the jail that day. I was the only woman in sight. This was my first day of work.

I'd been hired as a legal intern for the San Francisco Prisoner Legal Services unit. There were eight of us: five men and three women. The interns handled legal issues for prisoners for eveything but the crimes that had brought them to jail in the first place. They had their public defender for that. My colleagues and I spread out through the jails every day, going wherever we were assigned or needed. If a prisoner was accused of a rule violation in the jail, or if he wanted to accuse a deputy sheriff of harassment, or if he was getting evicted from the apartment where he lived, or if he was losing custody of his children, he talked to me or one of my colleagues. The legal interns were the catchall. I wasn't a lawyer, none of us were, but I was supposed to function like one.

I was twenty-six years old, had barely made it through high school and didn't have a college degree. I'd never been in a jail before, and had one day of training, which consisted of being told how to use the phones and how to file paperwork. I was told repeatedly not to give the prisoners gum because they'd use it to jam the locks, but I received no training on what to do if someone turned violent. I was handed a box of pens and a legal pad and told, in essence, to go save lives. "Wildly unprepared" would be the polite way of describing how I felt.

I'd been warned about walking Mainline my first day. Rita, a colleague I'd met during training, compared it to being a sheep in a pack of wolves. She'd recommended that I present my request at the front office and meet the prisoner in an interview room, at least until I got the hang of things. But I wanted to prove that I was strong enough to stare down the monsters without flinching. I was curious, too, wondering if the men were as scary as I'd heard.

The men crowded to the front of their tanks to watch me when I stepped onto the tier. The few inmate workers in the hall stopped in place and turned toward me, as if they were a compass and I was due north. The noise receded for a second, then there was an explosion of voices.

"Oooh baby, come over here. I won't hurt you."

"Hey, baby. What's the matter, you get lost?"

"Come here, I need some smokes."

"Hey, little girl, I got something you could smoke."

Some of the men smiled, some made a meal of me with their eyes, a few just stood there with pitiful looks, like little children trapped in men's bodies.

With each step, a jolt of fear coursed through me. But I was also growing angry. I singled out a jeering kid on my left, walked up to him and barked, "Are you addressing me? Do you need something?"

I surprised him. His face went blank. I went up to the bars. "If you whistle at me again, I will hurt you like a dog. How would you feel if your mother was walking down these tiers and she was treated like this?"

The guy's voice barely slipped out of him. "Uh, um, I dunno." His eyes were wide. The others were watching. I could see some were smiling, taking my measure.

I was there to interview my first client. His name was Martin Aguerro. I'd been handed his file with a pile of others that morning. His seemed like the most interesting case and so here I was, ready to work. I returned to Post 5 and told the deputy I wanted to interview Aguerro. He rolled his eyes at me. This was the second deputy sheriff I'd talked to and the second set of rolled eyes, and it was pissing me off. Moving at a glacial pace, he checked his books, got on the phone, and after a few grunts, hung up and said, unceremoniously, "No."

"What do you mean no?"

"Just what I said. No." He crossed his arms.

I expected to fight with the prisoners, but I hadn't expected to fight the deputies, too. "First of all, he filed a claim," I said through clenched teeth. "The only way to follow up on the claim is to meet the guy. Why can't I see him?"

"I'm just doing what I'm told, lady. They tell me he's too dangerous. You can't see him without a two-deputy security complement and I don't have the staff right now."

I knew the deputy was giving me the "weak girl" assessment. I didn't look older than my twenty-six years, but I was no Twiggy. I was five feet nine, solid and could handle myself. After all, I had two older brothers whose idea of nurturing was an unceasing flurry of full nelsons and charley horses. I liked to think that had made me tough.

"Listen," I said, "I don't care if he's the biggest gangbanger ya got. He has a right to see me and I am not leaving until I meet with him."

I got a tired stare. I stared back until finally, with a shake of his head, the deputy reached for the phone and called the chief . Twenty minutes later the chief deputy sauntered up with a smirk on his face. At six feet five and three hundred pounds, he towered over me. "You know your so-called client is a shot caller in the Mexican Mafia?" he said.

I was too green to know that the Mexican Mafia was one of the most powerful gangs operating behind bars in California, and they controlled large portions of the drug traffic coming up from Central and South America. What I did know was what any child of Chicago knew: anybody who came from *the* mafia, *any* mafia, was probably a tough SOB. I pushed on, breathing through my teeth. "I couldn't care less; this is my job."

"Well, Miss Schwartz, I want you to know, I can't guarantee your safety."

I rolled my eyes, told him I understood and sat down to wait and bring my heart rate down. I was sitting right outside the deputy's station. Prisoners periodically came up asking for things. They needed to get to the next tier for work detail. Someone's toilet was stopped up. Somebody else was complaining about his mail delivery. I caught pieces of conversations I didn't understand—the guys on D block were freaking out because they missed their commissary delivery, a sergeant was twitching because two code 3s had been called yesterday and he was buried under paperwork. (A code 3 was radio shorthand for a deputy needing assistance because a situation had turned violent, meaning the prisoners were fighting or there was an attack on a deputy.)

As I sat there, I was struck by the most unexpected thought. Even though this was my first time inside a jail, and I was far away from Chicago, where I'd grown up, and far from Tucson, where I'd spent the last eight years of my life, I felt like I was home. In the eyes of the inmates, in the cold stares of the men trying to be hard, in their vulnerability, in all the pathetic, twisted, mangled personalities on display on the walk down Mainline, I'd seen shadows of myself.

I could do something for these men.

I certainly felt more at home on Mainline than I did in a law school classroom. I'd been a first-year law student at this point for exactly three weeks. (How I managed to scam my way into law school without a college degree is a story I'll get to later.) The world of books and notes and tests and number-two pencils had always been a place of shame for me. My school transcripts were a minefield of truant reports, failing grades and discipline problems. I thought about the class I had that night—it was about contracts—and, honestly, I felt more comfortable in the jail.

Half an hour went by and there was still no sign of my client. Martin Aguerro had filed a claim accusing the San Francisco Police Department of shooting him in the back. The allegation was serious and could end up in court one day, but the rules said he had to file an administrative claim against the city first and exhaust that route, so that's where I came in. Out of the mountain of files I'd been handed that morning, his sparked my interest. Most claims were from inmates needing a defense after they'd broken some jail rule. They'd gotten into a fight or had refused to obey an order from the deputies. Penny-ante crap that might add a day or a week onto their sentence. This was different, something I could sink my teeth into.

Finally, I heard the echo of a gate opening and closing, and I saw a man in red who I presumed was my client at the end of the tier with two deputies flanking him. The color red was for the most dangerous inmates and escape risks. I watched Martin Aguerro come toward me. He was moving slowly, as if he were underwater, and it looked like he was pushing a cart. As he and the deputies came closer, I realized that this violent, dangerous prisoner, the man around whom they could not guarantee my safety, was dragging his legs behind a walker. He was trussed up in full belly chains that kept his hands secured at his waist so he could barely hold the walker. Martin Aguerro was a skinny Latino man with greasy hair that hung into his eyes. His file said he was my age, twenty-six, but he looked eighteen. He was no taller than I was and had to be a good twenty pounds lighter. When he got closer, I could see he had the trappings of toughness. He had *hate* tattooed on the fingers of one hand and *love* on the other. On his left arm, he had a Sacred Heart of Jesus, on his right, a half-naked woman. But yapping poodles have frightened me more. I suppose he could've whacked me with his walker, if he'd been able to lift his arms.

I introduced myself as we sat down at a table. He was polite, didn't bring any attitude. His voice was slight, his speech a little lispy. We talked about his claim. He said that there'd been a warrant for his arrest and the cops came for him. They surprised him at his apartment and he didn't know what was happening. He'd tried to run, and before anyone said anything, a cop had shot him in the back.

"They didn't say 'You're under arrest'?" I asked. "They didn't announce themselves, identify themselves as cops?"

"Nah, man, they just started firing. I get hit. The next thing I know, I'm in the fucking hospital. Man, I can't piss right. Can't walk. They really fucked me up."

Good, I was thinking, good. It was a miserable story, but if what he was saying was true, I had a case. I'd barely started law school, but I did know that the police had to announce themselves. They couldn't just come in firing.

I pushed on. I didn't know anything about Martin, didn't know his rap sheet and had no way of assessing if he was being truthful with me. Someone had told me during training that I didn't need to worry about what crime they'd committed. Our job was to deal with their grievances, not with the reason they were locked up. But I felt like I needed to know.

"What was the warrant for?" I asked.

"Oral copulation on a child and rape." He said it like he was wanted for traffic tickets. Here I'd been feeling sorry for the guy, ready to jump into his corner and fight it out. But in an instant that feeling was replaced with disgust. After a few more questions, I was shaking with rage. The girl he was accused of molesting was nine years old.

"I gotta tell you something." I coughed, my fist clenched. "I want to hurt you for committing such a horrible act of violence. So we're gonna have to talk about this 'cause I'm sickened."

Martin's eyebrows shot up. But he didn't say anything except "Yeah?"

I paused for a second, trying to find my words. "It's really unpleasant for me to be in the same room with someone who's done that to a child. So actually working on this complaint is going to be difficult for me."

Martin stared at me during my explanation, nursing his silence. He didn't try to defend himself. He didn't tell me he'd "been framed" or that there were "extenuating circumstances" or that everything was consensual. He just looked at me and answered my questions, as I tried to figure out how I was going to live with myself and work with him.

I was making it up as I went along. I made sure he knew how to read and assigned him a book report on Susan Brownmiller's *Against Our Will: Men, Women, and Rape*. I'd read Brownmiller's book a year earlier. It was a comprehensive history of rape and its place in Western culture. It wasn't full of academic jargon—*I* got through it, for God's sake—but it clocked in at around five hundred pages, and I was pretty sure Martin was never going to finish it, which worked for me. If he didn't do the assignment, then I wouldn't have to deal with him. He said he'd try and we set a time to meet.

A week later, when I sat down with him again, he'd made it through the first chapter. He'd even produced a book report. His writing was pathetic, looking like mine did in the fifth grade, full of misspellings, bad grammar and incomplete sentences, so his report didn't reveal much. But we talked about his insights, such as they were. He'd read the "Personal Statement," and chapter 1, "The Mass Psychology of Rape," which contained references to Freud and Marx. He didn't know who they were, but he did get the basic point of the chapter, which was that throughout history, women have had to contend with men defining what rape is. "It's like, these ladies came along and they said, rape ain't right, right?" he said, which was pretty close to the gist of the first chapter. I wanted to believe he was taking something away from our discussion, but honestly, I couldn't read the guy.

We met every week. He reported on the chapter he'd read and I learned about his case. He was so unguarded in everything he said to me. I didn't have any reason to disbelieve his story of the night of the arrest. But his account—that he received no warning, that he was unarmed, that he was running away scared when he was shot—was contradicted by the arresting officers and some of the physical evidence. The arrest reports said all the proper protocols were followed: officers had clearly identified themselves when they came through his door and he was shot going for a handgun found at the scene. Was he telling me the truth, or just trying to game the system? Eventually I decided I wasn't going to figure it out. If the cops were as disgusted as I was, I could picture them going in with guns drawn ready to fire.

The third time we met, he said to me, "Can you believe it, they're shackling me when I'm paralyzed. Where the hell am I going to go?" He complained all the time. "It's a jungle in here," he'd say. "I wanted to do the book report but they don't even let me have a pen to write with." Other times he told me, "I can't take a shower because they don't have any facilities for guys like me." They were all garden-variety complaints, and I couldn't disagree with him. The food sucked? Yup, no argument there. The doctors didn't care? True as well. He *was* being treated like an animal; who wouldn't complain? But eventually I just wanted to shake him, knock some sense into him. "You've got to be kidding me!" I wanted to tell him. "Whose fault is it that you raped a little girl?"

He read the book dutifully. Finally, after two months, even though he hadn't finished the book, I told him he'd done enough and I'd file his complaint. But I had him sign a contract, a contract I made up, that said if he heard someone joking about rape or objectifying women in any way, he would confront the man and tell him to knock it off. We'd been talking for weeks now, and when I asked him to do that, it was the first time I heard any interest from him, any sense that he was thinking about the ideas I'd been trying to put into his head.

"I can do that," he said over and over. "Man, I will do that." Either he was hustling me, or he really thought it was a good idea, or maybe he just liked the idea of telling other men what to do. Whatever the reason, he signed the contract and agreed to confront other men if they made women-hating jokes. He also agreed to try to start a study group in prison to figure out ways to help women and children who'd been raped.

Then and only then did I file his complaint. Even as I did, I pictured Martin back in his cell spouting off, "Get this—this bitch is crazy," and laughing with the other predators. I had no time to do follow-up with him, no way to call him out if he did go back to his cell to form a predator support group for his hideous views.

His complaint was summarily dismissed. Given the evidence against him, it didn't matter if he was right or wrong. He was a child predator resisting arrest and it was his word against the cops'. There wasn't much more to it than that. By the time the decision came down, I'd had at least sixty clients, and I'd realized that Aguerro's complaint was a fool's mission. Complaints from inmates passed through my hands every day, some about the quality of the food, others about the high phone bills inmates' families had to pay. Some were assault charges against deputy sheriffs. Some had merit, some didn't. There were a few I could actually win, many more I couldn't.

Martin's case was never anything but a long shot. But Martin himself was unique. He didn't excuse his crimes with me or claim he'd been framed or claim that there was a good explanation for what happened. Most other prisoners did that. But Martin *was* like the other prisoners in a specific way.

He had no remorse. He complained about jail conditions, complained about his lawyer, felt bad for himself, but never offered me one word of sorrow for the people he'd hurt, the pain he'd caused.

Oh brother, the child rapist doesn't like jail. That's how I felt most of the time. But his attitude nagged at me.

"How you live is how you die" is what my mother, Frieda, always said. She was a woman of sayings. This one was always declared with a sigh whenever someone's failings were on display. Every day in the jails, as the doors were opened onto a new set of problems, my mom's words rang in my ears as if they were on a loop. I heard them every time the doors clanged shut behind me on Mainline. Every week there were new faces staring out from the bars, faces showing the barest hints of beards. And standing beside them were men I recognized. Men who'd been released only to return for their third or fourth or tenth visit. Martin Aguerro soon was gone. He was offered a deal of ten years and went off to follow his walker around San Quentin before I lost track of him. There he probably still got shoddy medical care and filed complaints to fill his time and maybe, just maybe, he held court and told men to knock off the women-hating crap. But I doubt it.

Martin Aguerro didn't defeat me. I didn't give up on the prisoners because of him, but he did educate me on the limits of what I could do. I went on to meet murderers and petty thieves and everyone in between. Almost all of them hid behind an excuse. After six months on the job as a law intern, I'd heard them all. After a year I could recite them chapter and verse. I didn't stop asking prisoners why they were in jail. But I learned not to be surprised when very few could answer with the simple truth: they were in jail because they made the choice to commit a crime.

Many convicts used their past to justify their crimes. It was infuriating to listen to. But the past did matter. There are plenty of people with sad stories to tell who end up as good citizens, but I never met anyone behind bars who went through childhood unscathed. There are reasons why people end up behind bars. It's no coincidence, not for any of the inmates I've worked with, and not for me, either.

CHAPTER 2

1966

"Don't trust rich folks, Sunny," my dad, Seymour, said, wagging his finger at me. "You can't. They're full of shit."

He said this to me all the time. But in this particular instance, my dad was referring to Cindy's new in-laws, the Millers, whom my sister was bringing over for Passover seder. Seymour imparted this nugget of wisdom while banging the vacuum through the living room. He was a handsome, cranky piece of work, whom all my friends were afraid of. But my parents really loved each other despite all their problems, and that day he helped clean the living room so my mom wouldn't have a conniption. She had been wandering through the house for days, mumbling nonstop to herself.

"Look at this dreck!" Frieda pointed to the worn carpet. "It's dreck! And look at the stains on the furniture. *Oy vey,* I hate this peanut house," she said as she tried to rub the stains off the pink hand-me-down couch. I normally loved my mother's voice, the way it revved up and went bouncing along like an accordion. She was a talker. Everywhere she went, she had friends and confidants. I'd listen to her on the phone, kibitzing with her girlfriends, her voice breaking into peals of laughter. But as we prepared for Passover, she was a dark cloud, scowling at me if I dared tell her to relax. "Dolly," she'd bark, "go clean your room."

Our family lived in Marionette Manor, in the shadow of the South Works steel plant on Chicago's south side, in a roiling stew of working-class Jews and Catholics, Polish, Irish and African Americans. Cindy was my half sister and, since she was fourteen years older than me, more like a favorite aunt. She came from a mysterious time in my father's life, his short-lived first marriage to an alcoholic woman who was evidently so unfit that my father had been granted custody of Cindy. Where my two older brothers, Jerry and Stevie, were full of my father's bullying energy, Cindy was nurturing. When she still lived with us, her room was all lace and pillows and delicate things, a refuge from the tough-guy atmosphere in the rest of the house. Cindy had married a boy from a wealthy family and now lived in Hyde Park. And to my mother's ever-lasting embarrassment, had invited his parents to our Passover seder.

My mom had a rich, earthy family legacy, which suited her like an old housedress. She would have traded up for a more sophisticated model if only she could have. Frieda's mother lived with us. She was a lumbering old tank of a babushka who had fled a Russian pogrom. We called her Bubba. Bubba had never bothered to learn English beyond the basics, and I could barely understand what she said half the time because her dentures were the wrong size and wandered around her mouth. Bubba charred pieces of toast and saved them in the drawers of our kitchen to crush into her borscht. My mother would find the crusts and grit her teeth.

Uncle Harry, my mom's brother, lived nearby. He arrived that afternoon and parked himself in front of the chopped-liver appetizer. Uncle Harry was "touched," according to Frieda. "He got goofy from the war," she'd say with a sigh. "Ya know, war wound." And she'd look at me knowingly and tap her head. Illness seemed to be leaking out of his fingers where they were stained brown from his unfiltered Lucky Strikes. Frieda lovingly yelled at Harry a few times while waiting for the Millers to arrive. "Stop eating! Leave some for the company!" she'd beg. Liver was smeared all over Harry's fingers.

My father just nodded at Harry and snorted. He was on his best behavior that day. Seymour had an edge—a gruff, volcanic spirit that was always on the verge of erupting. On days when his temper did flare up, my mother would retreat to the kitchen to defrost the refrigerator, her mouth pressed into a thin line. The rest of us worked out our own methods to avoid him. Jerry would go do his homework. Stevie would go out to play baseball. I would mope in my room. Seymour was an orphan whose parents came from Eastern Europe, one from Russia, the other, we think, from Latvia. I'm not sure he really knew.

He never talked about it, except to say that he could remember that his mother was beautiful and that she had a voice like a nightingale. I'd catch him sometimes in his basement room going through old photos, his eyes misty. The photos were the only remnants of his mom and dad that he had. Whenever he talked about them, he seemed hurt, then quickly grew grumpy. If my mother's family was an embarrassment, my father's family was missing in action. But, in general, Seymour tried to make my mother happy, even if it meant being polite to some full-of-shit in-laws.

My sister and her husband, Bob, arrived in their Porsche. Bob's parents came in a chauffeur-driven Cadillac. They spoke so quietly, I can remember sitting in the living room, my mother shushing everyone, straining to make out what Mrs. Miller was saying.

"Frieda," she said, smiling, "you have such a warm home." My mother smiled back, desperate to be the perfect hostess, glaring at Stevie and me because we kept cracking up at Bubba's wandering dentures.

Jerry rarely laughed along with Stevie and me. We called him the Alderman. He was the oldest boy. He behaved. He did well in school. Stevie was two years behind him and trouble—trouble for the girls, who all loved him, and trouble for my father. Stevie just wouldn't fall into line with Seymour. It helped make us allies.

I was the kid sister, two years behind Stevie, and he and Jerry ganged up on me. There were the names—Dumbass, Fat Pig, Loser and Chubs (Stevie gave me that last one; I had a spare tire at age eight). There were also the attacks—being pinned down and sat on while one or both slapped my face until I went nuts; them spitting in my butterscotch pudding; being locked out of the house in winter while I shivered and pleaded with them to open the door. But when Jerry wasn't looking, Stevie would ask me what I was thinking. He sometimes even took my side against Jerry, and he taught me how to throw a curveball, too. When Harry started mumbling incoherently during the lighting of the candles, it was Stevie who got me laughing uncontrollably by mimicking it under his breath. I was always his best, easiest audience.

We got through it. My mother shushed us and smiled uncomfortably and the Millers seemed kind, not at all what my dad led me to expect. Seymour blessed the wine and we all got a sip. Stevie slipped some to Bubba, and by the end of the meal, she was smiling a little too broadly and spitting out her water. We washed our hands and ate the parsley dipped in salt water, my father intoning the prayers as a reminder, as if we needed any with the Millers sitting there, of our lowly origins and how we'd all been slaves in Egypt. Matzoh was passed. Bubba yelled out non sequiturs in quiet moments and my mother leaned over, finally giving up appearances, and stage-whispered "Ma—shhhh." Uncle Harry interrupted to ask my mom, "Fritzy, where's the chopped liver?" and everyone laughed, even the Millers. Finally we sang the Dayanu that concludes the Passover story. We were liberated from the seder and got down to eating my mom's amazing meal.

Those were the good times in our house. They were few and far between.

If there's one memory from my childhood that stands out, it's of my dad stretched out in the backseat of our Buick with the windows rolled down, fingering the stops on his cornet. Seymour Schwartz was a self-taught jazz cornet player and songwriter. My mother would say he'd gotten lost again when he'd retreat to the car. He played "God Bless the Child" slowly, mournfully, the notes expanding along the quiet residential streets. The old Billie Holiday standard was one of his favorites. Mine, too. I'd sit alone at the window, singing along with the melody.

> *Mama may have, Papa may have,*
> *But God bless the child that's got his own*

My dad was always scrambling for his big break but never quite making it. The closest he got was when he worked with Mahalia Jackson. They became friends in the early 1950s and our family went to her house for fried chicken dinners on a few Sunday nights. Seymour wrote a song for Mahalia called "The Holy Bible" and they performed it on the Studs Terkel radio show. My heart swelled with pride every time my mom cued up the reel-to-reel recording. But Mahalia moved on and my father's career stalled. His style was too schmaltzy, not original enough. He didn't have many live gigs, either. He fought with the other players. At some point it seemed, he always marched through the kitchen door referring to his bandleader as a "fucking Nazi bastard," and then he'd stalk off to the basement to write.

With Seymour you were either his enemy or you were his friend. There was no in between. His kids could fall into either category. I can remember poking around in the garage when I was nine. It was filled with milk crates of records and sheet music, my dad's work, along with junk that should've been thrown out, old broken chairs, a broken radio, tools for the garden. The garage was my father's domain. I spied some dusty records that had fallen behind a filing cabinet and on top of the pile was a 45-rpm recording I knew he'd been looking for. It was one of his schmaltz-soaked ballads, "No One Seems to Care." That evening, when I heard the car drive up, I ran out to meet him with the record in my hand.

"Daddy, look what I found!" I was all giddy energy.

He left the car with a scowl and wheeled on me. The 45 was there in my hand one second, and the next it was like a magic trick, my hand was empty.

He broke the record over his knee and threw it to the ground. "This is shit," he bellowed at me. "I never want to see this or any other record again. Fuck it!"

My mom saw the whole thing from the front porch and tried to stand up for me. "She didn't mean anything by it."

My dad huffed away, grumbling to himself, "Everything's bullshit."

I looked at my mother, my little fists clenching. She looked so powerless and sad in that moment. I ran off down the street, sobbing.

My father periodically would climb into bed with my brothers and me. He didn't molest us, he just needed us near him, needed the comfort of another body. I guess he did it when my mom got tired of him. He usually came around when he'd been moping in the basement over one of his songs. Jerry or Stevie would shout out from their room, "Don't Greek me, Dad! Jesus!" and I knew he would make his way to my room. When I got old enough to stand up for myself, I gave him the same line and kicked him out. I knew even then that he wasn't there to comfort me.

Truth be told, I didn't feel safe in my house. Between my dad and the torment of my two older brothers, I didn't feel safe. When we first moved into the house, I was around four, and my next-door neighbor, a chain-smoking Irish Catholic with the remarkable name of Laverne Liberty encountered me in the yard.

"I heard this tiny voice screaming bloody murder." Laverne would laugh as she recounted the story. "'Shit, goddamn, I'm gonna kick your ass!' And I came out into the driveway and it was you howling at your brothers, who were sitting on top of you and pummeling you. Just another day at the Schwartz house."

Laverne's house became my refuge after one too many charley horses or dead arms or taunts about how I was in the remedial classes with the retards. She'd make me Oscar Mayer hard-salami sandwiches with butter on white Silvercup bread. My dad would complain that I was spending too much time with the goyim.

The worst part about it was that I *was* in the remedial classes. I'd started to fall behind the other kids at the very beginning, sent home year after year with report cards burning a hole in my hand, never sure when I opened them if I had passed on to the next grade. In the sixth grade, I tested at a third-grade reading level. I yelled at the teachers, learning how to fight like my father, never learning how to deal with school, with the shame and fear I had that I might be a complete loser. The teachers liked to mark me for "Citizenship Failure" at Luella Elementary. I was mouthy. I came to know the principal's office intimately. Luella Elementary was two blocks from our house and every morning the walk felt like a death march. The torments of my father and brothers were well matched by the torments of geometry and the Battle of Hastings.

Those torments also competed with the Pulaski brothers, the scourge of the neighborhood. There were three of them and they were about the same ages as my brothers and me. I can't tell you how many times one of them and their punk friends chased me and cornered me up against the church that was between school and my street, taunting, "You killed Jesus! You killed our god! You killed Jesus! Go home, you dirty Jew!" The Pulaski brothers were greasers. They were big and tough. Each had slicked blond hair and wore green iridescent pants and pointy half boots. The Pulaskis were Polish Catholics, and I was too scared to shout back the Polack jokes I learned from my brothers.

Jerry stayed out of their way. He was a bookworm who walked around with black-rimmed glasses, oxford shirts, and kept to himself. He was no nerd, he was tough, but no one really knew who he was. Stevie was popular, and had a pair of iridescent pants, too, so was more of a target.

When I was ten, one of Stevie's girlfriends came running up to me after the last bell at school. She was out of breath, "Stevie's in a fight, and the guy has a knife." I ran to find Stevie cornered in the playground. Eddie Pulaski, the middle brother, was taunting him with a switchblade. A crowd of kids was watching. My brother was on the verge of tears, his eyes wide like a surprised rabbit. He was trying to keep it together, but tight short sobs kept spurting out. It was horrible.

I had a Trapper Keeper, one of those heavy, three-ring binders, in my hand. I sneaked up on Eddie and I brought it down on his head with a knee-buckling thwack. I grabbed Stevie and ran. He turned on me as soon as we were free, tears staining his checks. "Why did you do that? Why did you do that? Now they're gonna make fun of me because my kid sister protected me."

Summer was one of the only times I felt some freedom. I had my bicycle, a Schwinn with a white banana seat, and I had friends. I was mouthy after all, like my mother, a good talker, willing to walk up to almost anyone and give them a piece of my mind, or tell them to come riding with me to the beach.

I trailed after my brothers when I could but when they had no use for me, I took off with my girlfriends. There were no rules about where I could go or when. I just had to be back for dinner. My friends and I whirled like dervishes during the day—to the beach, to Pinzer's drugstore, where we'd hang out on the mechanical horse out front, or if it was hot enough and we had some money, to DeVito's bowling alley to roll a game—anywhere our bikes would take us.

July 1966 boiled. Biking on days that hovered in the nineties with ninety percent humidity felt like swimming through hot soup. The heat finally broke in the middle of the month, and when I went to bed on July 13, I didn't stick to the sheets. If I'd been paying attention to omens at age twelve, I might have thought good times were ahead, but then the morning came.

"Oh my God, oh my God, oh my God." A hysterical woman was yelling. It took me a minute to realize it was my mother. My eyes flicked open. I sat up in bed. It was early, I could tell by the light. There was another voice seeping in through my screen, our neighbor, Laverne Liberty. I felt disoriented, my stomach turned over.

My mother's voice scared me. She didn't say anything but "Oh my God." I could hear bits of what Laverne was saying, and her voice didn't sound much better. She kept whispering, "Keep the kids in the house. And keep them away from the town houses."

The town houses were six rental apartments two and a half blocks from the house, and right across the street from my school, Luella Elementary. I was just able to pick out a few phrases of the story Laverne was telling: "Just terrible . . . one tried to crawl out through a screen . . . they haven't caught the killer!"

My brothers and I all rushed to breakfast that morning, dying of curiosity. My mom, her face drained of color, wouldn't reveal anything.

"Hey, Mom, Mom," Stevie was begging. "What's going on?"

"Be quiet," she snapped. She never snapped at him. Stevie was her favorite. Jerry and I stopped moving.

"Stay near home today and don't you dare go near 100th Street. Don't go any further than the church." Our Lady Gate of Heaven was at the end of our block.

I tried to ask why and she shushed me. No one spoke much after that. The clinking of spoons in cereal bowls felt unnaturally loud. My brothers left me alone that morning. They kept to themselves, playing catch briefly in the backyard but giving up because a helicopter was hovering over the neighborhood. I watched it hang just over the tree outside the front window; I'd never seen a helicopter so close. I was antsy, watching the blades turn; I wanted to see everything for myself and was mad to be cooped up in the house. I told my mom I was going for a bike ride. She looked at me sideways. I'd never had to ask permission to go biking before, but she was preoccupied, so she just repeated her orders to stay away from 100th Street.

I went running out the back door and hopped onto my bike at a jog. Stevie was sitting on the front stoop as I peddled away. "Hey, Chubs, Chubs!" he yelled. "Where ya going?" I kept peddling. I wouldn't have known what to say if I'd stopped. Something had frightened my mother. I needed to see what had happened, needed to understand what had caused this sickening shudder down in the dark core of things. I couldn't have said this to Stevie. I was just going.

After a heartbeat, I passed the church. A block later, I was turning the corner onto 100th Street. A crowd of people was milling outside the town houses. Reporters and cops were still at the scene. I stopped at the edge of the crowd and stared up at a window on the second floor. People were talking around me and I picked out a few more awful details. Somebody had murdered the women in that apartment. They were all young student nurses. Somebody said three women had been killed; another person said there were over a dozen. A story was told of one woman trying and failing to escape through a window screen. I could see a screen torn back from its frame on the second floor. Every once in a while a figure, most likely a cop, would move behind it.

Just then, the front door opened and two men in white coats wheeled out a gurney. A bundle went by. I stopped breathing. A woman's arm had slipped out, as if its owner had fallen asleep. Everyone was quiet. The gurney wheels squeaked.

I looked at the people around me and suddenly wondered who had come out to watch. I realized (I don't know why I hadn't thought of it) that the killer could be there, too. The hair on the back of my neck prickled. I suddenly jerked my bike backward out of the crowd, knuckles white on the handlebars, afraid to look around me. I raced home, my legs working the pedals as hard as I could. I was scared for the first time, terrified of passing cars, of monsters lying in wait in our backyard. I went straight to my room and threw myself under the covers. I thought of the ripped screen and the night before, a woman tearing at the screen like a wild animal, her eyes glazed in terror, and then a man coming up behind her and catching her. My stomach kicked. I squeezed my eyes shut, trying to blot out the image.

I wished Cindy still lived with us. I could remember violent thunderstorms from when I was small and the sky would turn yellow, the color of death, and the leaves looked like they were standing upside down in the wind. I would run to my sister's bed to whimper under her covers. Cindy comforted me as the thunder crashed, saying, "Sunny, dear, there is nothing to be afraid of. The flowers need the rain." She'd put on a record, usually Rimsky-Korsakov's *Scheherazade*. She'd coax me out and we'd dance, and soon enough the rain and noise would stop.

But the storm that rolled through our neighborhood that summer night in 1966 did not end, and there was no one to make me feel better. The next day, I told my brothers that I'd gone to see the crime scene. I was half proud of myself for being brave, half needing to talk about it.

Jerry sneered, "That was stupid. What did you do that for?"

"Jesus, Sunny, you're crazy," Stevie chimed in. "I can't believe you did that." There was disapproval in his voice, but also a little admiration. I think he wished he'd done it himself.

"If that killer tried to come after us," Stevie confided, "you know I could take him. I bet I could beat him up. But Sun, you're crazy for going over there. You're an animal." He gave me a small nod. I grinned back.

That night, my mother lit the Shabbos candles as she did every Friday. I loved watching her do it. My brothers and my dad usually weren't interested but that night, everyone gathered around the kitchen table. Everyone knew the bare facts of what had happened. Eight women, all student nurses, had been murdered. Unspeakable things had been done to them, and the killer was still loose. My mother was more solemn than I'd ever seen her. She waved both hands over the flames three times as if she were lapping the light into her heart, her movements slow and deliberate, and then she covered her eyes for the blessing. My mom's little nose stuck out and turned bright red and her lips moved a little. The words of the prayer echoed in my head.

> *Baruch atah Adonai Eloheinu melech ha'olam*
> Blessed are you, Lord, our God, sovereign of the universe,
> *asher kideshanu bemitzvotav vetzivanu l'hadlik ner shel Shabbat.*
> who has sanctified us with His commandments and
>   commanded us to light the lights of Shabbat.

I knew my mom was praying for "those poor girls." It's what she'd been saying to herself the last two days. "Those poor girls, all they tried to do was help other people. What must their families be feeling?" She stood with her eyes covered for a long time. The house was quiet. Then she passed her hands over the candles a final time.

I was waiting for magic. If God, the sovereign of the universe, was ever going to demonstrate his power, I thought, it had to be now. I stared at the flames, waiting, hoping for something that would explain the horror committed against those women. The candles flickered. There were no signs, only an empty homesick feeling.

My mom opened her eyes. She sighed once, then said, mournfully, "May we all live and be well," and she kissed me on my forehead.

Within days we knew what to call what had happened—the Richard Speck murders. A troubled journeyman and carpenter, the product of an alcoholic, abusive family, Richard Speck followed a path from petty crimes to assaults and murder to the horror of July 13 and 14, 1966, when he had surprised nine student nurses in their apartment, then tortured and murdered eight of them over the course of the night. The ninth woman had managed to hide under a bed undetected, and later identified Speck at the trial. In its day, the Richard Speck case was called the "crime of the century."

For me, for my neighborhood, for Chicago, there was a before the Richard Speck murders, and an after. A shift happened at that moment in our behavior, in the way we saw the world. On my street, we locked our doors for the first time. We feared strangers. We were suspicious of our neighbors. Speck had been caught within days, put on trial and sent away to prison to live out the rest of his days. But the man had still tracked each of us into the deepest darkest recesses of our hearts, and settled there, a resident bogeyman, ready to jump out and come after us if we got too comfortable.

Richard Speck was the first true monster I can remember in my life. He was far from the last.

CHAPTER 3

1971–1980

Before he went crazy, Stevie saved me. Before his brain turned against him, he was the one who paved my way out of Chicago. He didn't know what he had done, and neither did I, but he saved me all the same.

Jerry, the obedient son, had already gone off to the University of Illinois as a pre-med major. Stevie had rushed out of high school a sports star, a passionate Roman candle of a kid, liable to go off at the least provocation. Ever since my Uncle Rolly gave him a set of golf clubs for his Bar Mitzvah, he'd obsessed over the game. If you could imagine golf as a ferocious game of blistering hits and violent tempers, that was how Stevie played. Always an indifferent student, he'd won a free ride to the University of Arizona in Tucson on a sports scholarship.

I brought up the rear in every sense of the word, ejected from high school with a pathetic whimper and an upraised middle finger. My sophomore year, my parents moved from the south side of Chicago to a small house in Glenview, Illinois, a white suburb with a growing Jewish population. My parents were following the crowds, joining the white flight of the time, complaining, in their sometimes narrow-minded way, how dangerous it had become since the *"shvartzes"* had taken over. *Shvartze* was the Yiddish derogatory term for a black person.

I'd gone from the back of the line at Bowen, the Chicago public high school where I was barely getting by in remedial classes, to the absolute bottom of New Trier West, a large, college preparatory powerhouse of a school. To the white well-to-do kids who were my new classmates, a mixed crowd of Catholics and Protestants and a few random Jews, I might as well have been a redneck from the hills of Appalachia, or a foreign-exchange student from India. And they seemed equally bizarre to me. They had chandeliers in their houses, maids who cleaned their bathrooms, and they took ski trips to Colorado over the Christmas break. The closest my friends and I got to downhill skiing was "skeeching," which was when we chased cars down the streets to grab their fenders and get dragged through the dirty slush. In Glenview, I learned phrases I'd never heard before: "I'm so depressed" and "I'm ambivalent about that." No one was ambivalent where I came from. They were either loyal to the ends of the earth or wanted to hit you upside the head with a two-by-four. What was there to be ambivalent about? I wasn't ambivalent about Glenview. I hated it every fucking second I lived there.

They tried to expel me a few weeks before graduation because I yelled at a teacher. (I did it so often I can't remember what I said.) I was sent home and told not to come back until my parents and I had a conference with the principal. My mother wouldn't come. She was mortified, afraid that I'd finally gone too far. My father put on a tie and jacket and I would've said he looked handsome, except the pulsing muscle at his jawline kept clenching with fearful regularity. He looked like he was chewing something unpleasant.

"Dammit, Sunny," he said as we drove to school. "You keep your trap shut today, you hear me! And you do whatever they tell you!" He slapped the steering wheel as he said it. He knew I was as liable to play the obedient daughter as he was to play the cool-headed dad, so he added, "You're almost done with this place, Sunny. I know you're miserable but it'll be over soon if you just follow the rules."

I'd been in the principal's office half a dozen times already but I couldn't pick the guy out of a lineup. He looked like one of those anonymous guys with a shit-eating grin from an Oldsmobile ad. He had on a suit and horn-rimmed glasses, and he told me I'd have to agree to behave and follow all the rules in order to return to school.

"I want you to come back, Sandra," he said, pouring salt in the wound by using my given name. No one called me that except my old truant officer from the south side. My father said that of course I'd behave, then they both looked at me. "Do we have your promise, young lady?" asked the principal. Behind him on his bookcase, I could see a photo of his smiling family skiing in some mountain paradise. In the photo he was wearing a hat with a pom-pom. I wish I could say I thought about my response, thought about what it would mean to go forward without a high school diploma, had some clue about what the phrase "the rest of my life" actually meant to the rest of my life, and come up with a reasoned, rational and engaged response. But I didn't.

"No, you'll have to throw me out. I'm not going to do it." My father groaned. I felt a sharp pain in my shin from where he kicked me with his wingtips. "God, Dad, what'd you do that for?" I yelped. He groaned again. The principal looked stunned, as if I'd plunked him on the head with a baseball.

"Of course she'll behave," my dad barked. "Don't listen to her; she's too dumb to know what she's saying. You tell him that you'll behave."

"No, I won't do it. I got a right to speak up when something is bull-shit."

My dad unloaded again on my shin. I gave a shout of pain. The principal looked scared, and then confused, and then just sad. He gave us both long, searching stares. I don't think he wanted me back for another year and I had enough credits to graduate. He finally gave a resigned shrug and said, "Get out of here. I'll expect you in class on Monday." I slammed the door on the way out. I refused to go to their damn graduation.

Two months later I was driving west. Stevie was entering his junior year at Arizona, and had grudgingly agreed to let me ride shot-gun. I left Chicago with fifty dollars in my pocket and no plan beyond escape and Tucson seemed like as good a place to land as any.

Stevie had grown, to use my mother's words, "a little goofy" since going off to college. He used to be full of confidence, a joker and a fighter. But now he was a brooder, all dark thunderclouds, and when he came home he kept to himself. He didn't laugh as much; his temper had grown to resemble my father's. The most popular boy I knew now barely left the house except to play golf. Still, I was his failure of a kid sister with no cash and no friends in Tucson, and he was willing to take me with him, which earned him big points in my book.

Out in the Sonoran Desert, I swear I felt like Neil Armstrong taking one giant scary leap. The exotic landscape mesmerized me—the saguaro cactus with its long arms waving in all directions, the ocotillo with its spinelike vines speckled with bright red flowers at the tips, the Palo Verde trees and jumping cholla and Gila monsters and tarantulas and mountains. Chicago is flat as a pancake and to wake up and see mountains surrounding the small city, I was my own personal astronaut.

In Tucson I kissed a girl for the first time and it was heaven. I discovered the theater, finding a voice with friends and a community that didn't know me as the dumb kid in the remedial classes. I went to free classical concerts at the University of Arizona. I painted with watercolors. I read and read and read for the first time in my life. I took ceramics classes, making myself the shadow of my teacher, an old man named Fay. He had one hand. The other he'd lost in an industrial accident. He was quiet, his brown face cracked and lined like a catcher's mitt, often lost in a cloud of Pall Malls. I kept up with him cigarette for cigarette with my Tareytons. I'd punch the clay and swear when it didn't spin into shape. Fay laughed at my short temper. "Sunny, life's too short," he'd murmur, without looking up from his wheel. "Life's way too short."

I made a paycheck. I paid rent. I took lovers. I broke hearts. I fought Nixon and the Vietnam War and myself, and, eventually, after much coaxing, I held my nose and went back to school. The students at Pima Community College were my kind of people—diverse, working class, all trying to figure out how to catch a break and some dignity. I took English and drama and feminist theory classes.

I'd gone to Tucson with Stevie, but I barely saw him. He slipped away. I'd go visit him and he'd seem agitated, distracted. One time he was convinced his philosophy professor, who happened to be Catholic, was deliberately trying to fail him because he was Jewish. Another time he told me that his golf teammates were conspiring against him. He was kicked off the team for fighting. He started playing only in the early morning, barefoot. I began to think he was doing peyote. Then he was gone, graduated, back to Chicago where he moved in with my parents.

I can see now that we were traveling different paths. He was beginning to explore his nightmares; I was starting to explore my dreams.

Back in high school I'd always been stuck in the classes with the castaways. "Sunny and the *shvartzes* and poor kids," as Seymour would say. My classmates and I danced to the Temptations and never talked about our grades. And then, regular as clockwork, we'd lose someone. They'd get into trouble, sent to the Cook County juvenile detention center, known as the Audi Home. I felt so awful for them, knowing that they had no one to help them, that they'd skated along the brink for years, facing abusive parents, or the abuses of poverty, until they finally slipped into the abyss and into a life of crime. Every time someone disappeared there was that shock to the system. Could it have been me? Could I ever fall so low? I also had another thought, a crazy one, little more than a whisper in my ear. I wished I could help them, almost as fervently as I wished I could help myself. I knew it was stupid, an impossible hope. But even so, I had a dream. I wanted to become a lawyer.

In Chicago I was too stupid to be a lawyer. But in Tucson, I became the shoot-from-the-hip feminist/lesbian-in-training with a big heart. And I didn't have to be embarrassed about it. And hell, if there was anything I knew how to do, it was talk. I was a shouter, and a toughie, and if you tried to stick a finger in my chest, I'd stick mine in your eye. With each class I took at Pima Community College, that pipe dream began to seem more and more possible. When a friend of mine told me about a law school that didn't require a college degree, I jumped.

My girlfriend, Debby, practically wrote my application and miraculously, terrifyingly, unaccountably, it worked. In the fall of 1980, I drove to San Francisco to start classes at the New College of California School of Law in San Francisco. This happened even though the dean had told me during my interview that she couldn't allow me to attend, couldn't take my money in good conscience, because she knew I'd wash out. She said it to me with a kind look and a gravelly voice that exuded wisdom. I told her I was coming with or without her blessing. I was going to show her, just like I was going to show the anonymous principal who tried to throw me out of New Trier, that I was going to do it my way.

My way was defiance. In San Francisco, all I had left was my defiance. My parents had finally stopped trying to change me and we rarely spoke now. Neither of them could accept that I was a lesbian. I hadn't told them. My father had discovered some letters from a girlfriend of mine when I'd come home for a visit. He'd confronted me and told me I'd betrayed every article of the faith, and that he could not accept this "horrible sinful phase" I was going through. I told him that he'd have to get used to it. He threatened to have a funeral for me, sitting Shiva to let everyone know I was symbolically dead to him. He only gave up on the idea when I told him I'd show up. My father now spoke to me only when my mother forced him to take the phone. My brothers couldn't figure out why their idiot of a kid sister thought she had to be a fruit. My mother was more forgiving, but troubled, throwing up when she found out, wondering what she'd done wrong, wondering if it was her fault.

But I long ago ceased to be the greatest heartbreak for my parents. In 1975, Jerry and Stevie took a pilgrimage to Israel and came home strict Orthodox and had convinced my parents to join them. Then, in 1977, Stevie went on a second pilgrimage to Israel. My parents thought it would do him some good, get him out of the house and challenge him. But in the streets of Jerusalem, Stevie started an argument with an Israeli Arab. By the time it was over, he had the man on the ground, and was kicking him in the head, calling him a "dirty Arab" and a "fucking anti-Semite." Stevie was sent home babbling incomprehensibly and heavily dosed on antipsychotic drugs. This was his first breakdown. We were lucky he hadn't been thrown in prison. Back in Chicago, Stevie was diagnosed as a paranoid schizophrenic with depressive tendencies. He now maintained his equilibrium only if his meds were calibrated just right.

He and I still talked. He still asked me what I thought. I still sought his approval. I still thought of him first when I wanted some family in my life, especially when I wanted to talk to someone about law school. Sometimes he would cheer me on. "You can do it, Sunny. You are the only one in the family who will make it!" he'd say when his energy was peaking. But sometimes, if I caught him on the wrong day, he'd launch into a tirade. "You are such a loser," he'd yell. "Are you crazy? You can't pass shit. You were the worst student in high school. This is law school. You need a college degree for that but you were too dumb to get one." I'd have to put the phone down and let the tears come. Even though I knew he was crazy, he was repeating my inner monologue, the one I'd carried with me from Chicago, which whispered, ever so cruelly, "Who the fuck do you think you are?"

Half the week I worked with prisoners in San Francisco's jails. The other half I attended class. Walking Mainline and walking into a law school lecture were almost equally scary to me. I almost lived up to the dean's predictions in my first year, but after getting three tutors, and studying like it was my new religion, I was allowed to come back for the next year. I barely made it, but I did *not* wash out.

On the first day of my second year, I rushed in from work late as usual. I pushed through the door for Criminal Trial Skills and was relieved that the professor hadn't arrived yet. Professor Paul Harris was supposed to be an amazing trial lawyer, and I'd actually been looking forward to this class. I dreaded contracts, felt like a complete moron in torts and legal analysis, but I had a new notebook and set of pens that I stole from the jails, and I felt ready.

I climbed the stairs to the back of the vaulted classroom. There was nothing particularly majestic about my law school. It wasn't *The Paper Chase*. There were no gargoyles and limestone. The place was bare-bones, with furniture that looked like it had fallen off the back of a truck. I felt comfortable in the New College student body. As I made my way to my seat, I passed discussions about Reagan's right-wing policies and the need to divest from South Africa. Most of my fellow students came from the liberal fringe of America, and that suited me fine. I settled in with eight other regular smokers whom I knew well. Our packs came out, lighters flicked, and soon we were in a cloud of smoke.

Professor Harris walked in as rumpled as they come—wrinkled shirt untucked in the back, glasses sliding haywire off his nose. He started to tell us about himself, and the kind of assignments we should expect, the usual drill. Then all of a sudden, he stopped and turned to a student in the front row.

"Excuse me," he said, annoyed. "I'm talking here. Could you please keep it down?"

The class shifted uncomfortably. I couldn't see what was happening, didn't hear anyone talking, either. But the moment passed and Harris returned to his talk. Five minutes later, Harris stopped again.

"I'm gonna ask you another time, please have some respect." He was more annoyed this time. "Please keep it down."

I exhaled a column of smoke and craned my neck, trying to see what was going on. I couldn't figure out who the guilty party was. I whispered to the guy next to me, "What the fuck?" He shrugged his shoulders and Harris again resumed his lecture.

Finally, a third time, Harris stopped. He was angry now. "I've asked you a couple times to stop talking. I want you to leave." His voice was brittle. He pointed to the door.

I could see the student now for the first time. He hadn't said anything, from what I could tell. Neither had anyone else. Again, Harris, his voice rising, repeated his demand.

"Listen, how long is this going to go on? I asked you to leave."

No one said anything until, all of a sudden, my mouth opened. "What the fuck is going on up there, man? I didn't hear that guy say anything."

There was a sickening silence. Everyone turned to stare at me, then back at Harris, who grinned.

"I've done this lecture countless times, at Stanford, Berkeley, all over the place, and . . . I can't see you back there in the fog, what's your name?"

"I'm Sunny Schwartz."

"Well, Sunny, I think we need to work on your delivery. That kind of language would never work with a judge. But congratulations. You're the first person who ever challenged me."

The guy he singled out hadn't been talking out of turn. He hadn't been doing anything, just sitting there. Harris was teaching a lesson in the power of authority, and people's willingness to suffer injustice in silence. The message was loud and clear, at least for me. Just about every day I'd questioned whether I would make it in law school, and whether anyone would take me seriously. This was the first time I was sure I was in the right place.

CHAPTER 4

1983

I sucked in a lungful of smoke, felt the kick in my blood, then opened my eyes. Fog hung over the hills. If I squinted hard enough to block out the road cutting across the hillside, I could imagine the world without people, a world with only deer, raccoons and seagulls wheeling overhead trying to find the ocean. The cigarette burned to the filter and I tossed it as I walked back into one of the greatest scars I could imagine people carving into the hillside. County Jail 3 was south of San Francisco, in San Bruno, on seven acres of beautiful, rolling, forested land. The jail was built during the Depression and embodied everything the time had to offer. The exterior looked like a giant concrete bunker. It smelled of mildew, even in the administration section, where the law interns had their office. Paint peeled off the ceiling in large ribbons. The few windows we had were smudged and cracked.

I checked the assignment clipboard, picked up my notebook and a file full of complaints and grudgingly headed into the belly of the beast. To talk about the life I faced every day in the jails, it's probably best to start with the language. There was a unique slang I'd had to learn in order to communicate. First, there were terms that deputies and civilians, like me, had for the inmates.

Baby banger: a young gang member who looks like a child and is often covered in menacing tattoos
Badass or **Hard-core convict** or **Gangbanger**: a major thug, often covered in menacing tattoos

Poocasso: a crazy person who uses his feces to draw on the cell walls

Sack a nuts, Roof job, 800, or **5150**: crazy person, someone who needs holes patched in his head. The numbers *800* and *5150* came from the penal codes and the health and safety codes respectively. Anyone who earned any of these terms was usually destined for the psych ward.

Shit-thrower: an inmate who throws shit, usually at deputy sheriffs

Spitter: an inmate who spits, usually at deputy sheriffs. "Be careful on rounds, there's a spitter in the second tank."

Then there were the terms that inmates had for one another, or for us.

Fish: a new inmate, a rookie, usually someone who has never been to jail

Narc: informer or snitch

Pig or **Turn-key**: a deputy sheriff. *Pig* was used more universally. A *turn-key* was a lazy know-nothing, only good for opening and shutting doors.

Public pretender: a public defender. "I don't want no public pretender, I want a real lawyer."

Punk: This was the worst put-down there was and it was pretty universal. A punk behind bars specifically meant a submissive homosexual—the receiver of anal sex. The term could be directed at anyone as a put-down, as in, "That guy's just a punk," or "a punk-ass bitch."

After four years on the job, I'd run into spitters and poocassos, and had prisoners complain about "public pretenders" and the "fucking pigs who threw me to the ground." It was a violent language to match a violent place. And every day on the tiers required stamina.

"Another day in paradise, hey, Sun?" Deputy Richard Drocco nodded at me as he pulled out a dirty brass key to open the bar door.

"Another day in paradise, Ricky," I said and smiled back. In my job I didn't have much interaction with deputy sheriffs but I'd managed to

befriend a few. They were protective of their turf, dismissive of anyone who was too soft on inmates, and that meant anyone who was a
legal intern. Too many times to count, deputies had said to me, "I
don't see why you bother. Bunch of liars, you can't do anything for
them." But there was no way to avoid them. The deputies were the
gatekeepers, in every sense of the word. If I wanted to do my rounds,
they had to open the door. Deputy Richard Drocco and I had a mutual
love affair with losers, both the Cubs and the San Francisco Giants, so
we had friendly gripe fests when we saw each other. Drocco was a
handsome bear of a man who could take a prisoner down in one second and in the next donate his paycheck to help get him back on track.
He didn't look at the inmates as his enemy, but that didn't mean he
loved them, either. He was fair, and he and I had a good relationship.
He was one of the exceptions.

Many deputies would barely look at me, much less talk to me. But
the law interns had a similarly dim view of deputies. We were like two
rival cliques in high school. To them, we were the dope-smuggling
hippie liberals, the prisoner lovers, the pillow fluffers. To us, they were
the sadistic, mean-spirited, right-wing thugs.

In my experience, some deputies were assholes, to be sure. They
talked to inmates as if they were cattle to be rounded up. A few seemed
to take pride in antagonizing inmates as much as they could. During
night rounds, they would take their keys and knock them against the
bars to wake up anyone who was sleeping. The worst deputies would
send inmates to lockdown for the most minor rule violation, and if a
prisoner said something even slightly disrespecting, they would wres-
tle the guy to the ground, stick a knee in his back and cold-cock him
with a forearm for good measure. But most deputy sheriffs I'd met
weren't like that. They were simply trying to survive an incredibly
stressful job. They spent their whole day with prisoners, many of
whom were infuriating, and some of whom were dangerous. They
had to manage intake, where men were stripped of their personal
belongings, given a number and a uniform, and had to squat and
cough during the strip search. They had to manage the prisoners'
complaints, search for contraband, confiscate weapons and drugs and
cut down the "string-ups," which was the euphemism we had for sui-
cides. Many deputies had short fuses but could be prevailed upon to

do the right thing, even if they were cynical about the results. Deputy Drocco swung the door wide and I walked in.

As I moved through the gate, the quality of the noise changed. The decibel level rose as I climbed the stairs to the fourth floor. The central stairwell in County Jail 3 climbed up through ten different living quarters, stacked five high on the south and north sides of the building. There were no sound barriers of any kind, and only bars separated the stairwell and each tier. The noise was so bad I'd started to lose my hearing. Many older deputies needed hearing aids. As I got to the top of the stairwell, the echoing voices grew shrill. I could hear cackles and shrieks by the time I made it to the entrance to 4 North, my assigned tier for the next few weeks. Four North was more commonly referred to as the Queens' Tank.

"Hey, Sunny! Who's the finest advocate this side of the Mississippi?" Barbara's high-pitched yelp cut through the noise. The Queens' Tank was a men's dorm, but most of the men were in some stage of preoperative transition. I tried to refer to them by the female pronouns *she* or *her* out of deference to their emotional self-identification. If they thought of themselves as "she," who was I to disagree? Barbara was giving me a limp-wristed wave from in front of the television. She was one of the more recognizable queens in the Queens' Tank. Her hormone treatments had given her these amazingly firm, full breasts that would be the envy of any biological woman. On the day we met, she'd introduced herself as Mark Toms and I'd replied, "I know that's your birth name, honey, but what do you want to be called?" She smiled wide and said, "Barbara," a little coyly. I had won an ally.

Barbara, with her slim figure, plucked-thin eyebrows and practiced flounce to her walk, was also, remarkably, the father of three children. Inside, off smack, she couldn't be more generous. She spent her days making picture frames out of cigarette packs to give to her kids. But outside she was a holy terror with no impulse control, losing her mind in drugs and prostitution. She rarely made it three months before she returned for another stay with us. Barbara sat with a bunch of other queens around the television watching *All My Children*. The volume was turned all the way up to compete with a radio that was blasting a talk show on the other side of the tier.

Transvestites and preoperative transsexuals made up the bulk of the population in the Queens' Tank, which was the dumping ground for the most vulnerable inmates in the San Francisco jail system. Snitches were housed here, as well as any inmate who had been raped and filed a claim. Their willingness to testify made them open to reprisal—especially out on the yard, where a hundred men at a time roamed the dirt-covered, hundred-foot-square field. Child molesters were also housed in the Queens' Tank. They were considered, in the class system of the jails, the lowest of the low, and the most likely to be singled out for "jailhouse justice" by the gangbangers on the yard. But looking around, you barely noticed the men. The queens drew all the light.

The way these inmates passed as women was ingenious. Makeup wasn't allowed inside. Everyone had a standard-issue uniform. But looking at the ladies crowded around the television, you'd think we were somewhere in the Bahamas. Most everyone had their T-shirts tied in a knot at their belly button. Their hair was twisted into ponytails, Farrah Fawcett feathered curls, Afro puffs, Zulu knots and braids in every variation. For curlers they used toilet paper rolls. Stuck behind their ears were glinting flowers constructed out of potato chip bags from the commissary. In their cells, a homemade frame might hold family photos.

Dawn wandered over as I settled down at one of the metal picnic tables. "How ya been, Sunny?" she growled at me. Dawn was like Barbara, also a preop transgender, but not nearly as successful at passing. She was about six feet two, 230 pounds, with dark black skin and intense flashing brown eyes. She was also more prone to violence.

"I'm good, Dawn. Whaddya know?"

"I know I'm getting out in a month because of you, honey. That's what I know." I'd helped Dawn get a few months knocked off her sentence. Many of my cases came from the miscalculation of sentences. If the inmate couldn't make bail, the time he or she served before being convicted was supposed to be subtracted from the sentence. But often someone forgot to write it down, and I had to get inmates like Dawn their time back. "You just let me know if there's anything Dawn can do for you," she said.

I smiled. Offers of help from inmates always had to be viewed in the most skeptical light. Sometimes they came with requests for special favors. Often they came with questions like "Where do you live?"

"How long ya been there?" and then, eventually, "You got a special someone at home?" These were barriers to be protected. I'd heard plenty of cautionary tales about deputies or civilians who had started relationships with prisoners. The power dynamic was too stark. Some of those people who crossed the line got involved in the criminal lives of the prisoners, often to sell drugs. Whatever the motivation, even if the relationship was completely innocent, there was nothing consensual about a relationship between an individual and the person he or she had locked up. But neither Dawn nor Barbara had ever crossed the line with me, so I just smiled at Dawn's offer.

I spread my papers out. I almost always worked in the common areas. It was either that or call my clients out one by one, and that was time-consuming. In the common area, I could cycle through men quickly, despite how unpleasantly loud it was. As I sat down, my clients began to assemble. I could feel a headache starting up behind my left eye. I spent the next four hours holding court—going over claims with inmates who had already filed them, and filling out new complaints for the prisoners who were illiterate or too lazy to do it themselves. I heard stories that ran the gamut. Some were about how they were being evicted and needed help, or how their wives had run off with their kids, or how they'd been given an eight-month sentence but that they'd already spent nine months in jail awaiting trial and "why haven't I been released?" Some stories were from inmates who'd been written up by a deputy for having contraband and now needed a defense. Other stories were more serious, about deputy sheriffs who they said beat them up, or raped them.

I wrote up each one in an Action Request Form. If the inmate was being accused of a rule violation, then I would represent him at the hearing in front of the watch commander, who ran the jail. If the inmate was having trouble out in the world, I functioned more like a social worker. If someone was being evicted, I might contact his leasing agent and try to work out a deal for payment. If the complaint was serious and could involve criminal action, I would normally go straight to the chief deputy or his boss, the sheriff, and Internal Affairs would need to be brought in.

Lately, I had been finding it hard to stay patient. I listened to an inmate named Ramón ramble on for twenty minutes about how he was about to be evicted from his apartment, and how all of his earthly belongings were going to be tossed into the street, and how his drug dealer had stolen his last three hundred dollars and all I could think was, If you didn't want to get robbed, you putz, you shouldn't have given your dealer your keys.

I glanced at the clock. Finally, my shift was drawing to a close. I was trying to finish up with Ramón. His voice was grating on me but then it was drowned out by a rush of voices from around the television. Maybe Erica Kane was getting married again. A group of inmates started this high-pitched screaming, like teenage girls in a lunchroom. "Oh my God!" "Girl, you didn't just do that!"

I shot out of my chair. "Jesus Christ, folks. I'm trying to work over here. Show some respect and keep it down!"

The group fell silent. I saw some irritated, childish looks, but they'd received the message. Good, I thought, I hadn't expected it to be so easy. I returned to my table.

As soon as I was back in my seat, a flutter crawled up my neck. There was a subtle, barely noticeable shift on the tier, like the wind was changing direction. Then I heard a grumbling sound. I looked up, and a man was walking toward me. He had the standard uniform on, nothing "queened out" about his orange T-shirt and pants, but his eyes were wild, as if his lids had been yanked open. In his hands, he had the only thing on the tier that wasn't bolted down, a mop wringer that he had just pulled off a bucket of filthy water. As he walked toward me, he lifted it over his head.

"What'd you say, bitch?" he mumbled. It was almost like he wasn't talking to me but it was clear he was. "You can't tell me what to do. Who the fuck do you think you are?"

I was totally on my own in the Queens' Tank. I had no whistle, no radio, no keys, nothing. That was true for every civilian who worked the jails. When I first started, the communication issues had scared me. But I'd grown complacent. The nearest deputy wasn't physically far away, maybe about fifty feet, but he was behind a gate, and behind a wall of sound. I wouldn't be heard if I screamed. An inmate with a mop wringer could crush my skull, and I would be powerless to stop him. I stumbled off the bench, stepped back and tried to speak.

"Wait a minute, wait a minute!" For a brief moment, I thought of

Stevie. I'd seen the same look in his eyes; the glassy madness that I knew meant that he could do anything. I was paralyzed, watching the guy come at me. There was nowhere to run except deeper into the tier.

All of a sudden, there was a flash of orange, and my attacker was on his back. The mop wringer clattered up against a cell door. Dawn had tackled him, and now lifted herself up over him, cocked her meaty fist and started raining down blows.

"That is *our* girl," Dawn yelled. She repeated it over and over, using it as a backbeat to her punches, until her knuckles were stained red. "That is our girl! That is our girl! That is our girl! Leave her alone!"

I finally came to my senses and realized Dawn could kill the man. "Dawn!" I shouted. "That's enough. *That's enough!*" The world around me smeared. There were deputies rushing in, inmates looking on. Ramón was cowering a few feet away. Dawn and my attacker were flattened beneath a pack of green uniforms. Then I was gone, hustled out of the tier, down the stairs and into the staff area. My colleague Rita was in our office and was startled when I barreled in with two deputy sheriffs as escorts. She brought me a glass of water.

I'd seen violence in the jails before. I'd gone out into the yard after one especially brutal fight. An inmate had turned a softball bat on an enemy, cracking open his head, staining the dirt around third base. I'd seen the victim being wheeled away. I'd heard the deputy sheriffs in the break room, talking about fights they'd broken up, beatings they'd had to dole out, or riots they'd been caught in. But it had never happened to me.

I sat there numb for a few minutes in the intern's office until I thought to take a sip of water. Deputy Drocco wandered in.

"You okay, Sun?" He gave me a pat on the back.

"I don't know, Ricky. I don't know."

Drocco looked at me kindly and gave me a sharp nod. "You oughta know that three or four inmates came rushing up to the gate yelling bloody murder, telling me to call the code three. They had your back."

I guess I was glad to hear it. There were two other deputies standing out in the hall. I could hear them laughing.

"Did you see the look on that guy's face?" one said. "He practically wet himself when we tackled him."

"Yeah, that asshole had it coming."

"And Dawn . . . that dyke can really dole out a beating! Imagine what she'd do to you in bed."

"That's sick, man, that's so sick."

There were reports to be filed but I got the hell out of there as soon as I could. I told people I was fine as I headed for the door, but the ground swam a little beneath my feet. My hands shook on the steering wheel. I was awash in adrenaline. It was a miracle I didn't get into an accident driving home. What would have happened if the man had reached me? Would I have reacted? Dawn hadn't hesitated. She turned her body into a weapon and rushed in. My car slid north from San Bruno back into San Francisco. The sun was setting and San Francisco Bay off to my right turned golden in the changing light.

I replayed the scene in my head. I gave myself another chance to react, picturing different ways for it to play out. In one scenario, I leaped from the table and ran around him, a base runner avoiding the tag. In another, I found my voice, and recruited the inmates around me to help. But in some, I took my fist and slammed it again and again into the man's face until my knuckles came away bloody just like Dawn's.

I went back to work the next day. My supervisor, Randy, told me not to come back for at least a week, but I wasn't going to let a lunatic with a mop wringer change my schedule. I went back to the Queens' Tank. Deputy Drocco gave me a smile as he let me in, and a warning. "They decided not to segregate Dawn. He's still in there."

Dawn and Barbara came to see me the minute I started my rounds.

"Hey darling," Barbara said, her eyes gentle and warm. "You doing okay today?" Dawn just nodded at me.

I smiled back and thought, Not yet, but I will be. I will be. I'm tougher than you think.

The guy who came after me was returned to the Queens' Tank later that afternoon. After a trip to the infirmary, he was sent back to his cell with two black eyes and a swollen lip. There wasn't anywhere else to send him. For a week he was in lockdown, which meant twenty-three hours a day in his cell, one hour out for supervised exercise.

I was still working the tier when his lockdown ended. One afternoon, he sidled up to the table where I was working, his face an unsightly mix of black and blue and green bruises. I jumped when I realized it was him. I looked around and saw that a table away, Dawn and Barbara were keeping a vigilant eye on me. The man looked sheepish.

"Sunny, Barbara said I should come talk to you," said the inmate. "I'm sorry about what happened last week. I guess I drank too much pruno, you know." Pruno was an illegal liquor the men brewed out of orange juice, sugar and bread in their toilets. I'd been told it was like drinking fermented gasoline.

"I drank too much, you know what I'm saying, and I lost it. I didn't mean it. If my head was straight, you know, I wouldn't have done it."

I looked at him. I was both touched that Barbara would have thought of this, and angry with what the man was saying.

"All right . . . what's your name?"

"Derek."

"Derek . . ." I hesitated, trying to find the words. "I accept your apology but you know what? I'm also disgusted. What kind of excuse is that?"

Derek's eyes widened. He blinked twice. "Excuse me?"

"'The booze made me do it'?" I answered him. "It's always someone else's fault. It's 'the drugs,' 'my old lady,' 'my abusive dad,' always someone else. When is it your responsibility?"

He seemed stunned. But he played his part, did what I expected him to do. He stayed hard, unreachable.

"Damn, I was just trying to apologize." He turned on his heel and stalked off.

At the end of the tier the TV blared. A table away, a man eyed me warily. An argument was echoing from the far end of the tier. A crowd of preops, looking a little like a football team in drag, were milling around waiting to meet with me, each with her own story to tell.

CHAPTER 5

1983

The phone rang in the law interns' office. It was Friday. I was the last one there for the day and should have known better than to pick it up. A mother was on the other end and she started pleading with me.

"Please," she said. "Please. My son is getting out on Monday, and he won't call. He returns my letters." The woman was desperate, which was unusual. Many of the family members I dealt with had checked out, had given up on their convict child or brother or father or mother. But she was begging. "I just want to help him but he's not right in the head. He's sick, you know, he's got mental problems. They've got him up on Three North." My heart sank.

The 3 North tier, otherwise known as the psych tier, was the only place in the jail system that creeped me out. I could get in a deputy sheriff's face and tell him I thought he was a grade-A asshole, or walk up to a group of thugs on 6 North or South, the hard-core felons, and confront them about being bullies, or walk through the Queens' Tank and pull down the sheets the men had slung up so they could have sex in private while the deputies looked the other way. I confronted the monsters every day. I didn't run from them. But the psych tier was the one place I could not face. The men on the tier were a random combination of paranoid schizophrenics, manic-depressives, addicts suffering drug-induced psychosis and Vietnam vets with posttraumatic stress. They were cutters, biters, spitters, men who pulled their own hair out and roof jobs. I hated it. The men shouted for no reason. They were calm one second, and the next they were screaming. Psych services was little more than a MASH unit doing crisis management.

The population was heavily dosed on antipsychotics. The men had what we called the "Prolixin and Thorazine shuffle" and every time I was there I thought of Stevie.

I think the woman who called me that Friday afternoon heard me hesitate, because her voice cracked as she pleaded with me. "If you could just please get a note to him. Don't tell him who it's from because he'll throw it away. Please just let him know that we'll be there to pick him up when he gets out. Please tell him we'll be waiting at the gates. Please."

I felt like I was talking to my mother. If I closed my eyes, I could picture Frieda, with the quivering lip she had whenever she talked about Stevie, her uncertainty over what to do about a son who was not her son anymore, not in any way she knew. My stomach was churning but I agreed to help.

I wrote the note and went to 3 North. I didn't go in. I couldn't. I asked the deputy, who was a friend of mine, if he could pull out the guy for me. "Really?" He looked at me skeptically. "That guy's kinda out of it." The inmate wandered out looking like the bottom of my shoe. His hair was a mop, a tangled dirty mess on top of a scraggly beard. His eyes were dead. He was one of the medicated zombies.

I handed him the note. "Please look at this right now," I said. "This is a very important message. I'm gonna stand here while you read it."

He opened it and stood there swaying. His eyes widened ever so slightly as he read it. Then he closed the note and popped it into his mouth. He chewed it with a quiet, angry intensity. His head bobbed forward, pigeonlike, as he swallowed. He glanced at me and then, without saying a word, shuffled back onto the tier.

Stevie had been living with my parents, on and off, for the past four years. He'd been unable to hold a job, and unable to find a doctor that could help him. When he was doing well, he was usually paralyzed on Prolixin. At one point, my dad called me up, sounding exhausted, to tell me Stevie had torn up all of his family photos. These photos were irreplaceable, and especially precious to my orphan dad. I'd visited Stevie and my parents a few times and came away worried. It seemed entirely possible that Stevie could take the next step and turn his anger not just on my dad's things, but on my dad. My parents were running out of money and ideas about what to do. The only time Stevie hadn't lived at home since his diagnosis was when he went to Los Angeles for a few months to try to become a boxer. No one had thought that was a good idea. He'd been beaten badly in the ring and came back to Chicago ranting about the *shvartzes* and goyim who had beaten him up.

I watched as the hairy roof job who'd just eaten the note disappeared back into the tier and I shivered. It might as well have been Stevie going back onto the tier. I did not know how to help my brother. I didn't know how to help this man.

I caught the Queens' Tank assignment more than my colleagues. It was tit for tat. They picked up slack for me on the psych tier; I took the Queens' Tank. It suited me. On good days, I felt like I could help the messy lives of the she-males.

That didn't mean I didn't feel like Sisyphus every time I walked in there, eternally pushing a rock up a hill. A four-hour rotation always left me with a headache and deep desire for a tequila shot, a cigarette and an empty-headed conversation with a lovely stranger at my neighborhood bar.

It was another Friday afternoon and I'd nearly hit the gate when a prisoner rushed up to me, sweating and anxious. I'd never met him but I'd seen him before. He was white, middle-aged, pudgy and wore horn-rimmed glasses, like a suburban dad or somebody's accountant. "Hey, hey, hey." He stepped into my path. "You need to help me. No one's paying any attention to me."

"Listen, buddy, my day is over. It's going to have to wait till Monday."

His eyes were darting around as if someone were chasing him. "I'm here on a child molestation conviction and was sentenced to a year in this hellhole. I've sent letters, letters to everyone, and nobody has answered."

I was on alert now. His desperation, his fidgetiness, his overall energy, was a warning sign. He took a deep breath and was practically spitting at me by the time he unloaded his full confession. "I'm getting out of jail in two weeks and I have been asking for help for a year and nobody has responded. I'm promising you I will do it again! There's a little girl whose mom is renting a room in the apartment where I live, and she will be my next victim."

I didn't want to be standing there, didn't want to be anywhere near him. But I swallowed, and tried to do my job.

"Okay, hold on, what are you saying?"

"What, you can't hear me? I promise you that the little girl living in my house will be my next victim."

My brain finally caught up with what he was saying. I didn't want him to clam up so I asked follow-up questions.

"Who is this girl? What is her mother's name?" He slowed down while I wrote down his answers. I looked back at him. "You need help. If I found a program that would help you, would you do it?"

He nodded yes.

I was trying to do the normal things I do in my job: write down the details, spend time with the client and set up a game plan. But I felt itchy, almost sick. I finally wrote down his name, Fred Johnson, and his inmate number and took off.

I went straight out the front door of the jail. I felt like I was drowning. I lit a cigarette and tried to clear my head. My job was to be that monster's advocate, to fight for him, almost like a defense attorney. But this was something different. He asked me for help but all I could think of was the girl living in his house. Who was her advocate? He wanted help; she needed it.

He was getting out in two weeks.

I jammed another cigarette into my mouth. Back in the front office, I pulled Fred Johnson's custody card. Johnson had been sentenced to a year in the county jail on child molestation charge 288 of the California penal code. His attorney must have struck a deal with the DA because he faced up to eight years. A defendant would get only a year under specific circumstances, such as if the victim couldn't or wouldn't testify because she was too young. It was as bad as I had imagined it.

I stewed over it all weekend, driving my girlfriend nuts. I had a mountain of homework to do for law school, including a presentation I was scheduled to give in my constitutional law class, but every time I tried to get started, all I could think of was Fred Johnson.

First thing Monday morning, I went to see my boss, San Francisco Sheriff Michael Hennessey, at City Hall, a beaux arts confection that is both majestic and imposing. It doesn't really fit Hennessey's style. He's an even-tempered, smart Irishman from Iowa, with an impish sparkle in his eye. I liked him. I was pretty low on the totem pole in the grand scheme of things. Legal interns were at about the same clout level as a cadet in the department, which was, if not at the bottom, very near it, but Hennessey didn't treat me that way. Hennessey created the office where I worked, and had a special place in his heart for the interns. He was a lawyer himself and liked talking through problems with us.

I gave him a quick nod as I walked in. But I was too anxious to chat and quickly spelled out the story.

"Sheriff, I'm at a loss," I told him as I finished. "We've gotta do something, right?" His lips pursed and settled into a scowl. Hennessey started twiddling his pen between his fingers, a nervous habit of his. He wasn't much for confrontation, and he did not speak hastily. So I kept going.

"Listen, I know my job is to advocate on his behalf. But I don't know what that means here. Am I supposed to try to have him brought up on charges for making a threat? His sentence is about to run out. How are we supposed to hold him longer?"

"Is that what you want to do? Hold him?"

"Hell yeah! I want to lock him up and never have to think about him again. But since that's not an option, I want to hold him at least until we can maybe get him some help, maybe get him into a program."

"Well, listen, Sunny, I agree that you're supposed to be helping these men, no matter what kind of crimes they've committed. But he asked you for help, so you've got a responsibility to pursue that." The pen twirled a few times in his fingers. "That being said, you have no *legal* obligation to report it. It's only a threat, and not exactly actionable. You know making a case on something like that would be a tough sell. But morally, that's another story, and that answer is easy: we've got to do something." The pen finally came to rest in his hand. He leaned back in his chair. Finally, he cleared his throat.

"Why don't you start with the sentencing judge? See what he has to say. Johnson's statement to you may represent a violation of the terms of his probation. Other than that, the law isn't really on your side. Trying to prove that what he told you is a criminal act is not easy. Intentions are not actions."

I got moving, heartened by what he said, but anxious. This was new territory for me. My colleagues and I in the Prisoner Legal Interns office had a specific identity. We were supposed to fight for the inmates' often overlooked rights. But here I was trying to bring the full weight of the system down on one of my clients, and that made me feel like a turncoat.

My next stop was San Francisco's Hall of Justice, the building that housed Mainline and most of the infrastructure of criminal justice in San Francisco County. It was built in 1958, a gigantic blank of a building, sheathed in marble, and utterly characterless. The top two floors were jail facilities, which included Mainline. The bottom floors housed the office of the district attorney and the adult probation offices, as well as various divisions of the San Francisco Police Department. Traffic court, some of the municipal courts, as well as the superior court rooms were there as well. Despite its having the charm of a big-box department store, I always liked going to the Hall of Justice because you saw more civilians. At County Jail 3, where our offices were, it was all deputy sheriffs and inmates. Orange and green made you depressed if that's all you saw. I was headed to the office of the honorable Judge Randall Scott, who had been Fred Johnson's trial judge. The judge's secretary, Mrs. Hendricks, knew me. I'd called her half a dozen times about inmates I was representing.

"Now who are you trying to set free this time?" She sighed.

I said it was an emergency, and she ushered me promptly into the judge's chambers. A veteran jurist, Scott looked like a Jewish Santa Claus, and had a reputation for combining compassion with toughness. He was respected by both prosecutors and defense attorneys, no easy feat. Hanging behind his desk was a large portrait of Martin Luther King Jr., and next to it, a hand-painted, framed replica of the Bill of Rights. I launched into my story about Fred Johnson, and he blanched as if I'd kicked him when I reached the heart of the story and Johnson's threat. There was a pause as he removed his glasses to massage the stress out of his brow.

"Ms. Schwartz, I appreciate you trying to do something here, but what can I do? His sentence was his sentence. Once it runs, he's served his debt. I'm not the jury. I've got no legal way to hold him."

"Judge, somebody has to do something. We are talking about a child. I can guarantee you he will hurt that little girl if he's released."

"I'm not arguing that point. I wish I could. I really do. But it's outside my authority."

"What do I do?"

He gave me a rueful smile. "You're doing what you can. You're trying. Try talking to the defense attorney. His advocate might know a way to work the system to protect everyone involved."

As I left, he looked as depressed as I felt. I wanted to argue with him but I knew it was pointless. A day later, I was back at the Hall of Justice, this time in the public defenders' corner of the building. This was the land of no empty surfaces. I don't know if I'd ever met a public defender with a tidy desk, and Fred Johnson's attorney, Susan, was no exception. Files teetered around as if she were a character in a Dr. Seuss book. I wondered if this was the life waiting for me when I finished law school. Susan gave me a haggard glance when I walked in, and I had to remind her who I was talking about. It didn't take long before her face scrunched together. "Augh, that pedophile. That guy was a creep."

"Right. Unfortunately, Susan, I hate to tell you but he is still a creep." I then told her my story, as I'd told the sheriff and the judge already.

"That guy really is a piece of work, huh?" she said.

"Yeah, so what do we do about him?"

Susan didn't skip a beat. "Listen, Sunny, if you try to raise any of this, or try to do anything to revoke his release date, I'll kick and scream about it in court."

I was afraid of this. "Why?" I asked.

"That's my job. It's not always pleasant, and I can tell you, this is about the least pleasant part of it. But if you want to hold him any longer, you have to convict him of something. No crime has been committed. He can't be held because of something he might do in the future."

I liked Susan. She was tough, juggling fifteen million things, and clearly a principled advocate. I'd been getting the same lessons in law school the last four years—every client deserves a vigorous defense, be a fighter, your job is not to sympathize, it's to strategize and win. I knew that even with a threat as specific as Fred Johnson's, any defense attorney worth their salt could have it bounced. There was no proof he had any intent to carry it out. In court, Johnson's attorney had only to claim it was idle chatter, something he said out of fear or anger, or better yet, just deny he said it, and the case would evaporate.

"There has to be something we can do, Susan," I said. "I think a true defense is to try to get your client the help he needs so he doesn't reoffend and end up doing harder time. Come on now, please, let's do something about this." At this point I sounded pathetic. Susan's eyes softened, but she didn't give me any rope.

"Sunny, listen, we're not social workers. I'm his lawyer. I can't go after him. It would be unethical. You know that." There was exhaustion in her voice but I knew this was the oath she took as a defense attorney and I didn't push it. The men and women we would be called on to defend would be despicable, most would be guilty, but the thing we were defending was the right to counsel. In my law school, and in law schools across the country, this idea was sacrosanct. I, too, held it dear to my heart. I looked at Susan, and she looked like a very weary crusader, but not one who was ready to lay down her sword.

By Friday, I felt beat up. All week I'd been told by the lawyers I consulted to drop it. Judge Scott had recused himself from Johnson's case, which I presumed was because my visit had biased him and he was no longer impartial. The case hadn't been reassigned yet but it was tough to lose a good judge. I was anxious about how much time this was taking away from my job and my schoolwork. My other colleagues were taking notice. I'd had to ask one to cover part of my shift the day I went to see the defense attorney and he'd agreed to do it begrudgingly. I felt like he was judging me. I knew I was judging me. The right thing, by the definition of my job as this monster's advocate, was to drop it.

Monday morning I sought out the last person I could think of— Fred Johnson's probation officer, or PO. I found the PO, Allen, in his office, a nondescript cubbyhole on the third floor of the Hall of Justice. I liked Allen from the moment I met him. His eyes were generous and warm, and he asked me questions. Many people who had a number of years under their belt in criminal justice were cynical, pushing their papers through the system, doing just enough to keep up with the workload. Allen had none of that attitude. He let me tell my story, and he didn't find a way to say no, or to complain that I was adding to his workload. Instead, he came up with solutions.

"Well, it's interesting, Johnson's release isn't a done deal, you know," Allen told me. "Johnson has to agree to two conditions. First, he has to register as a sex offender, and second, he has to enroll in a group to deal with his pedophilia. If he doesn't do both things, he would technically be in violation of his probation and I could send him back for that."

"Sounds pretty flimsy."

"Yeah, well, I bet he won't sign anything I give him. And I can guarantee he'll be a pain in the ass in court. It'd be flimsy, but it might be enough to do the trick."

I sat up in my chair and clapped my hands together. I wanted to hug the guy. This was the first sign of hope I'd had since this ordeal began. I told Allen that I'd found a locked facility in Los Angeles that worked primarily with sex offenders. It'd be the right place to send Johnson. Allen assured me that he would make sure that Johnson's confession to me was part of the record and that this thing would go to a hearing. Out on the steps of the Hall of Justice, I started a new pack of Tareytons and felt almost giddy.

Five days later, I was summoned back to the Hall of Justice, this time to the courtroom of Superior Court Judge Richard Daniels, who had taken over the case. As Allen had predicted, Johnson had refused to register as a sex offender and this was the probation revocation hearing. Judge Daniels was a law-and-order Republican who subscribed to the old saying "Justice moves with a leaden heel, but strikes with an iron fist." Normally, I would have been annoyed to be in his courtroom. But for this hearing, he seemed like the right SOB for the job.

It was just after 9 A.M. when I arrived. I went in through the back where the judges, defendants and bailiffs enter the building. I passed by the holding cells for the defendants who had a court date that morning. In the corridor, I passed a line of prisoners being transferred over. They were shackled together, ankle to ankle, waist to waist. Many knew me and called out, "Hey, Sunny, are you here to get me out?" "Hey, Sunny, whatchoo doin' for me today?" "I gotta talk to you, Sunny. I gotta get out of here . . . my woman's about to give birth."

I smiled weakly and hurried down the hall, feeling confused. Fred Johnson had asked me for help, but he hadn't asked me for more prison time, and that's what I was trying to give him.

When I got inside, I learned that, like the original judge, Johnson's attorney, Susan, was gone. A colleague was covering the case. I didn't know if it was the press of work or that she wanted out, but chose to believe it was the latter. That brightened my mood. There weren't many circumstances where a defense attorney, especially a public defender, would drop a client. It's hard to do; judges often won't allow it. A guy has to be pretty despicable for that to happen. I sat down in the gallery as the bailiff called out the introductions and Judge Daniels took his seat. Fred Johnson sat hunched over at the defense table with his new attorney, a man I didn't recognize.

After a few preliminaries, the new defense attorney said that contrary to what his client had told Allen, the probation officer, Fred Johnson would indeed register as a sex offender and was prepared to live up to the conditions of his release. The lawyer had the signed paperwork with him and Johnson told the court that this was all a big mistake.

It could have ended there, and Fred Johnson would have been released except, as the DA pointed out, there was my story to tell. I was sworn in by the bailiff. Johnson looked at me warily as I sat down in the witness box. I took a moment to give him the once-over. He seemed calm. I saw none of the panic that he had when I first met him. I caught his eye and he quickly looked down and wrote something on a legal pad. The DA walked me through the story leading up to Johnson's revelation to me two weeks earlier. When I explained how Johnson had begged for help and promised to molest a girl in his home, he jumped out of his chair.

"You're a liar!" he bellowed. "Why would you do this to me?" The judge started rapping his gavel. Johnson's new attorney was also on his feet yelling objections.

"Your Honor," he bellowed. "This testimony is outrageous hearsay and shouldn't be allowed."

The judge finally gained control of the courtroom and told the defense attorney to sit down. "Counsel, I'm going to overrule the objection for now." The judge then turned to me with an arched eyebrow. "All right, Ms. Schwartz. You're creating quite a stir. What are you suggesting we do?"

I knew this was probably going to be the one chance I had, so I took a deep breath, and dove in. "Fred Johnson asked me for help, Your Honor. He said he was going to get out and molest a young girl. I think he should be in a locked facility to deal with his problem and I've found one in Los Angeles that would do the job." As I said it, it didn't seem like such a long shot anymore; it seemed like common sense. Here, a child molester was saying he was going to molest again. I'd put a solution together. No one had to think about it. The judge just had to rubber-stamp it and you could almost call it justice. It was patched together, but at least the girl living in Johnson's house would be safe. But the defense attorney was having none of it and as I finished he started objecting like mad, almost screaming. Veins were bulging in his neck.

"Objection, Your Honor, this is irrelevant and so prejudicial that it outweighs any probative value. This testimony is also clearly outside the scope of this witness's expertise. Who is this person, Your Honor? She's only a law student. She's supposed to be his advocate?"

Now I got mad. "Wait a minute. I've spent more time with this man than anyone in this courtroom. And your client wasn't asking for help, he was screaming for help! If you want to do true defense, you'd make sure your client got the help he needed. You wouldn't be lecturing me about credentials. Everyone in this room is responsible, and if we don't do something now, we'll all have blood on our hands!" The judged rapped his gavel to shut us up.

He said he'd take it all under advisement and I stepped down. I'd barely gotten myself settled in the gallery when the prosecutor and defense attorney finished their summations. The judge paused for a moment, and then, without taking a break, announced his decision. I was stunned. What was I expecting? I thought he'd at least take a minute to think about it.

"On the issue of Fred Johnson's probation," the judge said, "I find that there is not enough evidence here to warrant a revocation of his probation. But I do want to put some safeguards in place." He did *not* send Fred Johnson to a locked facility. The safeguards he mentioned, from where I sat, sounded like a Band-Aid. The judge extended Johnson's probation from three to five years and imposed more court appearances and progress reports. Fred Johnson was released immediately.

I walked out of that courtroom boiling with rage and heartbroken, knowing for a fact that Fred Johnson was going to molest again, and I was pretty sure everyone else knew it, too. I stepped out onto the top stairs of the courthouse, which looked out at six bail bondsman storefronts and a mechanic's garage, a view as bleak as my mood. I lit up a cigarette.

On the side of the Hall of Justice is a plaque. It reads: TO THE FAITHFUL AND IMPARTIAL ENFORCEMENT OF THE LAWS WITH EQUAL AND EXACT JUSTICE TO ALL OF WHATEVER STATE OR PERSUASION. I ground out the cigarette under my heel. We'd followed the law "with equal and exact justice" that day but no wrongs were righted, no debts were repaid to society, everyone lost.

I kept thinking of something Susan had said when I met with her: "We're not social workers, Sunny." It was a line I'd heard from lawyers, judges, deputy sheriffs, almost everyone who worked with prisoners. In other words, it's not my job. In a fundamental way, Susan was right. Her job was not to help Johnson, but to protect his constitutional right to a defense. But I had to wonder whose job it was to fight for justice, to try to do what was best for everyone. It was no one's job.

I checked in with Allen over the next few months. He contacted the woman living with her daughter in Fred Johnson's house to warn her of the threat, and he did his best to try to keep track of Johnson. But he wasn't a babysitter, he had other clients he had to follow, and he couldn't watch the guy day and night. Three months later, he reported to me that Fred Johnson had been arrested for molesting a different girl, a six-year-old immigrant from Nicaragua.

CHAPTER 6

1985

The paint was bulging along a seam on the wall. There must have been a leak. County Jail 3 was old enough that there were leaks behind most walls. I was in one of the hearing rooms. Inmates did not get to testify in stately courtrooms with stained wood and moldings. They got dirty linoleum, fluorescent lights, uncomfortable chairs that were nailed down and no windows. Of course, that meant that's what we got, too—the law interns, deputy sheriffs and administrators who worked with them. I was desperate to get out of the jails.

A year earlier, after I finished my law school course work, Sheriff Hennessey put me on his legal counsel team. In one sense, it was a step up. I was paid a little more. But it was an unforgiving set of responsibilities. My job was to go after rogue deputy sheriffs and to act as something of a prosecutor in their administrative hearings. The deputies were accused of anything from sexual harassment to use of excessive force. When I was a legal intern, deputy sheriffs tended to eye me with suspicion. We were the liberal pinkos always taking the side of the prisoners. Now that my sole job was to go after deputies who broke the rules, I barely had any friends left among the deputized staff. I looked over at the deputy who was my target for the hearing. He was charged with an assault that left a prisoner with a permanent limp. I knew the deputy was a first-class bully who was just as likely to tell me to "move my fat ass" as he was to jack up an inmate for looking at him funny. The deputy stared back at me and smirked.

The bar exam results were coming that day. Some of my friends had received them that morning. A former classmate of mine had already reached me to say she'd passed and another friend had failed. Just the word *fail* made my stomach do flips. The California bar was one of the hardest in the country. I'd already failed it once along with two-thirds of all the other test takers in the state. I failed even though I studied ten hours a day and, near the end, barely slept. I promised myself I'd be healthier the second time around, and I gave myself a little more room to live. I went out, saw friends, studied six hours a day, slept a reasonable amount at night. Still, I walked out of the second test certain I'd failed again. I would have put money on it. My closest friends were helping me through it. I had three Hallmark cards by my bed, which were really condolence cards. "Whatever happens, we love you," one said. It might as well have said, "When you fail, we will still love you." If I thought about the test for more than a minute my monologue started up in the back of my head, an insistent jab, Who the fuck are you? Of course you're going to fail again, you always do.

I looked at the clock. Even if we won, the most the deputy would get was a suspension. It was highly unlikely he'd be fired, and even if he were, the cure might be worse than the disease. The fired deputy would become a martyr, the deputies would hold fund-raisers for his legal defense and the divisions would widen between the civilians like me who worked in the jails and the deputies.

I was fighting as hard as I could but it felt like I was accomplishing nothing. I thought often of the famous Stanford Prison Experiment, which I'd recently read about. In 1971, Stanford professor Philip Zimbardo had recruited male undergraduate students to populate a fake prison. Most were given the role of prisoner; a few were given the role of guard. On day two of the experiment, the prisoners revolted and the guards took extraordinary means to put down the rebellion. Over the next couple of days, "guards" withheld food, punished inmates with nudity or sexual humiliation, withheld bathroom privileges and took mattresses away from "bad" prisoners. Some prisoners started exhibiting such high levels of anxiety they had to be sent home. The experiment was supposed to run for two weeks. Zimbardo was forced to shut it down after six days. The methodology of the experiment has been questioned but one of the simplest conclusions was inescapable: captivity can create its own moral universe, and it doesn't take much to push even law-abiding citizens into despicable behavior.

I'd been an eyewitness to some of the worst behavior that captivity could provoke—the simple lack of respect some deputies showed toward inmates, and the disgusting behavior many inmates displayed toward the deputies. In the case I was working on, the inmate the deputy maimed was a world-class asshole himself whom I'd had to defend a few times for rule violations. Though no one deserved a beating, I was sure he'd done something to provoke it.

I'd listened to stories of men who'd been gang-raped while deputies looked the other way. I'd heard stories of men getting shanked in the yard because they'd disrespected an opposing gang member. I'd listened to stories of men who complained and complained and complained about being in jail but never once stopped to say anything about the people they'd hurt. I couldn't do anything about this culture in my job. It just was what it was. I needed out.

My roommate, Judith, was on the phone when I got home that night. I dropped my things, popped open a beer and made my way to the bedroom. My mail was on my bed. I wanted to sit down with the remote control, watch *The Cosby Show* and zone out for the night. But there it was, a letter from the State Bar of California.

I reached over and shut the door. I sat on the edge of my bed, stopping myself from throwing things around the room. I dug my fingernails into my hand, released them, took a breath and slit open the envelope.

I went running out into the living room, tears streaming down my cheeks. I gave Judith one of those ridiculous crazy-person looks.

"Sunny, what is it? What is it?"

I shoved the card at her. "Read it, Judith. Does it say what I think it says? Please read it out loud in case I'm hallucinating."

She gave me a queer look. "Okay, this one is from the California State Bar Test Committee. And, oh my God, Sunny, oh my God! *The committee of the State Bar of the State of California is pleased to inform you that you passed the bar of California!*"

She let out a squeal of delight for me. I almost fainted.

"They made a mistake," I finally managed to say.

"No, they didn't, Sunny. But even if they did"—she winked at me— "looks like you're a lawyer now!"

I sat down on the couch and let out an enormous, chest-heaving sob.

As soon as I collected myself I picked up the phone and called my dearest friends in the city and told them to come over.

I called my sister, Cindy. I called my mom and dad. Frieda laughed and without embellishment said, "Dolly, we are so proud of you." I called my friends in Tucson, my friends everywhere, anyone who knew where I'd been, how I'd tried to change the grades on my elementary school report cards with a pencil before bringing them home to my parents, how I'd gotten onto a first-name basis with my truant officer in high school, how every paper I turned in came back with so much red on it, it looked like someone had died. I called them to tell them how I'd finally pushed away all of the shame and fear and brutal self-doubt. I told them a miracle had happened.

And soon my friends were at my door, bewildered because I didn't tell them why they had to come, just that they did, and before you knew it we were pulling out champagne, hugging and crying and laughing, whooping it up. The music went on and we were dancing to James Brown and Prince, and life, for once, was fine. I had a way out of the jails. I had a way, I thought, to really help people.

After everyone went home, after I collected the empty bottles and cleared out the ashtrays, and the apartment was quiet and peaceful, I called Stevie.

It was late in Chicago, past one in the morning. He was still living with my parents. (I'd asked them not to tell.) I was half hoping my mother would pick up and that Stevie had already gone to bed. The phone rang a few times before the line clicked.

"Who's there?" It was Stevie. He sounded timid.

"Stevie, it's Sunny. It's your sister."

"Hey, Sun, what's happening?" I could hear sleep in his voice.

"Stevie, you're not gonna believe it. I got some great news today."

"Well then, go on and tell me, Sun. You got me up out here, it's like the middle of the night." He said it with vinegar in his voice, a hint of the old Stevie. I smiled and got to it.

"Stevie, I passed the California bar exam."

"Wow, Sunny, wow! But help me out here. What's that mean?"

"It means I'm a lawyer, Stevie. I'm a professional."

My brother laughed. I hadn't heard him laugh in a long time. "That's great, Sunny. Really . . ." He paused for a second. There was a catch in his voice. "You really stuck it to them, didn't ya? You showed 'em what's what."

I could feel time tick by and wanted to bottle it, save it for when I lost Stevie again. He felt present, the old Stevie. My brother. I was grinning, and calm, and giddy.

"Stevie, if I can do this, you can get better," I told him. I really believed it, too. I was supposed to fail, to reach and reach but be disappointed. But there I was, in a new world, a brand-new, unexpected world where my old identity didn't matter.

"You really think so, Sun? I'd like that. I would."

"Yeah, Stevie. If I can do this, I am telling you, why not you? We can take care of each other, do this together."

I closed my eyes and in that moment, I believed it, too. It was easier for me to remember my brother the way he was when he was healthy. He'd already been in and out of most of the psychiatric facilities in Chicago. Most wouldn't take him back because of his "violent tendencies." My mother said it was the boxing that changed him, "made him goofy," and that he must have been injured in the ring. I didn't have the heart to argue with her that he was sick long before that. I'd stopped believing I'd get Stevie back. But that night, I had hope.

A few months later, Stevie called me in a panic. I picked up and he was on the other end, out of breath. "Don't tell anyone, you have to promise not to tell!" he whispered.

"Stevie, is that you? What is it?"

"Sunny, Jesus, Sunny, you have to help me. I can't live here anymore. It's Dad. I can't live with him anymore!" His voice sounded almost like he was in a nightmare. I tried, gently, to wake him up.

"Hey, Stevie, it's all right, it's all right. Just take a deep breath."

"*No,* Sunny, you don't understand." His voice dipped and shook. "You have to listen to me."

"Okay, okay, just talk to me." Some of the panic left his voice and he started explaining to me how it was Dad who was the sick one. It was Dad who needed help and how he didn't feel safe living with him.

"You know him, Sunny. You know how he gets, how he stomps around the house, and is always so selfish. Well, it's a hundred times worse than it was. I'm afraid he might hurt me." Stevie almost sounded reasonable. I always thought Dad was a lunatic anyway, so why couldn't Stevie be right about this one? I desperately wanted it to be true, for Stevie's sake. I wanted to believe him.

"He's trying to hurt me, Sunny. You've got to get me out of here. I think it's in the food."

"What's that, Stevie?"

"I think it's in the food. I think Dad is trying to poison me." I came back down to earth. This was another one of Stevie's delusions.

"Stevie, you have to try to believe me. I know Dad is tough to be with, he can be a real creep. But I know he's not trying to poison you."

Stevie wigged out. I'd challenged him, and he couldn't stand being challenged.

"Sunny, God damn it, you are nothing. You are queer and abnormal and a loser and sick. Who the hell do you think you are, telling me anything?"

"Hey, Stevie, come on."

"You think God's gonna have mercy on your sick, queer-ass ways? He's gonna punish you, torture your arrogant stupid ass! Fuck you, you stupid queer fuck."

I knew he was sick. I knew it. I knew he wasn't responsible for what he was saying. His illness was talking.

I hung up.

Later that night, I went to my desk and opened my stationery drawer. I had a stack of Ansel Adams cards with Arizona landscapes, pictures that always calmed me down. Hopefully, they would do the same for Stevie. I picked one out and wrote: *I believe in you, Stevie. I believe you can get better. I want you to believe it, too. I will try to do better myself, keep calm, not push you. I just want you to know how much I care about you. Love, Sunny.*

I never knew whether he read the card.

*   *   *

On January 12, 1987, right before I went to sleep, I wrote this in my journal:

> *I feel so sad.*
> *I feel such guilt.*
> *I feel scared.*
> *I want so much to be normal—consistent—normal, God damn it.*
> *I want so much to rid myself of my past, my crazy family.*
> *I've felt too many times this year about wanting to end my life, something I never could relate to in the past. Such self-hatred.*

I'd been fighting with my girlfriend again. I fought with all my girlfriends. I fought and raged, and threw things until I hated myself and them. Even as it was happening, I knew I was imitating my father. I could stand back from the argument, and feel his shadow. "You don't love me," I'd yell, and I might as well have been saying it to him. I could feel the power of my anger as I let myself catch fire, that animal ferocity, and I felt addicted to it, and ashamed by it. The exuberance of the bar exam had not erased everything else going on in my life. It turned out I was still myself, an angry fighter who wasn't quite sure who or what I was fighting.

The next morning, I had to be up and in the office early. I had joined a small civil litigation firm that was a world away from the jails and the inmates. We did sexual harassment cases, job discrimination and civil rights claims. It was a good firm, tight-knit, and the partners' hearts were in the right place.

I couldn't have been more miserable.

One client we had was suing her former employer for discrimination. She worked at a bank for ten years and made forty percent less than her male counterparts who had the same responsibilities and less seniority. If I'd seen it in a law school case study, I would have been fired up. But trying the case had made me question everything I ever believed about the law. My senior partners were fed up with the client because she complained all the time, and the posturing on both sides made me want to gag. We sat in these meetings with opposing counsel and no one could look another person in the eye and say, Let's just make this right. I knew there was a game to be played. I knew this was what I had signed up for but it felt counterproductive. Truly resolving the situation, trying to make this woman whole, was not going to be accomplished with lawyers. I'd been sitting in our conference room the other day, one I'd been in countless times before, when I started staring at the painting on the wall. It was an abstract, squiggly lines in browns and blacks. I saw the title for the first time: *In the Company of Wolves.* Someone's idea of a joke, I guess. I didn't think it was funny.

I fell asleep that night with my mind racing. I wanted to escape into my dreams and wake up somewhere else, where Stevie was well, where my parents knew how to respect me, and where I knew how to love and be patient and went to work in a place where people's lives actually got better.

I woke up in a foul mood, banging things in my apartment as I made coffee and took a shower. The ringing phone broke through the blast of my hair dryer. It was seven-thirty in the morning. No one called me at seven-thirty. I let it ring an extra time before I moved to pick it up.

"Sunny?" It was my father but somehow not my father. His voice sounded strange.

"Yeah? Dad, what is it?"

"Sunny, Stevie's gone."

"What?"

"Stevie's gone. He took his own life."

Stevie's gone; he took his own life. I fell to my knees. The room turned gray and the floor came rushing at me. I was a puddle, a damp mess, a ruin, and then I was flying to Chicago.

CHAPTER 7

1987

Stevie had gone to live in Baltimore with Jerry, who was a resident at Johns Hopkins medical school. Jerry's wife had just had their first child, they'd moved to a bigger place, and Stevie took their old apartment. My parents were worried, but they'd exhausted every resource in Chicago, and in Baltimore they were able to set him up with a nurse for twelve hours a day through a Jewish charity. One morning, the caretaker for the morning shift hadn't been able to get into the bedroom. My brother's body was blocking the door. He'd hung himself in his room.

Going home hadn't been easy for me since I'd left for Tucson. Cindy was the only one in my family who had come to terms with my sexuality. My father always circled around to the same subject when I talked to him. "Sunny," he'd say, "it's a waste. You're too good for this. You'll make a man very happy and you'd be a great mother." After he finished that speech he'd almost always move on to the questions. "Did anything ever happen to you?" he'd ask.

"What do you mean?"

"Did anyone ever hurt you? Is this my fault?"

"Dad, if it was your doing then I thank you for it!" I'd shout back while he scowled. My mom never brought it up, and she never asked me about girlfriends, either. Jerry stopped talking to me, and barely acknowledged me when I did see him. He was living in an Orthodox community in Baltimore. His wife, when she left the house, wore a wig or *sheitl*. They didn't use electricity on Saturdays. He believed God had abandoned me. He didn't let me meet his child.

I stood in front of my parents' door for a minute before I worked up the courage to go inside. The mirror in the front room was covered, the custom during Shiva. There was an instant where it felt like if I turned and ran, I could escape the grief, leave the mirror and its horrible meaning behind. Tears started in my eyes. Then my mother found me and threw herself on me. She was wailing, "My baby, my baby." I gripped tight and tried to ride out her grief for her lost child, her favorite child. My father was a wreck. He sat on the floor in the corner, his mouth slack. My mother hung on to me until I could deposit her on a couch and she fell asleep. Jerry and his wife came. They were polite to me. They'd brought their second child, a newborn girl, because she was still nursing. It was the first time I'd met one of his children. The baby looked like my mother.

I slept in Stevie's old room. In the drawer of his desk I found his grammar school autograph book with its fading pages and ribbons. All the girls had signed it. Felicia from two blocks away wrote, "Don't forget me, ever!" I fell asleep sobbing.

The next day we buried Stevie in a pine box at the Jewish cemetery. Chicago's January sky was slate gray, the wind a jagged saw. I hung on to my mother, and she to me, and kept my face shielded from the wind. Stevie had left a note. Most of it was illegible, no matter how hard we tried to decipher it. The only line we could make out only served to remind us that his mind was broken. *The maharishi told me to kill myself.* Stevie used to tell my mom not to worry. "I will take care of you," he'd say. "I'll make money and get you out of this neighborhood and buy you a white Cadillac with red patent leather seats." He said it all the time. I will take care of you. I'd told him the same thing a year ago.

There are so many ways for life to fall apart. When I'd moved to San Francisco, I was full of hope. I was full of fear, too, but mostly I was full of this sense that I could fight through it all, conquer my demons and slough off the uncertain legacy of my family—my father's fiery anger, my mother's embarrassment, the insensitivity of my brother Jerry, and Stevie's madness. I still carried a needy rage that I used to attack every woman I'd ever let get close to me but I'd also managed to cultivate another lesson from my parents. For all of their faults, they had always sent my brothers and me out the door with a simple instruction: "Be a mensch." Be a good person. Do the right thing. That was the legacy

I'd carried into the jails and into law school, and that I'd used to pass the bar. I'd conquered the worst parts of my shame, I'd become a lawyer. I'd fulfilled my dreams. And I still felt awful.

Back when I worked in the jails, I'd had to stand by and watch the horror show—the men stewing in their sick crimes, left idle to learn nothing and do nothing but wait for their release. I'd watched deputy sheriffs, a few who were sick bastards, taking out their frustrations on inmates by jacking them up, squeezing them with rule violations, taking away privileges. I'd watched some try, just as I was trying, to help someone here, another one there. But I watched many punch the clock, believing there wasn't anything to do except ride it out until retirement. I'd felt like a collaborator, that all of us—civilians, prisoners and deputy sheriffs—were collaborators in a system that accepted and invested in failure. When I became a lawyer, that feeling, much to my frustration, remained the same. I felt like I was trying to win battles that shouldn't be won.

Standing there, burying my brother on that terrible winter day in Chicago, I could feel the last of my dreams collapsing like leaky balloons.

Before they gave me the cocktail of Valium and Demerol they asked me what I wanted to listen to. When my eyes wedged open, Bach's "Brandenburg Concerto" was playing in the background. My head hurt as if someone had whacked it with a two-by-four. I opened my mouth. A shard of pain greeted me. Could I still talk? Dr. Hiashima had said anything could happen. This was brain surgery after all.

I'd had a cold. That's how it started. One of those wet, damp colds where everything was running. I'd finished a deposition, and was collecting my papers and found myself staring at the painting again. *In the Company of Wolves.*

Am I the wolf, or am I the prey? I asked myself.

I blew my nose. A mild thumping started in the back of my head. The pounding started behind my right ear, and it beat in time to my heart.

The sound was still there when I woke up in the morning. It was there when I went to work, as I sat through endless meetings, and went home in the evening. I had a washing machine in my ear, spinning and swirling without pause. At first I was annoyed, but after two days, I began to feel nervous.

I received eardrops from an ear, nose and throat doctor but the Laundromat was in my head so I booked an appointment with a neurologist. I got MRIs. I got CT scans. I got almost every picture they could take of my brain and I was soon sitting with a radiologist, Dr. Hiashima. Pictures of my brain were spread around the examination room and the doctor had a grave expression on his face. I'd brought my girlfriend, Jan, along for moral support. We'd been dating for about a year and we fought like cats and dogs. But she was there when Stevie died. She'd helped me push my life back into shape and so she came with me to the hospital.

The doctor was straightforward. He told me I'd developed a leak in my vertebral artery at the base of my brain. It probably happened when I'd sneezed. The blood vessels were weak, he said, and could burst.

"Okay, fine, doctor, I'm with you. Let's fix it," I told him.

I looked at Jan. She was crying. I realized that maybe I might be missing something.

"Wait a minute. Am I hearing what you're hearing?" Jan whimpered a little.

"The problem you've got is very serious," Dr. Hiashima told me solemnly. "It can be attacked using a procedure that snakes a small latex balloon the size of a grain of rice up to your brain. It's experimental, but far better than the alternative: open brain surgery."

That was the good news. Then came the bad. It was still brain surgery. It was experimental. I had to sign a waiver saying I understood that as a result, I could become deaf, blind and paralyzed. In other words, if something went wrong, death might be a blessing.

I had two weeks until the surgery. It had to happen immediately. I was supposed to leave in a few days to go to Hawaii for a vacation with Jan. The doctor said I should go.

"Just don't do anything overly strenuous or stressful," he said.

I looked at Jan. She'd come with me for all of these doctor visits. She was also the focus of a good deal of the stress in my life. How was this going to work?

I'd told myself we fought so much because of Stevie, because I didn't know how to deal with his suicide. But she'd finally gotten the guts to point out to me that I was angry before he killed himself.

We went to Hawaii. I stumbled off the plane into the salty island air and learned to float. I'd been afraid of the water most of my life. I was a poor swimmer, and got nervous in the deep end of pools. But in the ocean, the fear inexplicably disappeared and I swam out past the break without hesitating. I snorkeled over reefs and got lost in the teeming world beneath me. I kicked gently, finding my way into protected coves, watching the flashing kaleidoscope of life scatter at my approach. I saw the same magical displays out in the open air, too. Even waiting in line at the supermarket was beautiful to me. It was then that I started bargaining with God.

For years, I had been too angry to pray, angry about Stevie, about my family, about how alone I felt. But standing there while three perfectly ripe mangoes were lifted into a paper sack, the misery I carried through so much of my life seemed, at least for a moment, very far away, brain leak or no brain leak. I gave thanks for the beauty right in front of me, and prayed that God might let me hang on to life for a little while longer.

When they snaked the tube up into my brain a week later, I was daydreaming about Stevie. Questions a ten-year-old might ask invaded my thoughts. Both our brains had malfunctioned. Why was he shifted from hospital to hospital, a burden to my parents and a lost cause? Why couldn't they have just gone up into his brain, and replaced a pipe, tightened some screws, and shut some doors that had been left open?

That afternoon, after I was out of surgery, my doctor dropped by my hospital room to check on me. Jan was there, and a bunch of other friends. Dr. Hiashima smiled and sat down.

"I have just three don'ts you've got to avoid to make sure this operation holds and you remain healthy. You with me?"

"Sure, doc."

"Number one: quit smoking. Number two: don't get angry because when you get angry your blood vessels expand and contract and that will be bad for the balloon I just put in your head. Number three: reduce stress in your life. That's all I ask," Then the doctor gave me a wink. "Simple, right?"

Some of my friends cracked up. A few wiseasses clapped.

"Doc, everything you just said I shouldn't do are the most habitual things I do as a human being. Anger and smoking and stress . . . those are my three middle names!" Dr. Hiashima looked me right in the eyes, he was good at that, to respond.

"Sunny, if you want to live, you need to figure out a way to stop."

After my first follow-up appointment I quit the law firm. The cigarettes went into the garbage. I'd already left the San Francisco Sheriff's Department and the jails and the criminals far behind. I made a promise to myself not to go back to a system that invested in people's failure. I wanted to work to heal divisions the way I was working to heal myself, not drive them apart.

I needed new dreams.

CHAPTER 8

1988–1990

I was smoking on the front steps of a brand-new jail, San Francisco County Jail 7, and a refrain from a Talking Heads song was running through my head: *How did I get here?* Life can take some funny turns if you let it.

One year earlier, I'd been on a bus in Thailand. I was terrified and alone and in a foreign country for the first time in my life. I was headed to the beach to float some more in solitude. Jan and I had broken up months before, just one of the many things that had come to an end after my surgery.

The bus was rumbling over a deeply rutted mountain road. Chickens were running up the aisle, having leapt from the arms of their dozing owners. Sinewy Thai men jumped off and on the bus at each stop, clinging to the side even after it started up. The people were patient in a way I wasn't used to. The bus stopped sometimes and did not move for half an hour. No explanation was given, and no one asked for one. Time was a meandering stream.

We were moving again when the bus lurched and I bounced against the window. While I swore under my breath, howls of surprise started up from the front. We ground to a halt. Another bus, coming from the other direction, had run off the road and rolled into a ditch. It lay in the tall grass, twenty feet down the hillside, twisted and broken like a bird that had slammed into a plate-glass window. Everyone around me started praying. Their hands went up, their heads lowered, their combined murmuring created an oddly musical chant, a gentle surface of sound. Then the bus doors flew open and everyone in a single motion stood up and filed out of the bus, and clambered down the hillside to help. No one talked about it. No one complained. Knowledge became action.

I went from Thailand to Seattle, where I worked for a hospice program as a part-time caretaker for the sick and dying, making macaroni and cheese and giving foot massages to old folks. But I'd missed San Francisco and had returned to take a part-time job at ALRP, the AIDS Legal Referral Project. It provided end-of-life legal assistance to people dying of AIDS.

It made sense to me that in my last two jobs I'd been working with terminal patients. The way I figured it, I didn't get to say good-bye to Stevie and this was my way to try to make it up to someone. Stevie had performed this long exit, as if he were bowing and backing out of a room, and I felt as if I'd just sat there and watched him go. He'd taught me how to throw a curveball, he made jokes just for me, he was the best ally I'd had. But he didn't let me say good-bye, so I was left trying to help his replacements die.

I came back to the jails during a bomb scare. It was just after lunch and someone had called in a threat to our office. This happened periodically. Even in San Francisco, there were plenty of folks who didn't like homosexuals, even ones who were dying. I'd grabbed my smokes and the messages from my mailbox. There on the top was one from Ray Towbis, Sheriff Hennessey's right-hand man at the Sheriff's Department. It was marked urgent and underlined three times. Ray was a piece of work. I don't know how the guy managed to yell at me through a "missed call" note but he did. I called him from the pay phone out front.

"Ray, what's happening? Where's the fire?"

"Schwartzy. Whatcha doing right this minute?" Ray barked at me. Ray Towbis was one of the most unusual-looking human beings I'd ever met. He stood about five feet three, had huge Coke-bottle tinted glasses, a flyaway comb-over and a potbelly that was almost perfectly spherical. But his energy was infectious. I got to know Ray when I had joined Hennessey's legal counsel, and he and I became fast friends. After I passed the bar, he had even hired me and my law firm to help him with some personal legal matters. I knew he had my back, and I had his.

"I'm in a phone booth waiting out a bomb scare I'm sure you called in," I told him, teasing him. "Why are you trying to scare me? What're *you* doing?"

"Sandra." He called me Sandra when he wanted to get my attention. "Get here now, we want to talk to you."

"Who's 'we'?" I replied, but I'd already asked too many questions.

"Sandra! Don't ask questions. Just get here. You're going to like this!"

I looked around. The fire fighters were just pulling up, and no one seemed to be in a hurry. I figured, why not?

"Schwartzy!" Ray yelled out as I stepped through the door, and he lumbered to his feet. He gave me a slap on the back. "Sandra, Sandra. This is perfect. We need you. We need someone with moxie. We've got a job that was made for you!" Ray was up for the sale that day. His tactics were pure. He'd happily sell you something you didn't want, but only if he thought it was for the greater good.

"Ray, what are you talking about? I'm a big-shot lawyer, you sure you can afford me?" I winked at him.

"C'mon, Schwartzy, we need someone with real vision about what to do for the prisoners." Ray was leading me into the sheriff's office. I gave Hennessey a wide-eyed stare when I saw him but didn't say anything. Both he and I knew not to interrupt Ray when he was on a tear. "The sheriff and I are throwing out the old rules. We need someone with your courage to do this. Get the deputy sheriffs working with you, and get the inmates ready to work and join society when they get out."

Ray went on like this for five minutes and I still had no idea why I was there. Then Hennessey piped in. "Sunny, we want you to take over all the programs in the jails. We've decided to overhaul how we're doing it, and we're putting all the programs into the new jail that just opened. We're taking a big risk on this jail, and we don't want to blow it. That's why we want you."

They made a good pitch, these two. I'd listened, and despite every voice in my head telling me to walk away, I agreed to go visit the jail. And that's how I found myself stubbing out a cigarette on the steps of County Jail 7, which had just been opened in San Bruno, and which happened to be a few hundred feet down the hill from County Jail 3, my old stomping grounds.

I felt a familiarity that was bloodcurdling. I'd spent four years tramping up and down the tiers of the San Francisco system. I'd inhaled enough smoke on steps like these to kill a horse. I'd tried quitting but the dirty habit crept back into my life. Did I want to add the stress and heartbreak and devastation of the prisoners and deputy sheriffs and this whole twisted industry, too? I looked around. No one thought of landscaping when they built a jail. They just dug a pit and dumped in the concrete. Of course, I got it. Why make it pretty for the criminals? But that was the question, wasn't it? Why not make it pretty? Why withhold easy grace? The view was here, the glory of God spread in the valley around us, but it was not intended for the men and women inside.

I was going to meet with the most unexpected director of a jail facility ever appointed, a guy named Michael Marcum, whom I'd known only slightly in my days as a legal intern. Marcum had been part of Ray and the sheriff's sell. He was a civilian in an industry where jail directors *always* came up through the ranks of the deputy sheriffs. They'd paid their dues, and if they'd shown a talent for administration, they'd been given a jail to run. Marcum was the first civilian ever appointed to run a jail in San Francisco County, and he wasn't just any civilian. Marcum was also a former inmate who had served time for a murder he committed when he was nineteen. He had shot and killed his father, an abusive drunk who'd abused Marcum and his mother for years. He'd worked in the jails ever since his release.

I'd had only one memorable interaction with Marcum when I was a law intern. He was the director of prisoner services, which meant he managed the staff members who taught classes in the jails, and the social workers who did postrelease programs. One of his employees was a jackass, a social worker named Hank. Every time I passed him, and I wasn't the only woman to have this happen, Hank said something vile. One day, I'd had it and barged into Marcum's office.

"Hey, Marcum, I got a complaint about Hank. You have to tell him to knock it off because I'm about to kick his ass." Marcum was as even-keeled as they came, and all business.

"Uh, first of all, hi, Sunny. What happened?"

It was a quick story. I'd walked by Hank's desk and he'd smacked his lips at me, and told me he was ready to "treat me like a real woman." Marcum listened patiently and, to my surprise, asked follow-up questions. I'd run into plenty of men in his position who considered my complaints a hassle.

"Did you tell him anything?" he asked.

"I told him if he ever did that again, I would break his feet." Marcum stifled a laugh. I think he was impressed. Hank had the build of a bar bouncer. A few months later, Hank was gone. Marcum was good people.

I found his office in the administration section. He wasn't there so I took a seat to wait. On his walls, there was a giant poster of Angela Davis alongside pictures of Jean-Paul Sartre, Roland Barthes and Michel Foucault. I smirked. This guy was running a jail? Another poster hung on his door—a picture of Woody Guthrie's guitar with the famous words written on the side: "This machine kills fascists."

Marcum rushed in looking exactly as I remembered him. He was a skinny, fastidious man with flipped-back, impeccably groomed hair. He always sat up straight, making no inefficient moves. He graced me with a big smile.

"Sunny, sorry to keep you waiting. It's great to see you."

I grinned back at him. "This is crazy, Marcum. Talk about putting the lunatics in charge of the asylum!" Marcum reached out to give me a hug. He was all right angles, like hugging a two-by-four.

"I'm glad you're here. So tell me the truth, are you really thinking of coming back?" Marcum didn't want to waste time with me if I wasn't serious and he had no reason to believe I was. When I'd left the Sheriff's Department four years ago, it was the no-looking-back kind of exit.

"You know, before I talked to Ray and the sheriff, I would have told you no, flat out. But they sold me pretty well. Now you gotta level with me. Are the deputy sheriffs going to play ball? Are they really gonna let you do anything?" Deputy sheriffs had always held the power in the jails. They controlled the culture of the place. If they didn't like you or what you were doing in programs, then you weren't going to succeed. It didn't matter if you had developed a pill that would solve all the prisoners' problems in one swallow. If they thought prisoners were animals who deserved to be treated like garbage, then that's how they were treated.

Marcum gave me a piercing look. "I know what I want to do, Sunny," Marcum replied. "I want to pull the jail culture down, down to the studs, and rebuild so it might actually help prisoners and make it a better place to work. And if the deputy sheriffs who are here won't play ball, I'll get some who will. What do you think?"

I shook my head in disbelief. There weren't many people who could leave me speechless. Marcum beckoned me and I followed him out the door and down the hall. He pressed a button on the wall leading into the prisoner section, and a speaker squawked at us from the wall. This jail was much more high-tech than County Jail 3. Here there was an interconnected camera and speaker system. Many doors were unlocked remotely by a deputy in a security room. But the smell of fresh paint didn't obscure the institutional assault of this place. This was still a building of gray cinder-block walls, glaring fluorescent lights and hard edges. It was the kind of place where dreams went to die. We went through a set of doors into a wide hallway with a couple of doors scattered at wide intervals down the right side. Marcum motioned me to one of the doors.

Inside was a giant dormitory, almost like an airplane hangar with gray walls and open bunks spread throughout. Prisoners filled the space. In the middle of the room, up on a slightly raised square pedestal, was a large console where a deputy sheriff was sitting.

Marcum explained, "You know the long tiers from County Jail 3 where you have the deputies at one end, and who knows what's happening at the other end? There's none of that in here. This is the new direct supervision model. The dorms are designed so that the deputy can see what is going on throughout the dorm. It's helping us."

It actually looked like a huge step up from County Jail 3. In the old system, the deputy posted outside the tier couldn't see into any of the cells. The men were on their own except for certain times of day—counts, bed checks and the like. The only other time they had contact was when a fight broke out. Then, the riot unit of eight to ten deputies was sent in to control the situation. It always seemed to me like having a high school detention hall filled with the worst bullies you could imagine, and putting the teacher out in the hall to wait for something to go wrong. Or as one deputy described it to me, it was the "warm water, fish-head soup, lock the door, forget about them" approach to corrections. This new design handed control of living areas, which had been in the hands of the biggest thugs in the dorm, to the deputies.

"Come on," Marcum said, keeping to his schedule. "Let me show you what we're trying to do. This is a top-down overhaul. We're assessing every deputy and we're assessing every prisoner, and making sure everyone is accountable for what goes on in here."

That got my attention. "Accountability, huh, Marcum?"

"Yeah," he said. "Absolutely. I want prisoners to feel like they are living in a humane society here, same as deputies. So we're watching everyone's behavior. This doesn't mean we're going to be nice to the prisoners, you know that. But I sure would love it if the punishment was productive, that these men could come away from this experience having learned something." Marcum then started ticking off his ideas. He wanted domestic violence prevention programs, new high school and college classes, as well as an array of counseling resources.

I was listening and thinking, This man has been smoking something. Either that, or Allen Funt was about to jump out from a secret hole in the wall and announce I was on *Candid Camera*. Back when I was a legal intern we'd talked about what we would do if we controlled the jails. But we never got much further than the light-a-match-and-burn-it-all-down approach. We all had dreams, ways we wanted to make a difference in the lives of everybody who lived and worked here. But they seemed like such an impossibility, why waste your breath talking about it? But here I was, hell was freezing over. Was it possible to do something good here?

"Come on," Marcum said. "I've got something good to show you." He looked at me with a mischievous glint in his eyes.

We wound our way through the halls until we arrived outside Pod A. It looked like the other dorm I had seen—an industrial gray airplane hangar. This was the workers' dorm. The workers had better discipline records than the general population and received special privileges to work in the mailroom or cafeteria.

"All right, Marcum, what are we up to?"

"Last night, we had an incident here, and this is the dorm meeting to deal with it." Dorm meeting? I'd never heard of such a thing. No one held meetings with prisoners. I'd seen deputies yell at them, or avoid them, and civilians meet with them individually, but never anything like a group meeting.

Marcum told me that they had a meeting every week to handle routine business, but this one had been scheduled specifically to deal with the incident. He told me about it as we stepped inside. The night before, a female rookie deputy named Teena Franklin had been harassed after lights-out. She'd been walking up and down the rows of bunks doing night rounds. This was a routine check to make sure everyone was still breathing and no one was escaping. In the middle of her rounds, a few men started yelling from the other side of the dorm.

"Hey, dyke bitch, you wanna come tuck me in?"

"Yeah, lady, why don't you try men for a change?"

There'd been more catcalls and homophobic jeers. This was the run-of-the-mill bullshit that was common in the old jails. We called guys who did that "cell soldiers" because they only got tough when their cell door was locked, or in this case, when the lights were out and they were anonymous in the dark. In my day, if the deputies figured out who did it, they might restrict some privileges, maybe even bump the prisoners from the dorm. But more likely the whole incident would pass unnoticed. Living with that kind of verbal abuse was considered standard operating procedure, something you had to get used to when you worked on the tiers. But Marcum was telling me that this was precisely the kind of thing that he wanted to change.

"We're going to confront it. These guys are the workers; they can't be behaving like this."

"But, I don't get it." I was feeling dumb. "How's it going to work?"

"You'll see." And he left me to go say hello to the deputy sheriff. The men were gathering at the bolted-down metal picnic tables in their common area and I decided to sit down with them. I parked myself at a table full of Latino men, who looked up at me a bit stunned. I stared them down, and then said, *"Hola."* They smirked.

The staff assembled. Lieutenant Becky Benoit stalked into the room. When Marcum had mentioned that she was the watch commander, I'd raised my eyebrows. I'd barely known her before but what I did remember was that she was a hard-ass who rarely smiled and was not very approachable. She was also about five feet two and petite. I wondered how she survived. Marcum had sung her praises but I wasn't so sure.

The men were assembling. I could see they'd done this before. To my amazement, with almost no prompting, they quieted down when Benoit walked out to start the meeting. She was carrying a book with her and she opened it and started to read. Her voice was quiet, a bit gruff, but it carried.

"After climbing a great hill, one only finds that there are many more hills to climb. I have taken a moment here to rest . . . But I can rest only for a moment, for with freedom comes responsibilities, and I dare not linger, for my long walk is not yet ended." She closed the book. "Nelson Mandela said that. Who knows who Nelson Mandela is?" A scattering of hands went up.

"Well," Becky continued, "Nelson Mandela is a great leader in South Africa. He was once imprisoned for many, many years because he was black. He hadn't done anything, hadn't committed any crime. But he kept his dignity, and after he was released, he went on to become president of his country. He is coming to visit San Francisco next week and I think you ought to know about him. He is a man who understands and talks constantly about how hate corrodes the spirit. It's like a poison. Mandela knew that he could hate the men who imprisoned him, but if he lost himself in that hate he would lose his soul.

"Now I want to talk about what happened in here last night. Some of you took it upon yourselves to yell homophobic language at Deputy Franklin. Those words were designed to do nothing but humiliate. We do not tolerate that kind of behavior here. We don't tolerate racism, we don't tolerate homophobia. We do not tolerate it in ourselves; we do not tolerate it in you. Our covenant with you is that we will treat you with respect and dignity. But we expect the same treatment in return. I want you to think of Nelson Mandela, a role model for all of us, and how he would have responded to this kind of behavior, and what he would have said to the men who said it."

The men had sat quietly through Becky's speech. Some looked bored, some were rocking back in their chairs, a few were falling asleep, but most were paying attention. My jaw was on the floor. Marcum joined in when Becky finished.

"This is our community," Marcum said. "It is everyone's problem if hate is tolerated." Marcum asked if anybody had anything to say. I was stunned to see a few hands go up. Raising their hands? In a jail? I looked at Marcum. He was looking at me as if to say, "See? I told you." He called on three of the men. They stood and apologized for not stepping up to stop the foul language. Finally, two more hands went up in the back of the crowd. They stood up together.

"Hey, we just want to apologize, and apologize to Deputy Franklin. We were the ones who did it."

"Yeah, we're sorry."

Both men looked like they were in their late twenties. They were scraggly, unremarkable. Both would have looked at home in a dive bar or a methadone clinic. I'd never seen anyone stand up and take responsibility in any corner of the criminal justice system where they weren't being offered a deal. I'd never seen such simple, healthy communication in a jail setting. Marcum was now talking to the two who had confessed.

"Thanks for your honesty, gentlemen. Thanks for standing up like real men."

There was scattered clapping in the dorm, which Marcum stopped. "This is not a show. This is not an exercise. This is serious, painful stuff. Your words have an impact, the pain you put out into the world is on you. And it's up to you to stop it."

Now he looked at everyone in the room, taking in the civilian staff and the deputy sheriffs in the room. "And that's on everyone. We all are making an agreement to stop hateful speech, to stop abuse of any kind. If we have to play cops and robbers, we will. If you act like criminals, you'll be treated like criminals, but if you act like men, you will be treated like men." Marcum then turned to other announcements, and even that incredibly pedestrian activity felt revolutionary. In the world, this was ordinary, ho-hum stuff. It was just a meeting. But here, a meeting meant something. It meant there were standards, a schedule, a community, and not just a roomful of lost souls waiting for their lives to resume.

Marcum made sure there were consequences for the two men who'd come forward. He gave them extra work shifts and a writing assignment. I was laughing when he finally circled back to me.

"Did you set this whole thing up for me or what?"

He smiled and then turned serious. "Listen, Sunny, I'm about as surprised as you are that we're getting this chance. But we need you to make it work. This was a good meeting today. They all aren't quite so dramatic, I promise you that. But these are the first steps. We want to build a respectful, dignified community so people are more prepared to go back to society. We need programs, we need you here, and . . ."

Marcum was no longer looking at me. He was giving a stump speech, the kind of speech I'd always wanted to hear from a boss or supervisor. They say you don't get too many fat pitches up over the plate. You have to swing when they come your way. I knew this was my pitch. I just needed to pick the bat off my shoulder and swing.

"Marcum, shut up for a second, would ya, and *count me in*!"

CHAPTER 9

1990

I had my own office. There were windows. Okay, so they were narrow slats of glass but I still had a view better than any I had when I was a lawyer. From my office chair, I could see a pristine patch of the San Bruno Mountains. I felt lucky when I wasn't feeling scared.

It was my second day on the job and my phone wasn't ringing. I'd looked at it at least fifteen times, wondering when someone would call. I had a scribbled list of priorities that Marcum had rattled off to me this morning, and I was hoping someone would tell me how to start. I'd checked in with Becky (Lieutenant Benoit to everyone else) to say hello but I hadn't seen either of them since. There had been a fight in the dorms this morning. We'd had a lot of fights since the place opened, and there were deputy sheriffs to debrief, a dorm meeting to hold, paperwork to fill out. This place was new to everyone, and until the inmates and staff got used to it, there would be fights.

No one knew yet what to call me. No one had ever had my position. I was in charge of programs for County Jail 7, and I was starting with Marcum's short unfinished to-do list:

1. Get a school back in the jails.
2. Start a parenting class.
3. Get a Domestic Violence (DV) group going.

The list wasn't supposed to be exhaustive, just a place to start. And we were starting from almost zero. The jail had a GED program that could accommodate twenty inmates at a time. There was an auto shop and a print shop that taught vocational skills. There were a few inmate worker positions in the kitchen, laundry room and library. The best program we had was the horticulture project, run by a woman named Cathrine Sneed. Sneed took out forty inmates at a time to work in an organic garden we had on the south end of the property. Planting seeds, weeding, fertilizing and tending a garden was a pretty good metaphor for what men had to do in their own lives. That was a heroic project, but all in all, we didn't have much more to offer. The city colleges had been teaching a few courses but Marcum had fired them recently. They'd been sending their worst teachers. We'd caught some sleeping on their desks during class, and one sold drugs to his inmate students. The vast majority of the 362 men and women in County Jail 7 did nothing all day, which was no different than any other jail or prison in the country. I glanced at my phone again, still nothing.

Deputy Richard Drocco stuck his head into my office at around eleven.

"Hey, babe. Good to have ya back in the fold." We caught up a little, then Ricky told me he needed to let me in on what people were thinking.

"Those knucklehead deputies," he said. "They think you're a prisoner lover and a cop hater. That's the rumor, at least." He was talking about the chatter in the deputy locker room. Drocco was smiling, making dramatic gestures with his hands, giving me an insistent finger waggle. "Don't pay any attention to them! I told them you're for real. But listen, babe," Drocco crossed his arms, turning conspiratorial. "We hear you're planning on doing all this stuff for the prisoners, planning to bring in a lot of programs. Don't be planning all these bullshit-type programs. Make sure these guys get some straight talking to. There are some real assholes downstairs." I knew what he meant by bullshit programs. There were a lot of flaky people in the prisoner services world, as well as plenty of con artists and good-for-nothings, trying to suck some easy money out of the correctional bureaucracy. They peddled self-esteem classes, addiction programs and anger management classes that were as effective as a Band-Aid on a broken leg.

"I hear ya, Ricky. Got any ideas?"

"Get these guys jobs. They need to make a living and start paying taxes instead of mooching off all of us." He was punching his palm with his fist. "And maybe you can get some classes for us, too?" He said it as a joke, but I loved the idea. To change the culture, everyone would need new training, including the deputies.

Drocco high-fived me on the way out. Seeing him was a good reminder. When I first started in the jails in 1980, my view on deputy sheriffs wasn't that much different from the inmates'. I saw them as the enemy. I knew one of the things I would have to do in my job was to break down the wall between civilians and deputy sheriffs, and get us all to work like we were on the same team. Luckily, Marcum had been able to pick and choose staff over here. But earlier this morning I'd seen Lieutenant Bill Hunsucker stalking the halls. I remembered Hunsucker as a mean, snarling bulldog of a deputy whose temper had reminded me of that of my father. I had asked Marcum about him and he just rolled his eyes.

"Yeah, I know, Sunny. Hennessey sent him over, told me I needed to give him a second look." I'd have to watch him. And then there was Lieutenant Becky Benoit, the watch commander. In every other jail, her position would have meant she was running the place, but here she was reporting to Marcum, as was I. I'd met her only a few times and hadn't figured her out. She was a quiet Cajun (an oxymoron if I'd ever heard one) from the bayous of Louisiana who managed the impressive feat of being feared and respected by both the other deputy sheriffs and the prisoners. I was her opposite—hugging and snarling and living as large as I could. Yesterday, we had already had our first confrontation. I had lit up a cigarette in the staff dining room. She told me to put it out. I told her that wasn't going to happen. The deputy sheriffs at the next table looked up alarmed, but Becky let it go and walked off. Deputy Hunsucker had motioned me over. "Never seen anyone stand up to Benoit like that. She freaks a lot of people out. Nice going." I was willing to give Becky the benefit of the doubt after the presentation she'd made in the dorm meeting, but I was wary. I'll admit it. I didn't trust the deputy sheriffs and I was dreading the fights we would have.

But they weren't the only ones I was working with. I had ten inherited staff members who reported to me and were waiting for me to set an agenda. I knew a few of them. They were long-serving prisoner service counselors, a job that bore some resemblance to what I used to do

as a legal intern. Prisoner service counselors were liaisons to the outside world, but didn't handle any of the legal stuff that I used to. They
were a mixed lot, just like the deputy sheriffs. Some were amazingly
dedicated and hardworking. Others were collecting a paycheck—
clock-punchers and do-nothings.

But I was grateful not to be surrounded by a bunch of bullshit
lawyers. I felt recharged by Thailand and Seattle, and was profoundly
thankful to be alive and not a vegetable in a wheelchair. I thought of
the balloon in my brain every day, a finger in the dam holding back the
flood. I wanted a second chance with this strange community of people. I wanted to be in this fight.

At the same time I had to swallow the fear creeping up in my chest.
Beyond the three action items Marcum had given me, I didn't have a
game plan. I had ideas, certainly, but I didn't have a list of programs I
wanted to see in the jail by year's end. What I knew for certain was that
no one else was going to show me what to do because we were making it up as we went along.

I began by cracking a book. Marcum had handed me *Jails, Reform,
and the New Generation Philosophy,* by Linda Zupan, the day before. It
wasn't going to be on the bestseller list anytime soon. It was by corrections people for corrections people. But it described the jail I was sitting in, which was new to the staff and me and relatively new in the
world of corrections. Reading it made me hopeful. Compared to the
normal "control and coerce" vibe you get in a lot of prison literature,
there were good intentions in Zupan's words. She wrote that in direct
supervision, contrary to older models,

> *The rules are similar to the standards and practices of a civilized society.
> When rules are violated, management must promptly respond in an intel-
> ligent and equitable way. The housing unit should always be viewed as
> the "deputy's space" with the inmates in the role of the visitor; not vice
> versa, as is so often the case. The housing areas are divided into manage-
> able units with the cells arranged around a common multi-purpose area.*

It sounded good to me, I thought, and shut the book. I needed to
force myself back into the monster factory, take its measure after a few
years away, and I'd been dawdling.

Another door, another wait. I looked through the window into Pod B. Inside, I could see men playing Ping-Pong. Some were sleeping in their bunks. Others were playing cards. It was eleven-thirty in the morning. The men looked the same as I remembered them: an unsettling combination of innocence and experience swaddled in orange. It was always strange to see a crowd of grown men who all looked like they were wearing pajamas. They had the practiced stance I remembered. Emotion was missing from their faces. They held their arms away from their bodies, stuck their chests out, making themselves bigger. The door grumbled and slid open. A familiar soundscape rolled out to meet me. There was a radio playing too loudly, to compete with the television. Not everything had changed. I sighed.

The pod I was in was designed like the workers' dorm I'd visited when I first met with Marcum. Greeting me on the way in were four showers, four phones and eight open toilets. Men were sitting there doing their business and I made a mental note never to look there again. In the far corner of the room was a weight set. Clanging metal punctuated the constant chatter. The deputy sheriff was sitting at his desk at the foot of the door. I didn't know him. He was about 240 pounds with a buzz cut. Like the men in orange around him, he sat with his chest out, a face of stone, and his arms held out ever so slightly from his body. I introduced myself.

"Deputy Powers," he said. "Yeah, I know who you are. I heard you were starting this week." I told him I was doing rounds to talk to the men about programs.

"Be my guest." There was a touch of exhaustion in his voice. I picked out the nearest table, where a card game was going on. As I approached, the four men looked up. There was a loosely veiled menace in their eyes. I sat down and asked them what they were playing.

"Spades." It was little more than a grunt. They were near the end of a hand, so I waited them out. They'd been talking and laughing before I sat down, but now they were mostly quiet. The guy to my left, an older black man with glasses and deep creases at the corners of his eyes, seemed the most at ease. He was still whooping it up as the tricks turned his way and he made his bid. Once all the cards were out and the dealer was shuffling I started asking questions.

"So what do you do here all day?"

"You're looking at it," the older man said. The other three men snickered.

"What would you rather be doing?"

At this point, the guy to my right chimed in. He was a skinny inmate with baggy clothes.

"Getting out, man. What do you think? Can you get me outta here?" He gave me a poor-puppy stare. There were more scattered chuckles.

"What would you be doing out there?"

"Getting high," Skinny said, and the whole table roared. But the laughter died quickly, because I wasn't going along with it.

"Why?" I asked, as serious as I could. No one answered.

"Hey, why do you want to know? Who are you?" This came from the older guy.

"I'm Sunny Schwartz. I just started working here. I'm in charge of getting programs into the jail."

A third guy piped in. "Hey, are you Indian?"

"No, I'm Jewish."

"Oh." He looked bewildered. I don't think he knew what to make of that. The fourth guy wasn't looking at me. He was shuffling the cards.

"So, who has kids here?"

It turned out they all did. Cedric, the older guy, was fifty, and a grandfather. I couldn't believe Skinny. He barely looked fifteen. But he said he had two boys, ages four and seven.

"What was your last job?" I asked.

At this point, Cedric became exasperated.

"Lady, you ask too many questions. All I want is to do my time and get outta here. It ain't more complicated than that."

I wasn't going to let him off the hook.

"I get it. I do. I'd want to get out of here, too. But my job is to help you guys for when you *do* get out. So what classes would you take if we started some?"

"I need a job," the third one said.

"That's what we all need," Cedric chimed in. "But ain't nobody gonna hire us."

"Bullshit," I said.

"Oh yeah?" Old guy fought back. "They'd hire you. They won't want to deal with convicts."

"Some don't, but you're assuming that all you can do is commit crimes. You're also assuming who I am right now, aren't you?"

"Fair enough, young lady, fair enough." Cedric wasn't fighting me anymore. The others look annoyed, but they were listening. The fourth guy had stopped shuffling.

"You need jobs, okay. Have you thought about what kind of jobs you want to have?"

"Damn, lady." Skinny replied. "You think a motherfucker like me can be choosy about a job?" Normally, I wouldn't have let that kind of language pass, but today I only wanted to provoke so much.

"Come on, now. I'm not saying you get to do excatly what you want when you're released, but it's good to have dreams. What are your dreams for the future once you get out?"

There was silence at the table. Skinny folded his arms. Cedric looked down. The fourth guy, the guy who'd been shuffling the cards, set them in front of him, and quietly, almost angrily, said, "Shit, what's a dream, man? I don't know what that is."

I went from dorm A to B to C. The men spent their time watching *Jerry Springer* and slasher movies. They were dealing cards, playing dominoes and pumping iron. I could count on one hand the number of men who were reading a book, or writing a letter. The women's dorms—E and F—weren't any better. Some of the women were drawing cartoon figures on envelopes, which they would trade for candy bars. Others were doing each other's hair in front of a row of mirrors that gave off weak, cloudy reflections. Everyone said they wanted a job. No one had dreams.

I sat down with Deputy Powers at the end of the day in the break room. He was just getting off his shift in Pod A. I asked him how long he'd been working here. He replied that he'd been "in theater for a little over three weeks," and gave a short grunt of a laugh. He was funny in a hard-boiled sort of way. He also said he was scared shitless of Lieutenant Benoit. This last response I'd found to be pretty universal. The woman was beginning to impress me. I asked him if he thought the place was working and he threw up his hands.

"I don't know. I still don't get it. We can't get a break to go to the bathroom, you know. We're stuck in the dorm, and the inmates have nothing to do. Why the hell do they call this the 'program facility'?" Prisoners were saying this, too, though not quite so directly.

"What's with all the fighting?" I asked. "Direct supervision" was supposed to discourage fighting but so far there had been just as many fights as we used to have on Mainline or in County Jail 3.

"Yeah, well, there are some things that are better over here. The fights are short-lived and more controllable. They happen right in front of us, so it never has time to spread and get out of control. It's not like Mainline, where someone could be getting his ass kicked and we wouldn't know. We get to step in quicker, and that's better, I guess."

"But?"

"But it all happens right in front of us. We don't have any barrier. And there's no place to put them."

"What do you mean?"

"There are only two holding cells in this whole place. Fights happen, and we can't lock those guys down in their cells, 'cause they don't have cells. They either go to the holding cells for a few hours, and that's if no one's in them, or they stay in their dorms, watching TV with the guy they just had a beef with."

Two holding cells. Two holding cells for 362 inmates. That was incredible. That didn't allow for many options.

"Whoa, what happens if you lose a dorm?"

"Exactly, what happens if we lose a dorm?" "Losing a dorm" was our euphemism for a riot. Riots were the worst thing that could happen in a jail. We all feared them. I'd never been in one and I hoped I never would. The horror stories were enough. The deputies were vulnerable here in County Jail 7 in a way I hadn't imagined. There weren't the fallback positions, the way to isolate everyone for a mandatory cooldown like we had in the old tiers. If a riot happened, if you lost a dorm, you had to hope you got out. If the dorm was at maximum occupancy—sixty-two inmates—that was enough to make any deputy sheriff think twice about running in there. There was a twisted genius to it. Deputies couldn't jack someone up just to teach them a lesson, because the inmates would be watching. Still, it seemed burnout was a real threat here and I asked Powers about it.

"I don't really feel better at the end of the day, if that's what you mean. This wasn't just an assignment over here. They asked for volunteers and I raised my hand. Ray Towbis and Marcum said this was going to be a better working environment. It was going to be better for us and for the inmates. I liked that. The inmate should have more to do. And I'm not gonna argue if someone thinks it should be better for us. But right now, these guys, they've got nothing going on, so they give us problems. So I go home, and you can ask my wife, I'm as big a son of a bitch as I always was."

"So far, it's not better?"

"The only thing that's really changed is that I get to watch these guys take a dump all day."

I told him that I was responsible for programs now. And then, having listened to suggestions and complaints all day, I said something crazy. I knew it was crazy when I opened my mouth, and yet, I believed it ought to be true, so I said it anyway.

"Mark my words—this place will have each and every prisoner in class every day for most of the day—all three hundred sixty-two of them will be in some program!"

He nodded at me as if I were nuts. Neither of us had ever seen anything like that in the jails. He had no reason to believe I could deliver on my promise. Neither did I. But it should've been true. These men and women needed things to do. They needed to learn something before going back out into the world, and it needed to be something different from the rage and frustration they normally came out with. They owed it to us to get to work, to make something of themselves. I was going to demand it of them.

CHAPTER 10

1990

We took control of the televisions. I'd come to that decision early on. One day, I was talking to a deputy sheriff in one of the pods when a prisoner started whistling at the far end.

"What's that for?" I asked. It was loud and, strangely, no one seemed pissed. It was the middle of the afternoon. Prisoners began to gather around the television.

"That's the Woody Woodpecker alarm," the deputy sheriff told me. "Someone does that every day at four."

"It's the what?"

"The Woody Woodpecker alarm." He looked at me for a few more beats and then explained. "For the cartoons. It's the one thing the 'bangers all agree on, actually. You know, Woody Woodpecker, Chilly Willy, those guys. It's about the only thing that gives me any peace in a day."

"Well Jesus, that's just sad." The men had spent all day doing nothing. Now, in the only organized activity of the day, they were going to spend another half hour watching cartoons. That pretty much made my decision. Changing a culture takes a thousand small steps, and this was one of the first. But this step provoked a pitched battle against an especially annoying adversary whom I came to know intimately, an inmate named Leroy Clinton.

Clinton's arrest record was extensive, depressing and entirely typical of the men we had in the program facility. Leroy was what we called a retread. He was caught in a vicious cycle of incarceration interrupted by brief moments of freedom. Leroy had begun committing crimes in his teens and followed a predictable path from minor to major offenses. In the three years before I met him, he did three stints in our jails on drug and car theft charges:

- 3/87: Vandalism/property damage. Fine and probation.
- 7/87: Malicious mischief to a vehicle. Dismissed.
- 8/87: Malicious mischief. Convicted. Ninety days in jail and three years probation.
- 3/88: Possession and sale of cocaine. Dropped for lack of probable cause.
- 8/88: Vehicle theft. Dismissed for lack of evidence.
- 11/88: Vehicle theft. Dismissed for lack of evidence.
- 12/88: Grand theft auto. Dismissed for lack of evidence.
- 4/89: Numerous counts of possession and sale of cocaine. Convicted and sentenced to ninety days in jail and three years probation.
- 12/89: Probation violation. Remanded to one year in County Jail 7.

Leroy entered the program facility when he was thirty-four and quickly became one of our most notorious inmates. It wasn't that he was stabbing people in the bathroom, or smuggling drugs, or setting fire to his mattress. But Leroy was consistently, infuriatingly defiant. If the staff said yes, he said no. He was five feet eight, balding in front, and he had dreadlocks down his back so thick they could be used to tie up a boat. Leroy must have been at least 350 pounds, and he was a giant pain in my ass.

We announced the new television policy at our weekly dorm meeting. All the details had yet to be decided but the bottom line was that the deputy sheriff in the pod would now supervise the remote, and prisoners would no longer choose what was playing. *Jerry Springer* was out. Educational programs were in, as well as some occasional entertainment, but none of the slasher-film screamfests the prisoners liked.

That afternoon, I was in Leroy's dorm talking with the deputy about a schedule change. I was in midsentence when Leroy's voice leapt above the din.

"They are a bunch of dictators. These people are trying to control everything we do. We have a right to watch *Jerry Springer*," he yelled. "Hell, these fascist fools won't even let us go outside!" (That last complaint was purely Leroy's issue. Marcum had denied his request to join the organic gardening program because, as Marcum said, he had "too much rabbit in him.") Other men were joining the cry.

"Yeah. What the hell is this?"

"Fuck this shit!"

Just then, by chance, Lieutenant Benoit came into the dorm. She and Deputy Drocco and I all exchanged angry looks. We decided, on the spot, to have another dorm meeting. We collected the men from around the television. Most peeled off from the protest easily. When he was nearly deserted, Leroy finally gave way and came over.

I introduced myself again. This time, unlike the morning, I heard people sighing, I saw some rolling their eyes. Disrespect. Respect is a currency in jail and if you give it up, it is not easy to win back. My voice took on an angry edge.

"I worked with some of you in the early eighties. Some of you younger kids, I actually worked with your parents. I was your law advocate, and I know I don't deserve the kind of reception I just got." Stillness settled over the room. "I have now been here for a month and I've been talking to everyone I can. Let me tell you, you are all saying the same thing! You want to get out of here. You want a job. You want to be with your family. I would have to be deaf not to hear it!" I was stalking up and down, my hand beating time to drive my points home.

"You're protesting the way the television is programmed? I can hear that, too. Let me make it very clear to you what I think. It is not my job to ensure that you enjoy your time here. My job is to make your time constructive." I told them that over the next few months, we'd be bringing education back to the program facility. I'd made good progress in my search for a school to come in with high school equivalency and college courses.

"You are going to have an opportunity to read. Learn how to talk to a potential employer. Learn how to raise your kids." I could hear more sighs and angry chatter. Most of it was coming from Leroy. The next thing I said I addressed directly to him.

"Who here thinks they are perfect parents? Anyone? Do you, Leroy? These classes are for your benefit." Now I pointed toward the television in the corner. "That box is not interested in whether you have a job, whether you have your dignity. It does not care about you or your kids. So before we start talking about your constitutional right to watch *Jerry Springer,* I want you to think about what it will really take for you to leave this place and not come back. I want you to figure out how you can show your loved ones, your community and yourself that you are in fact serious about getting the hell out of here!"

I opened the floor to comments. Leroy shot to his feet. He was steaming.

"Ms. Schwartz, we have a guarantee. Title Fifteen of the California code gives us the right to watch TV and if we want to watch *Jerry Springer—*"

I cut him off. "Look, Mr. Clinton. This is not a debate or a contest." The Title 15 regulations were California's minimum standards for jails in the state. It did not guarantee Leroy the right to watch whatever television program he wanted. But I wasn't going to get into that argument with him. "We are talking about matters of life and death. Your life. Your death. But one thing that is not yours is this jail . . . just as much as it's not my jail. And I will remind you what Mr. Marcum likes to say all the time." I liked to invoke Marcum. He had credibility with the men as an ex-con. "This is the taxpayers' jail. They pay for your room and board. They hired me to help decide how it is run. This is not your home, that's not your bed, and that is definitely not your TV. I would ask you to be the leader that you are so very capable of being. Recognize that this is a program facility. The programs we're putting together are for your benefit, and one thing that is definitely not benefiting you is *Jerry Springer.* So bury this idea about your right to watch his awful show."

I won a chorus of men singing "Ooooh, she got you, man," as if we were in the seventh grade. It was enough to put down Leroy's insurrection for today. In the end, we formed committees of deputized staff with inmates' input to select the TV and radio programming. This was how we managed most of the changes in the dorm. We sought buy-in, enforced discipline, and treated the men with respect until they did something to lose it.

After that second dorm meeting, Becky Benoit took Leroy aside to talk to him. She actually took him to the staff conference room. No prisoners were ever allowed in there but that's where she felt she could deliver the strongest message. She sat him down, and told him he was a pain in the ass, and that she wasn't happy she had to take time out of her day to deal with his petty complaints. But she also told him she respected him as a human being, and that she saw potential in him, and that, if he chose to, he could be a leader in the dorm.

She told me about the conversation at the end of the day. "Sunny, you should see the grievances I get from him. He's always going on and on about the food, or the deputies, the phones, the clothes. But you know what? It means the guy is alive. Leroy knows that this is no way for a man to live. That says something! I think he will be easier to deal with."

Leroy didn't stop fighting us, but Becky's intervention had changed him. He softened. The dorm deputies started asking me, "What did she do to him? Slip him a Quaalude?" I learned from Becky that day. I looked at the fire in her eyes, and thought about the other deputized staff I was working with, and I realized I might have to give up on some of my prejudices against deputy sheriffs.

Becky and Marcum both turned out to be remarkable colleagues. They were unstinting advocates for the jail, and for the essential dignity of everyone there—staff and inmates alike. Marcum became like my brother, or at least, the brother I always wished I had. He kept a tight lock on his emotions, was absolutely loyal and was a cunning administrator who played politics like a champ. He called me Sunshine; I called him Pencil Dick when I thought he was wimping out with the City Hall big shots. Becky scared everyone, she never backed down from a fight, and her attacks could be withering. She was fierce in her support for the dignity of prisoners, and did not compromise on their obligation to make amends for what they'd done. We shared these two desires, and it turned out, a lot more besides.

Many months after I started in County Jail, Becky and I found ourselves becoming intimate, drawn together by the passion we both shared for the work. She was the opposite of every woman I'd dated. I usually went for the mothering, nurturing types who took care of me, and overlooked or excused my temper. Becky was a cop, and a hard-ass, who had a temper and needs of her own. Plus I didn't want to mess up what we had at work. County Jail 7 was too important to screw it up with one of my patented dysfunctional romances. But Becky was persistent, and attractive, and so damn passionate about the work. That was a turn-on. We moved in together after seven months, though we fought like banshees. She was jealous. I was needy. I tried to bully her into submission, but she spit fire right back at me. We also fought equally hard for our programs in County Jail 7. Together with Marcum, the three of us kept taking each one of the thousand steps forward, trying to redefine what a jail could be.

One big step had happened before I even started. Marcum instituted a social contract for all new inmates. It was probably the single most important part of County Jail 7 in those early days, the thing that set it apart from other jails:

SAN FRANCISCO
SHERIFF'S DEPARTMENT
Prisoner Contract

As a participant in the San Francisco County Jail Programs, deputized and counseling staff will be available to assist you in your adjustment to dorm living, your participation in programs and assignments, and in understanding the basic philosophy of human decency and self-respect. The programs of this Facility are designed to help you take responsibility for your life and actions while you are in jail and when you are released.

- I _____ state and agree to the following:
- I have been informed of every Jail Rule and Regulation.
- I will obey the rules and regulations.
- I will participate in good faith in all assigned programs.
- I will attend all assignments on time.
- I will discuss problems with other prisoners and staff in a positive manner.

- I will work sincerely toward meeting the goals I establish to prepare for a positive reentry in the community.
- I will follow the Rules of Student Conduct.
- In addition, I agree to participate in _____.

I understand that I am required to treat others and myself with respect and dignity; and that my positive participation in Programs and Work Assignments will enable me to earn work time credits applicable toward my release date. I understand that racism, sexism, anti-gay/transgender/lesbian remarks, glorification of substance abuse or criminal behaviors and any other form of antisocial behavior will result in loss of privileges, extra work duty or removal from the Program Facility.

Inmate _____
Date _____
Staff Signature _____

The contract underwent permutations over the years but the intent stayed the same. It helped define the environment that we all wanted to live in, an environment that promoted the best in people rather than the worst. The contract was accompanied by a rigorous orientation process. In most correctional institutions, entering a jail was a hazing. Inmates were strip-searched and barked at and then flung into the general population to sink or swim. In our jail, civilian staff and deputized staff worked with new inmates for their first three days in the system. We went over jail rules with them, and put together a set of goals for them to pursue, which we checked on every couple of weeks. From the beginning, we set high expectations for their behavior. Leroy had signed the contract. So did everyone else in the jail.

Of course, my miserable contracts class in law school had taught me that a contract was just a piece of paper unless all parties entered into it in good faith. If we were going to expect a higher level of behavior from our inmates, we had to hold ourselves to a higher standard as well. This applied to both civilians and deputized staff. Everyone grumbled at the changes we introduced on swearing.

"No swearing? What the fuck?" Lieutenant Hunsucker yelled out from the back of one meeting, provoking laughter. Hunsucker had proved to be a thorn in all of our sides, a loose cannon of a deputy whose emotions swung in unpredictable swaths. In meetings, he'd lob rhetorical javelins like an Olympic champ, often complaining about how we were throwing money away, or about the good-for-nothing prisoners. But turned out to be a good kind of thorn because he was often the first person to say what other people were thinking.

A prohibition against swearing had been in the deputy sheriffs' manuals from ancient times, but it had been treated like "no spitting" laws in small towns, a quaint relic. We resurrected many of those rules: no swearing, no disrespect, no favoritism toward inmates, and everyone was recruited to enforce the rules. In the past, civilians wouldn't write up inmates for violations. Now, they were required to. It was a mind-set as much as a practice. My staff complained about having to play disciplinarian, but that at least put them and the deputy sheriffs on the same team. No one was allowed to say, "that isn't my job."

We also tried to break the hierarchy that existed among prisoners. This meant we did away with "trustees." Trustees, in the old system, were prisoners appointed by deputy sheriffs as their eyes and ears on the tier. The trustees received special privileges and helped manage the place. Often, the most Machiavellian figures would get the position because they could keep order. It was a bargain with the devil and encouraged corruption. We replaced the trustee system with a rotating work board so that every prisoner had the chance to be in a position of leadership.

Changing the rules inside, however, was a small part of my job. I had to make good on the promise of constructive programs, and my first big push went to getting a school in the jail.

I discovered that our neighbor to the north, just behind the razor-wire fence and a stand of trees, was Skyline Community College. I gave them the hard sell, told them our population needed their classes more than anyone else, and they'd said they would try. We were able to get state funding for the students because our inmates counted as students as much as the next person did. One of the first things the college did was help us perform a survey of our population's needs so I would know what kind of programs I should start:

- 75 percent were reading somewhere between the fourth- and sixth-grade levels.
- 90 percent never had a legal job.
- 90 percent were self-identified addicts.
- 80 percent were self-identified victims of sexual or physical violence as a child.
- 65 percent had been placed in a special-education class at some point.
- 75 percent were high school dropouts.

It was dismal. If there was ever a set of numbers that spoke more plainly to the need for some alternative to warehousing people, I hadn't seen it. Even I was surprised that 80 percent said they had been abused in the past, and I was stunned that 90 percent had never had a legal job. These were incredible obstacles. If I thought about it for too long, I got depressed. I focused instead on designing a curriculum. With Skyline's approval, we started twelve basic classes. Writing, reading and math were among the basics. I also insisted on geography because many inmates had never been out of their neighborhood except to go to jail. We offered two levels of English as a second language; basic health education (which included information about drug addiction and sexually transmitted diseases); a class called Life Skills, which taught job interview fundamentals; and another on cultural awareness (which was elementary sociology and anthropology). These joined the auto mechanic and print shop I'd inherited, which taught vocational skills. Finally, the wild-card class I brought in was physics. When I was a remedial-class dummy, I liked the experiments my boyfriend Danny got to do in his physics class, and I figured some of the men and women wanted the challenge.

Just before we got the full slate of programs up and running, I made another decision. Classes in the San Francisco jails, and in many jails and prisons across the country, had always been voluntary. But after looking at the results of our assessment, I knew this population could not afford to opt out or they would be right back in our jails within months. So we made an announcement at a staff meeting, and then in the dorms: classes would be mandatory.

Leroy led another protest. That much I expected. The inmates really got into calling us dictators. But what I didn't expect was how much resistance I received from deputy sheriffs. For them, the problem was that any change that made the prisoners unhappy also made them unhappy. A deputy sheriff's job is to keep the peace and it's harder to do when the prisoners are pissed off. Most deputies predicted there would be riots if we made the men go to classes. Deputy Powers, who had practically begged me for classes, said I was crazy to try it. Lieutenant Hunsucker made a threat every time I saw him, whether we were in a meeting or out in the hallways. "Just you wait," he'd say with a sneer. "I pray I'm not on duty when you institute this disaster."

I received resistance from my own staff. Some of them thought it was unconstitutional—that we couldn't force the inmates to learn if they didn't want to. If any argument bothered me, it was that one. It seemed horribly narrow-minded. Every day in the jails, we strip-searched people, forced them to spread their cheeks, squat and cough, while a deputy sheriff inspected their anal cavity. None of the staff complained about the constitutional rights of inmates because of *that* security measure. But we couldn't force inmates to open a book and learn to read? We could only force them to do things that were humiliating? It made no sense. Others argued that it just wouldn't work. People who didn't want to learn couldn't be forced to learn. I told them to just wait and see.

Becky and Marcum were worried about riots. Marcum, as a former inmate, knew the inmate mind-set. Any new thing that they were told to do was often one new thing too many. But to anyone who questioned the program, and this included Becky and Marcum, I made a guarantee. I guaranteed that within three months the inmates wouldn't be complaining about the classes, they would be complaining about the lack of classes, and demand more.

After two months of mandatory classes, Lieutenant Hunsucker found me in my office. Just before the class policy changed, he had switched himself to the four-to-eleven swing watch shift so he wouldn't have to deal with the programs. I braced myself for another unpleasant exchange.

"Hey, Sunny, you got a minute?"

"Sure," I said eyeing him warily. Hunsucker had been a complicated character to deal with. By his own account, he'd left blood in every jail in the county before he'd come over to County Jail 7. He had started his career on Mainline, then went to maximum security with the hard-core felons, then over to Administrative Segregation, where everyone was on lockdown. He told me he hadn't intended to become hardened and cynical, it was just a survival mechanism. You cracked heads, and locked them up and went home for the day.

"I've got to tell you, everyone on swing watch has been talking about how the day shift's horrible. They're saying there's too much activity. And you have to know that I was saying the same thing." He'd told me as much on a dozen different occasions. I began to grit my teeth. I nodded at Hunsucker but didn't interrupt.

"Last week I substituted a few days on the day shift. I was prepared to blow a fucking gasket. But ya know what? And I really hate having to tell you this but . . . it was one of the best shifts I ever had. It was much simpler than what we face before those guys go to bed. During the day, the inmates are busy! When I get them, they've got downtime. They're always asking me for shit. I get no peace until lights-out." He was looking at his shoes the whole time. "I gotta give you some credit, Sunny. In the old jail, all I did was yell and curse at people all day. Then, I would go home and sit on the couch, drink beer and not talk to anyone. Last week, I talked to my wife, if you can believe it. I had a goddamn conversation with my wife." I kept nodding, feeling smug.

"And you know what, Sunny, deputies don't live into their retirement. I just found this out during salary negotiations. The union rep told me we all keel over from a heart attack before we ever get to sixty-five. I bet that's one reason our retirement fund is so goddamn rich." He now fixed me with a rueful smile. "I can't believe I'm saying this, but it's true. If this keeps up, I'm going to live longer working here. I'm switching back to the day shift."

After a year, County Jail 7 began to work as I wanted it to. We developed training for the staff, both sworn and civilian, so that they could run programs more effectively. We had outside consultants come in to evaluate our programs, look at their effectiveness and help us to improve. We had countless staff meetings where Marcum or

Becky or I talked about turning prisoners into taxpayers. A lot of this had knocked the deputy sheriffs and civilians out of their comfort zones. We were asking them to be role models for how to act in civilized society. Some had resisted, and we had transferred a bunch of them to new assignments, but the ones who stayed with us had, for the most part, embraced the new culture. We were investing in inmates' success rather than their failure. That was more or less our motto.

After a year, I could walk into a dorm and everyone was in a class, or doing work, or taking downtime. I rarely received grievances complaining about mandatory classes. Now the most frequent petition that inmates made was about classes they thought we should implement. Staff committees planned the music and TV schedule. During television period, from four P.M. to six P.M., we might play a *National Geographic* special, or *Oprah,* or reruns of *The Cosby Show.* The radio might be playing a Beethoven symphony. One prisoner, listening to a string quartet, yelled out, "Hey, what's with the shoplifting music!?"

It wasn't paradise. Men still fought one another over absolutely nothing. On a monthly basis, we would still confiscate shanks, and drugs, and pruno. But the jail was better than it had been before.

To take an antisocial institution and try to make it human was a never-ending war. The battles I won, I won because I had Marcum and Becky fighting with me. They were nervous about some of my schemes and I couldn't blame them. Marcum especially would catch heat if something blew up. But they both said yes even when they were scared, and no if they honestly believed it was a bad idea.

Leroy Clinton made all of our lives miserable while he was with us. He was a practicing Muslim, and many of the grievances he filed had to do with our alleged failure to respect his religious beliefs. During Ramadan, he demanded his food be served to him hot after sundown, which was well after our scheduled mealtime of 4:30 P.M. That request we tried to honor, but nothing we did was ever good enough. The food wasn't hot, he said, it was lukewarm. The time and space we allotted for his daily prayers weren't acceptable. He led hunger strikes in the dorm because we were bigots. He organized protests because

we were forcing them to rotate work schedules. He would write grievance letters about the water temperature, about not getting his mail on
time, about not having a jail uniform that fit his substantial girth. Over
and over, he would yell that "this is a violation of Title Fifteen and you
people should know better. We may be convicts but we have our
rights, too." Then, under his breath, he'd whisper, "Redneck mother-
fuckers."

Some days, I boiled at the mere mention of his name. But Marcum, Becky and I kept faith with our mission, to hand out effective
punishment. In some correctional institutions, Leroy would have
been dumped in solitary confinement and forgotten, until he had
grown so angry he would have taken out his rage on the next person
he could get his hands on. We took each of his grievances on its own
merits, and denied or honored each one after as fair a review as we
could muster. On occasion, this meant doing things for the prisoners
that some law-and-order types might consider coddling. For the jail
uniform issue, we sent a deputy out to a paint store to pick up an
XXXL orange jumpsuit.

But after Becky sat him down in the staff break room, slowly,
surely, the tenor of his protests changed. When I would go into Leroy's
dorm, he didn't barrel up to me. He would approach me calmly, and
hand me a page of suggestions about a class he thought should be
offered. We eventually allowed Leroy to organize men in his dorm to
do a presentation to at-risk boys and girls who were bused to the jail.
Leroy came to me afterward, excitedly proclaiming, "Sunny, Sunny,
we really got at those kids, man. I touched them. I really touched
them. I ain't jiving you, my hand to God. I felt something in there I
ain't never felt before."

The dorm deputies began reporting that Leroy was keeping more
to himself and writing. He was also getting routine visits from Reverend Billy Ware, a soft-spoken minister from San Francisco's Third
Baptist Church, who did rounds in the jails. Reverend Ware looked
out for everyone, not just the Baptists, and would gently remind us
of an upcoming holiday, be it Passover, Ramadan, or even Diwali, the
Hindu festival of lights. Leroy sought him out and Reverend Ware
became his mentor. Ware would stop by my office periodically and
tell me in a whisper, as if it were a secret, "Sunny, he's trying, and he's

struggling, but you really got to him, especially Lieutenant Benoit. She got to him. I think we'll see a different Leroy when he gets out."

After about a year, Leroy came to me. He was about to be shipped off to San Quentin. His trial date had come and gone and he'd been found guilty of selling cocaine, which was no surprise to him or anyone else. He received a three-year sentence. He'd already spent over a year with us awaiting trial, and with time off for good behavior, he had only another couple of months to go. He approached me when I was doing rounds and delivered a promise I had heard many times before from other prisoners on their way out the door.

"Sunny, God bless you. I'm gonna do better. I promise you that. I ain't coming back here. My hand to God, I ain't coming back."

As a legal intern, I'd heard this promise enough to be able to recite it in my sleep. Inevitably, I would encounter the man a month or a year later, after his arrest for another drug deal, or domestic violence incident. Many days in County Jail 7 I was filled with doubt, with worry and with rage over the jail and what wasn't getting done, the deputies who fought me at every turn, the inmates who lied and lied and lied. But something in Leroy felt real to me. I had to believe he could turn his life around. I had to believe that. There was no reason to do this work if I didn't. I shook Leroy's hand, wished him luck and walked off.

Change is difficult. How many of us have set out to get more exercise, watch less TV, or lose weight, and failed to do it? Men like Leroy have to go through changes so gut-wrenching it can be like tearing off limbs. They have to change who they hang out with, how they support themselves, where they live, and most of them have to kick a habit, too (90 percent are addicted to something). It takes pulling yourself apart piece by piece, and rebuilding yourself as a new person. But I knew it could be done. I knew it. If I ever found myself doubting it, all I had to do was look at my bar exam results, or at what happened with Leroy after he got out of San Quentin.

Ten months later, Marcum, Becky and I walked into the Third Baptist Church of San Francisco for Sunday morning services. Leroy had asked us to come. By all reports, he had kept on track at San Quentin, finished his sentence, and had been released on good behavior. Leroy Clinton was now here, apprenticing to be a preacher himself. None of us knew what had happened to his Muslim faith, but anything that kept him from dealing coke and boosting cars was something we could get behind.

We found room in a pew about two-thirds of the way from the back. There had to be about three hundred people in the church. It was pulsing with energy. Kids were running around, giggling. A gospel band was noodling around, waiting for the service to start. People came and filled in around us, pushing us to the middle of the row, and I grew anxious. Ever since I was a kid, Christian services had made me uncomfortable. It was the memories of the Pulaski brothers, taunting me in the playground about killing Jesus. I turned to Becky and said, "There is no way I'm going to kneel down."

"That's the Catholic church, Sun," she whispered. "Don't freak out. These are the Baptists. You can stand up whenever you want."

The choir started up, and the congregation joined in, full-throated. Everyone was clapping, the organist took a solo, and I tried to relax. We never got to move like this in temple. I could feel the surge of joy that moved through the people, and to me it was like a sudden rainstorm in the desert. Leroy was a test case for our jail. He had been one of the first inmates admitted into the program facility, and had probably come the most distance in the program, from angry rabble-rouser to advocate. He had natural skills that should serve him well. He was a born leader, not frightened of speaking out, and possessed a stubborn streak. If he failed, if he fell on his face, then, in some ways, our program was a failure. We were trying to institute a largely untested jail philosophy— create a humane atmosphere, give criminals some opportunities, make them responsible and accountable for their behavior, and some will turn around. But if a fighter like Leroy couldn't turn around, then I would have to rethink everything I was doing.

The preacher, Pastor Amos Brown, was giving a welcoming prayer. He had a bass drum of a voice, and was getting the congregation revved up. "We've got a new man here today," he roared. "He's seen the light. He's been to prison but today he is transformed. He's going to come up and preach to us this morning."

People said "Amen" all around us. Michael, Becky and I exchanged looks. What exactly were we going to get this morning? Marcum shrugged at me as if to say, Wait and see, Schwartzy, wait and see.

Leroy bounded to the podium, his unmistakable dreadlocks still framing his face. He looked dapper, having traded in his orange uniform for a coat and tie. He pulled out some note cards, placed them on the podium and took a moment to survey the crowd. His eyes flashed with the fire I remembered. Fire I always had a hard time reading. Was he angry, or glad? He cleared his throat and began. "I want to testify today, testify to my journey, how I got here. I want to testify today about my story. I was living in hell."

Leroy talked about how he had come up on the streets. How he and his friends had started stealing cars as a way to get by. "I wanted to get ahead, you know, and I didn't know any better, my dad was gone, my mom was high all the time. I thought I could take something for myself."

He said he had started selling coke, and had pimped a little even though he'd never been convicted for that. He said he knew how to be mean and tough in order to do his drug deals, to maintain his status, to be hard. He talked about how the cocaine he'd sold had destroyed lives. I looked around. The audience was paying attention. Leroy had the preacher's touch. The voice that I remembered so well, complaining and shouting and yelling, was now raised to witness, witness his sins.

The women fanning themselves were saying, "Amen, go on brother, we're with you." I was nodding with him, knowing a little about the sin of anger, the sin of violence and something about shame.

"But I have to say that I was *saved*." Leroy landed on this last word like a hammer on a nail. "I was saved. God came and saved me. And you know God is great, don't you?"

The congregation was picking up speed. More voices were raised in affirmation. "Yes, yes. Amen, brother."

"I need to tell you how I was saved." Leroy paused again, and he started in on the next part of the story. This part was about the police.

"You know the police have never been good to us." His voice was rising. He was catching fire now. "Some white folks really hate us. They hate us, they take our children and throw them in the backs of squad cars because they're black, throw them in prison because they're black."

"Yes, yes," the congregation yelled back.

"Now, I have always thought that the police are out to get us. They destroy us, they terrorize us in our communities."

At this point he had really gotten the crowd going. I was beginning to remember the Leroy of old, the pain in the ass, staging protests to piss off as many people as he could. My heart was pounding. I wanted to crawl under a pew.

"I got a new story to tell you." Leroy was working up to a climax. "I got something to say about the Sheriff's Department, and we got three members of the Sheriff's Department here with us today. We got three of the people that ran the jail where I was held sitting with us in the congregation."

Everyone turned in their seats and stared at us. Some seemed surprised; they hadn't seen us come in. And the heat from all that attention wasn't completely friendly. I represented, after all, a symbol of so much that had gone wrong in the black community. I looked at Michael, who had a hint of a smile on his face. He met my anxious gaze, and gave me a little nod. Why the hell was he so calm?

Leroy had taken the church with him on his journey, whipped them into a frenzy, and now he was going to shock them, as he was going to shock us.

"If it wasn't for the Sheriff's Department, and those three law enforcement members who are sitting among you today, I would be dead or on death row. My world has changed. I was saved. I was saved by the loving power of Jesus Christ, but he didn't come to me directly. He was working through the Sheriff's Department and was working through Becky Benoit, Sunny Schwartz and Michael Marcum. Because without them, without them, I would be dead. I wouldn't be with my children or my wife today if it wasn't for the Sheriff's Department. I wouldn't be standing here with you and working with the youth to help them get on the right path if it weren't for the Sheriff's Department. Those three people are my family. They worked with me when I was low, when I was down with Daniel in the lion's den. They never gave up on me when everyone else had left me for dead. They are here on a Sunday morning on their day off because God worked through them, my hand to God, he was there working in them. And I tell you, this is the law I am talking about. They are here and I love them and thank them from the bottom of my heart."

People were rocking and amening and clapping and staring back at us and smiling. The air was buzzing and my heart took flight. Here was a day to celebrate a man who had pulled himself up. I knew every day would be a test for him. The habits of criminality, once learned, are hard to break. But each day that he made it, he was living a good life.

CHAPTER 11

1992

There was a Jewish woman in County Jail 7, a Jewish woman besides myself, I mean. It wasn't too often that we got a member of the tribe in the slammer. I don't know why. The old corny Jewish joke doesn't really cut it. How come there are no Jews in jail? Because they eat lox. There were plenty of black folks and white folks who came through the jails, a big population of Latinos, even some Asians. But Jews, whatever the reason, were an anomaly, and I was curious about Tanya Horowitz.

I caught sight of her on rounds in Dorm F. She was a slight woman with dyed orange hair that looked like straw. Tanya's eyes, which were ringed by large dark circles, looked blank in the way writer Annie Dillard described cows, all stew back there. I watched her wander aimlessly through the dorm for half an hour. Then, Tanya's bunkmate said something under her breath, and in an instant, she found a different gear: rage. She lashed out, calling the woman a motherfucker and yelling, "Who do you think you are?" A shoving match started and the deputy and I rushed over to intervene. But Tanya's anger had no reserves. By the time we arrived, her energy was spent, and all I could see was stew again. She had disappeared again. Tanya looked like a lost child.

I approached her after the altercation, when she'd had a few minutes to herself. She seemed shell-shocked and fidgety, a sign her withdrawal hadn't fully set in yet. In a few more days, Tanya would probably be itching at coke bugs and climbing the walls, and might have to be sent to the infirmary to detox fully. I asked her how things were going.

"I got a baby in foster care, and I'm working to get her back," she told me. Her daughter, Trudy, was four years old. "Trudy needs me, you know, I'm her mother. But I failed a drug test so it's good I'm here." Tanya was gnawing at her thumb, which she'd chewed to a bloody stump. I didn't doubt her intentions, but I knew she had no sense of the obstacles she faced. She was addicted to heroin and crack, her dealer pimped her and beat her, and she had sold drugs herself.

Tanya had a college degree and had received her master's from the University of Southern California's creative writing department. That put her light years ahead of her fellow inmates, most of whom were reading at a fifth-grade level. But she kept complaining about the deputies, and all the rules in the program dorm, and how she was worried about people hustling her for her commissary credits. These were all warning signs. When you complain about the hustle too much, you're still in it. Both physically and mentally, Tanya seemed much worse off than many of the other women, and that meant she was in trouble, because the women's dorms were a disaster.

Other staff members or deputies would always fix me with a sad stare when they heard I was going to the women's dorms. "Spending time with the heathens, huh? Hope you survive." With the women, there was always something flaring up—an argument, a fight, a confrontation with the deputies. Someone was always complaining about how she missed her man even if he hit her, or how she couldn't get a job, or, most painfully, how she missed her kids. Small fights erupted constantly. Burnout among deputies assigned there was much higher than in the men's dorms. With the men, it was just quieter. They didn't ask for attention or melt down emotionally as much as the women did.

For the longest time, I couldn't explain why this was so. It seemed counterintuitive. Men were more violent, more advanced criminals on every level, and yet the women were far more difficult to manage, especially in the direct supervision dormitories of County Jail 7.

In many respects, the male and female populations were similar. Whatever their crimes were, 80 percent were addicts, and had been forced to go cold turkey by incarceration. In addition, many were survivors of abuse (sexual abuse was higher among the women, but the majority of both populations had suffered physical and/or sexual abuse as children). Women did have an added burden most men did not. Eighty-five percent of them were the sole providers for their children. But this did not explain why working in the women's dorms was so much harder than working in the men's.

I don't think it was because the women's needs were more profound, or because the men were better adjusted. The differences, I came to believe, had to do with gender, and specifically, how men and women dealt with their emotions. The men tended to bury their feelings. There was just no socially acceptable way for them to express the shame, humiliation and fear they felt about their situation. Men who did were sissies or punks. Working with the men was like working next to a boiler that was slowly building up pressure. It could be days or weeks or months before anything went wrong, but when it did, there was an explosion. Women had fewer emotional barriers. They blew off steam constantly; their emotions were on display all the time. Even with classes, the women's dorms were difficult places to be.

I caught up with Tanya a few weeks later and her eyes were clearer, there was a spark there. She told me she had started taking classes but she was bored and didn't like all the rules. "I just want to serve my time, you know, and get out. The more time I'm in here, the less time I get to spend trying to get Trudy back."

"Tanya, what's going to stop you from getting high once you're free?" I asked. "Nothing's stopped you yet."

"C'mon, Sunny, I'll figure it out. I can't get Trudy back if I'm using. I know that."

"You knew it before," I said. Tanya didn't reply. Her thumb went back to her mouth; she looked at her shoes. Tanya was in on a possession charge, which ran out after a few months. She made it for two months on the streets, then was processed back into our dorms, a typical retread, on a charge of possession with intent to distribute. When I saw her again, she was strung out, her hair now dyed green, and she desperately needed a bath.

"Cunning, baffling, powerful." That's a catchphrase in the recovery community for the struggles of addiction. It was on posters in our jail and since nine out of ten inmates had an addiction, it applied to almost everyone. In my first couple of years in charge of programs, fighting addiction was one of my top missions.

I started with the women mostly because they needed it more. We were going to start losing deputies if the women's dorms didn't calm down. But starting a program for women was not as simple as starting one for men. On the outside, there were plenty of successful addiction programs. These were "tough-love" programs that had been developed with men and their triggers in mind. The "therapeutic community" model was one of the more popular treatment programs. Depending on who ran it, it could be very confrontational, using a military mind-set almost like boot camp. Facilitators sought to break down the participants through ridicule and hostile confrontation. The theory was you had to destroy the old addictive personality in order to replace it with something healthier.

But there were few recovery programs that had been designed specifically for women. Nationwide, women's addiction had largely been ignored as a social issue until recently. This was due, in part, to the fact that women had only had a minor role in the criminal side of the country's drug problem until the 1980s, when get-tough-on-crime programs helped cause a spike in women's incarceration rates nationwide. Treatment programs lagged well behind men's programs. But thankfully, by the time Tanya came back for her second hitch with us in 1993, we had launched a program to address her needs.

We called it the SISTER Project, for Sisters in Sober Treatment Empowered by Recovery. The model was the therapeutic community, but the SISTER Project was designed by women for women. Where men tended to respond well to military discipline, women did not. The tough love in men's treatment programs too closely resembled the way women had been treated by abusive parents or partners. There were many similarities between the SISTER Project and Roads to Recovery, the men's program we set up six months later. Sure, the SISTER Project was a disciplined place to be, but there was less of an emphasis on hierarchy and more of an emphasis on sisterhood.

Tanya did not want to be moved into the SISTER dorm. "I just want to do my time," she insisted. "I don't like sitting in a group and talking about my problems." It was a universal reaction, true for men and women. I understood. Who likes sitting down in a group of total strangers and talking about her worst memories? But Tanya responded to our prodding, and early in her second hitch with us, was processed into the dorm.

For her first week there, she was a watcher, barely saying a word. She was assigned a big sister, a woman who had been in the program longer, but Tanya didn't talk much to her, either. The women participated in groups for large parts of the day under the guidance of a counselor. They sought to understand the individual triggers that led them to seek refuge in drugs, and build defense mechanisms against them. Time was set aside for journaling and individual meetings with counselors. A typical day was:

6 *A.M.* Breakfast

7 *A.M.* Acupuncture

8 *A.M.* Morning dorm meeting

8:30 *A.M.* Morning meeting for SISTER—positive announcements, awareness games, news and so on.

9 *A.M.* Women attended school (adult basic education or GED classes) and/or met individually with their counselors. They were also encouraged to take care of their needs and write letters to lawyers or their children.

11 *A.M.* Lunch

12–3 *P.M.* Recovery groups and relapse prevention, which looked at various issues, including triggers for addictive behavior and creating a safe environment for women to disclose their problems. Other issues covered during these times were parenting concerns, health education and dynamics in the dorm. Individuals were pulled out for more specialized groups such as survivors of sexual abuse, or family dynamics.

3 *P.M.* Quiet time on bunks. The women were encouraged to write in their journal (daily narratives were mandatory and the counselors reviewed them weekly).

5 *P.M.* Dinner

6 *P.M.* Cleanup

7–9 *P.M.* Therapeutic groups and special events

Tanya sat at the edge of her group all day long, barely in the circle, looking bored. She stared at the ceiling. I even saw her nodding off. Her group had some strong inmate leaders, three older women, who mothered the younger ones in the group. There were also four younger black women who had bonded over their love of their children and Michael Jordan. But Tanya kept to herself.

Michelle, Tanya's counselor, was a gruff New Yorker from Queens. She told me Tanya was in a critical stage. "She could go either way right now. She's still trying to decide whether to trust this. Just gotta hope and pray that she gives in."

After lunch one day, a new member of Tanya's circle spoke up. Shantell had only been in County Jail 7 for a week. She was a fair-skinned black woman with freckles framing a round face and looked to be in her twenties. Her features were almost childlike, but her voice sounded too old for her. She talked about being raped by her father when she was five years old. She was honest and angry and hurt and talked about how she blamed herself for her father's assault and had buried that guilt in heroin and relationships with vicious men who robbed her and pimped her and raped her. She was crying so hard her voice disappeared in wracking sobs. She had snot all over her face. A woman next to her took her hand.

At the beginning of her story, Tanya had been staring at the ceiling, fidgeting with the drawstring on her pants, a vacant look in her eyes. But as Shantell spoke, Tanya's fidgeting stopped, her eyes focused. When the woman finished, Tanya was leaning forward, her chin on her hands, tears streaming down her face.

If there was anything I'd learned by that point, it was that stories could bind broken people together, and help stitch up their wounds. Every time I listened to a disclosure, I felt hints of connection, a sense that the anger I had when I yelled at Becky because I was hurt or ashamed was something many people struggled with, criminals and citizens alike. Shantell that day kicked open a door for Tanya through her story. In the days that followed, Tanya edged her way into the circle. She started voicing some of the affirmations that every inmate in the recovery dorms was taught to use. "I want to use the group" or "I need all of your support" and the women in the group would respond in unison, "You got it." It can seem mechanical, the call and response. But it serves a purpose. These women had very little support on the outside and few communication skills. They needed the basics. So we taught them how to support people in group discussions. It's a first step in accepting a program, in agreeing to join the path to recovery. Tanya started on the journey with one step, saying, "I support you." She started to answer questions and engage in class sessions. Then, one Thursday afternoon, Tanya told her story.

The group started with the elders leading the way. A stocky Latino woman with a wide smile began. "We have a new sister joining us," she said, gesturing to a mousy woman who had just made it through orientation. "We welcome her here and support her with an open heart. Why don't we introduce ourselves."

The women went around the group saying their names. Tanya was staring at her hands. She was so quiet when her turn came that someone had to ask her to try again.

With the introductions finished, Michelle, our staff counselor, opened the floor. "This is the time to speak up, let people know what's on your mind, share the struggles you're going through." Michelle was all Mother Earth, her arms falling open as if she wanted to hug everyone there. Women leaped in with quick reflections. One asked the others to pray because her grandmother, who was taking care of her kids, was sick, and she didn't know what would happen if she didn't get better. Another woman shared a poem. Then Tanya spoke: "I want to use the group." Her voice was small.

"We're here for you," said the woman sitting next to Tanya. The others echoed her.

Tanya raised her eyes. She didn't look at anyone but she took a deep breath, held it, and then the dam broke. "I'm nine, I think. I don't remember anymore if I was nine or ten. It was just before Thanksgiving, I knew, because we had just come home from school with turkeys that you make out of hands. Where you trace the outline of your hand, and your thumb is the turkey's head." Some of the other women smiled.

"I'd done three of them. One for my mom, one for my little sister and one for my dad. I'd come home so proud, wanting to put them up on the refrigerator. It was also my birthday. Of course, it's easy to remember when it happened because of that. My birthday is just a few days before Thanksgiving. No one really wants to throw a party for you. They're so busy getting ready for the holidays, and you kind of get lost in all of that . . ." Tanya trailed off and looked around. There was a glimmer of fear in her eyes. I was worried she might stop, but she didn't.

"So I brought home these three turkey pictures as presents. I was thinking maybe if I gave presents then I would get great presents on my birthday. I don't know, I guess I was a big believer in karma or something." She smiled.

"I walk in from school and I'm all excited. I guess I knew my mom and dad fought a lot. But you know, I was nine. I didn't know what 'a lot' meant. I knew that I didn't like it when they fought. I'd find my mom crying. She'd have a black eye. When I asked her what happened she wouldn't answer me. She wouldn't lie about it; she just wouldn't look at me. The funny thing is I never saw him hit her. I don't remember ever seeing him hit her. I always hid in my room with my sister. You'd hear things banging. But I tried to put pillows over my head so I wouldn't hear it. Made it feel like it wasn't happening.

"When I walk in with these turkeys, sure enough, they're yelling at each other. He's yelling about my birthday cake, of all things. My dad is screaming, calling my mom lazy, and ugly—all sorts of stuff. He's saying how he'd just worked all day and she still hadn't picked up the cake. My mom looks horrible. She's just sitting in the kitchen with her purse in her lap, she's crying but not moving. Finally my dad calls her a lazy whore and slams the door to their room."

Tanya caught herself then, and a sob broke from her. The women around her murmured, "Go on, baby. You'll be all right." Tanya fought her emotions and finally regained her breath.

"It's like she was barely there. I started walking toward her but I stopped because I was afraid. I still had those goddamn turkeys in my hand. I just stood there like an idiot. Then my mom stood up and walked out. She didn't say anything to me. She didn't look at me. I ran to my room. That was the last time I saw her. She took off going to get my birthday cake."

Tanya was shaking. When she spoke again her voice came out clear and strong.

"I hate my birthday. I've hated it since that day. I thought that if I'd never had a birthday, that she wouldn't have left. I've replayed that scene again and again, imagining my saying something and getting her to stay. I kept telling myself if I just hadn't wanted presents and a party so much, then my parents wouldn't have fought and my mom would have stayed. I really was an idiot. I blamed myself that she left. I blamed myself for when my dad began hitting us. I blamed myself for when he started going to my sister's room at night. I blamed myself saying that if I'd just said something, anything, then maybe Mom wouldn't have left."

Tanya sobbed, finally giving way to anguish for a good long minute. A couple of other women in the group were crying, too. When Tanya continued, she told the group how she started drinking when she was eleven, sneaking liquor from her dad's cabinet. How she started shoplifting when she was thirteen. How the drinking turned to drugs, how recreational use turned to addiction. How she made it through college and wanted to be a screenwriter but finally the heroin took hold. She said her life was a slow, continual, downward slide.

"When I landed in the gutter, it was like I was supposed to be there. I didn't feel like something had gone horribly wrong, it was just the logical step from where I'd been the day before. I had friends in the gutter. It wasn't like I woke up and realized I shouldn't be there. It just seemed like where I belonged. And my boyfriend!" Now she sneers. "He's the father of my child, and he's the one that keeps me high!"

Other stories flooded out of Tanya, a jumbled collection of her life today. She talked about the shame she felt over going to jail and abandoning her daughter, Trudy, just as her mother had abandoned her. Tanya talked about the men who had abused her, the men she'd lied to and stolen from. "It scares me to death to say all of this out loud. I don't want to be here. I don't want to be telling this story. I've wanted for so long for it to just go away. For this story to be someone else's. But you know what. It's my life. It's my life. It's my life."

She finally ran out of words. As she finished, she sat up straighter, tension dissolved from her face. The woman in front of me said a quiet "Amen."

I thought about Tanya for the rest of the day. How many times had I heard a story like hers. These men and women we locked up, they are supposed to be the perpetrators, not the victims. And Tanya certainly was a perpetrator. I'd come to know her record well. She'd been involved in grand theft auto, home invasion and drug dealing. Her daughter had lived through her mother's three trips to jail. She'd been dropped off countless times with relatives, lived with a junkie mother who could barely take care of herself much less a child and been shuttled in and out of foster care. When I thought of what that child had been through I wanted to lock Tanya up and throw away the key. But Tanya had a story, too, a history of damage that fueled the damage she inflicted on her child. I despaired thinking about this long line of tragedy, like someone staring into a set of mirrors that faced each other, seeing her image reflected back on itself into infinity. How could you possibly stop it?

I felt lucky. My parents hadn't molested me, they'd worked hard and had provided a roof over my head, a home for me and my brothers. They fed me and loved me the way they knew how. But there were parts of Tanya's story that resonated with me. I could tell these women of my father's overwhelming temper, how I wished my mother could have stood up for me about my brothers' bullying, and the shame I felt being sent to the dumbest of the dummy classes, and how today, I couldn't stand it when lovers didn't agree with me. How I channeled my father when I fought with Becky. I could talk about how I had learned to focus my anger to a sharp point, and jab it until I felt I'd hurt her as much as she'd hurt me. I could talk to these women of the struggles I had and how I feel at home here.

Two years later, we gave Tanya a job. Karen, the point person in my office for women's issues, had an administrative position open. Tanya had been out and clean for eight months, and had just graduated from her postrelease halfway house. She had the most education—a master's degree in creative writing meant she was overqualified—and more basic skills than any other applicant. The only reason we wouldn't have hired her was because she was an ex-con.

I ran it by the sheriff to be sure he didn't have a problem. Hennessey gave me the go-ahead, saying it was a good example of us putting our money where our mouth was. I checked with Tanya's probation officer. The job would require Tanya to have some contact with prisoners, inmates with whom she might have done time. Probation departments don't like putting felons around other felons, believing it's like an alcoholic trying to work in a bar, but her probation officer thought this was a good opportunity and that Tanya wouldn't have any problems. We hired her.

Tanya was an extremely good writer, well organized, got all her tasks done on time. At first, she had attitude problems. She could be defiant, and questioned Karen's authority. Karen allowed her no wiggle room; she knew employers on the outside had to be pushed to hire ex-offenders. If an ex-con started questioning a boss's direction and their work assignments, they could quickly find themselves looking for another job. Still, Tanya's clashes with us were short-lived. She rarely questioned the same thing twice, and she learned from her mistakes. Within weeks, Karen and I were delegating critical work to her, asking her to write letters for grant requests and interdepartmental correspondence. She exceeded my expectations.

But not everyone was as happy as I was. I knew people would grumble. Some of the hard-line deputies still complained about Marcum being put in charge of a jail. For them, ex-cons couldn't be trusted, they shouldn't get a second chance, at least not in the jails. I knew this. But I was still shocked at how angry the responses were. Soon after we hired Tanya, I got a call from Undersheriff Frank Adams. Adams handled all labor issues in the department and I had always considered him an ally. He came from the private sector, not up from the ranks of the deputized staff, and he was a singularly smart and passionate civil servant. But I sometimes thought he was too slick for his own good. I'd first met him when I was a legal intern, and he liked to question my motives. "Hey Sunny, why do you advocate for this person so much?" he'd ask me. "Is she gay or something? Jewish maybe? She related somehow?" He never could believe I was working on general principle.

When he called me, he was coy about why. "Sunny, now why do you think I'm calling?" He barked at me over the line.

"Jesus, Frank, what is this, twenty questions?"

"The Deputy Sheriffs' Association is very upset with the Tanya Horowitz hire. You couldn't guess that?" Frank was the first to review complaints from the Deputy Sheriffs' Association, or DSA. It was a powerful union, and maintaining a working relationship with them was critical to keeping the jails running smoothly. I didn't like where this was going, so I played dumb.

"I'm not sure I get you, Frank. The DSA is angry that we hired an ex-offender to do secretarial work? Why?"

"Come on, Sunny, you know why."

"No, I don't. You're gonna have to explain it to me."

"Sunny, the deputies are offended that they have to eat in the same lunchroom with a former inmate they supervised a year ago. You need to think about who you hire and bring into this department. The DSA has their code of honor, too, ya know."

I tried to explain to Frank that our sole mission with programs was to get prisoners to enter the workforce as functional citizens. "The deputies ought to know this," I said.

"Cut the crap, Sunny. It's about respect. You're telling these deputies you think they're no better than the inmates they've got locked up when you send one of them into their lunchroom to eat with them. This shouldn't be a surprise to you."

I was furious. "Frank, tell me, would you and the deputies rather have me fire Tanya Horowitz so she can collect welfare and start acting like a real ex-con? You want me to hand her a few syringes with her pink slip so she can get a head start on the whole thing? What's wrong with you? Right now, people ought to be happy for Tanya. She came in and earned herself a job from the people who locked her up. That takes guts."

"Well, don't blame me," Frank yelled back at me. "The deputy sheriffs are mad, they might file a grievance, and I would have to respond to—"

I was shaking by this point, screaming into the phone like a howler monkey. "Fuck them," I yelled. "Let them file a grievance. I'd love to read it. Nothing would expose their twisted priorities more. I would love to personally represent the department on this one if you're so worried about it!"

At that point Frank pivoted, and tried to give me an inch. "Look, here's a compromise. Let's just limit Tanya Horowitz's clearance to the administrative offices instead of giving her full access." This would mean that in addition to not being allowed into the prisoner areas, which was no big deal, she also would have been forbidden access to the staff lunchroom. The offer was insulting. It would have hung a scarlet letter on Tanya.

"Forget it, Frank, you should know better. Separate is not equal. Is this coming from the sheriff?"

"No," Frank said, which was a relief. If Hennessey didn't have my back on this, I was the one in trouble. But knowing it was just Frank, I felt okay finishing it off. "Tell the deputies to go fuck themselves and I'll see them in court!"

I called the sheriff as soon as I got off the phone with Frank. Hennessey didn't skip a beat. "Hey Sunny, you did the right thing by hiring her," he told me. "And listen, if anyone else complains, you tell them this story." Hennessey went on to tell me a parable. It was an old Russian fable. "A farmer finds a genie in a bottle," he said. "The genie offers the farmer one wish. The farmer was a poor man barely able to get by. The farmer thinks for a minute and says, 'My neighbor has a cow, and I have none. Therefore what I want you to do is kill my neighbor's cow!'"

"You think that story will work?" I laughed.

"I don't know, Sunny. It should. Say hi to Tanya for me while you're at it." I loved the man. If he had been in the room with me I'd have given him a big wet one.

The deputies never did file a grievance. I guess they realized how ugly it would look on paper. But many found other ways to send their message. Many wouldn't talk to her, wouldn't even look at her. And it turned out it wasn't just deputies who were angry. Even some of the civilian staff treated her with thinly disguised disdain. The shop manager for their union, a lifer in the department named Harold, complained to me that hiring Tanya "cheapened all of their jobs."

"Look, people are complaining," Harold told me. "These are people with master's degrees. They're professionals. You're asking them to be on the same level as an addict who just got out." I tried telling him Hennessey's story about the cow. Harold didn't get it.

One day, I was out doing rounds at County Jail 2, which was in the Hall of Justice. We were introducing some classes over there, and I was going to meet with the staff. When I walked in, a colleague of mine approached me with a concerned look on her face and placed a flyer in my hands. It had Tanya's mug shot on it and typed underneath was this message:

Meet your new co-worker.
Employee of the month.
She will deliver good tricks and treats whenever you want!
Make sure to welcome her!

"Sunny," my colleague said, "this was faxed here today. I think you ought to know about it." It was a prank, a stupid prank pulled by a bully. Then I saw that it had been faxed from the Sheriff's Work Alternative Program office, which was across the street from the Hall of Justice. I walked right over there spitting fire to find out who sent it. Alternative Program had some of the more progressive postrelease programs and staff members in the Sheriff's Department. The deputies and civilians there all functioned a little like social workers, helping inmates make the difficult transition into the world after their release. It was supposedly a place of tolerant thinking. Marcum and I, who oversaw the site, made sure to bring in deputies who enjoyed working with the inmates, who didn't believe they were trash.

If I've learned anything about bullies, whether it was bullies in my family, bullies who were inmates in the jail, or bullies who were deputies, it's that the story was never just black and white. Few people were ever just the bad guy. When I walked into the Alternative Program office, the person who had made the flyer approached me immediately to apologize. I didn't have to issue threats or do an investigation. He looked up, saw me with the flyer in my hand and came right over. He was a deputy sheriff named Jamie Perez, a quiet, gentle guy who had worked with us at County Jail 7 in the past. I'd always thought of him as a deputy who cared, who tried to do the right thing by the inmates, was tough where he needed to be, but not malicious. We went to a private room.

"Why, Jamie? I don't get it."

"I don't know, Sunny." He looked deflated. "A bunch of us were sitting around talking about Tanya Horowitz being hired and some of the deputies were really mad. I thought I'd make up something to get them to lighten up and laugh about it."

"Jamie, I'm hurt by this. Do you know how awful something like this would be to Tanya if she saw it?"

"Has she seen it?" He looked pained.

"I'm not sure, Jamie. I haven't been back to the office yet, but I sure wouldn't show it to her. I got to tell you, Tanya Horowitz is having a hard time. How do you think she feels every day coming to work with this kind of crap going around? What did she ever do to you?" Jamie started crying.

He was shook up, saying over and over, "Sunny, I don't know why I did it. I am so sorry. This is not me. I loved working with you and Marcum and Benoit. I loved working at the program facility."

I believed him, too. Deputies usually didn't cry.

"What should I do?" he asked.

"What do you want to do?" He thought for a second, then said that he wanted to take the lead and apologize to Tanya himself.

Jamie told me he had faxed the flyer to a couple of the jails in the system. Some people had probably thrown it out. I heard it had been distributed in a few places. I tried to send out the message that I wanted it destroyed, but it probably made the rounds anyway. Part of me wanted to find a way to humiliate Jamie, the same way he had tried to humiliate Tanya. But I resisted the feeling, trying to treat Jamie the way I would have treated an inmate who was trying to make amends. I didn't want to excuse his behavior, but I also wanted to try to give him a chance to make it right. I told him I'd push for a write-up in his file and he said that was fair. He told me that he would apologize to Tanya, and that he would also raise the issue with the other deputies who had egged him on to make the flyer. He accomplished the second part long before he accomplished the first. His supervisor reported to me that week that they'd had a meeting about the flyer and that Jamie had made good on his promise. His apology to Tanya took longer. He never sought her out. But he did run across her a few months later and apologized.

Tanya never saw the flyer and when we talked about it, she said she didn't want to. She told me that the day-to-day cold shoulders from the people in our office were worse than a prank from someone she didn't know.

"I feel like a marked woman some days. Like I'll never be able to live down my past no matter what I do. People won't talk to me, you know. It's like I'm back in the eighth grade and the cool kids have decided to freeze me out."

It was hard to miss the toll this was taking on her. On days when it was bad, her shoulders would slump, she would walk the halls staring at her shoes, avoiding eye contact with anyone. I would ask her to go to the lunchroom, but she'd make any excuse not to go with me. I asked her what she wanted to do and she smiled.

"Sunny, this is part of my recovery right now. I need to learn to not feel ashamed no matter what other people say or do. There are a lot of good people here. They helped pull me out of the gutter. There are assholes everywhere."

In that moment, I knew Tanya was going to make it. I just had a feeling. Two years later, after being clean and sober since her release, Tanya won back custody of her daughter, Trudy. The girl grew up to attend the University of California at Santa Barbara.

CHAPTER 12

1994

I had closed the door to my office and for a day and a half had looked through custody cards. We had one for every prisoner in County Jail 7. Each card had a photo, contact information and a list of priors. I was also going through intake interviews. In them the prisoners were asked about past crimes and past violence and often revealed incidents that weren't on their rap sheets. I was going through everything because I was stubborn. Our violence numbers had been dropping at the jail. When County Jail 7 had opened, our numbers had been about even with the other jails in the system. In those early days, we had about five violent incidents per week. After our programs got rolling, the numbers had dropped to about three violent incidents per week. I'd touted the numbers to the sheriff to show that we were on to something. But I kept hearing excuses undermining our results. People thought we were getting the easy criminals, the small-time guys who wanted to go to class and weren't violent to begin with.

"These results aren't a fair comparison," one watch commander said to me. "We have to deal with the thugs who won't go to school."

"Bullshit," I shot back. I knew we didn't select our prisoners. We did take the people who wanted programs, but about half our prisoners came to us randomly. People didn't want to admit that the programs were working. I wanted to prove them wrong.

I went through almost five hundred custody cards and intake interviews in two days. I reviewed the information we had on the current prisoners as well as any who had been released in the last six months. Marcum came in and laughed at me on the second afternoon.

"Is this really a good use of your time, Sunshine?"

I scowled. "Look." I showed him the chart I was keeping. "We're completely right. We have the same number of bad guys as the rest of the system. We've got the same number of robberies, assaults, assaults with a deadly weapon. The same number of addicts. It's all the same. It's not that we're getting the choirboys, the jail is making the difference."

Marcum looked at my pages of scribbled numbers, then back at me. "Can you stop now?"

"I dunno, Marcum, there are some things I'm seeing in here." I showed him a second page. "I started to keep a list of violent crimes. How many people are in here on a violent arrest or have a violent incident in their past."

"Okay."

"They're all men."

"Okay." He wasn't impressed. I wasn't saying anything surprising. Conventional wisdom said men perpetrated the vast majority of violent crimes.

"No, I mean, they're *all* men. Sure, occasionally you've got a woman in here who got into a fight in a bar. Or someone who was beating her children, but it's this tiny number. These women . . ." I held up a stack of custody cards for the female inmates. "It's all dealing, or prostitution, a few robberies. I've been going through this stuff and something like eighty percent of the men have some violent crime in their past—a fight, an assault, something. Who do you think they're beating up? Women mostly, their wives, people like Tanya, or their kids, who then grow up to do drugs or join gangs or—"

"Sunny," Marcum interrupted me. "This isn't exactly a headline."

"I know, Marcum. I'm just depressed, I guess. I feel like we've got this war going on. All these men are at war. They're angry and ashamed, and is getting them off drugs, or teaching them how to read really going to do anything?"

"What are you talking about, Sun?"

"How are they going to stop being violent?"

We both sat there. Neither of us had an answer.

*   *   *

Stevie was talking to me. Where were we? New Mexico? Somewhere
in Oklahoma? All I could see out the car window was big, open, starry
sky, headlight glow and blackness.

"Let's say a bear is caught in a trap, and you came across it in the
forest," Stevie was saying. "This is a big, mean, angry bear. It's been
there long enough to go crazy with pain. What would you do?"

"Stevie, I don't know. Listen, where are we?"

Stevie didn't answer me. It was like he was a mile away in the
driver's seat. I got the impression he didn't even hear me. He repeated
his question.

"If a bear is caught in a trap. And you're the only one that can free
it. What would you do?"

He could be so frustrating! I needed to know where we were. It
suddenly seemed incredibly important. I could see the car leaping forward into the darkness and I was afraid that the road might end in an
instant, that we might pitch off a cliff, that a brick wall might materi-
alize in front of us. The dark became more and more impenetrable
until it seemed like the world disappeared.

"C'mon, Chubs, answer the question. A bear, a trap, it's up to you."

I hated it when he called me Chubs. I was annoyed that he wasn't
listening to me, he wasn't worried about the road, he just wanted to
know about the bear. Free the bear and risk having it turn on me, or
leave it there in agony and walk away. I felt trapped.

"Damn it, Stevie, I don't know, I don't know."

"Answer it, Sun, just answer the question."

"Free the bear, I guess. I'd free the bear."

"Why?"

I racked my brain. I wanted to say something smart but I just felt
dumb. Finally, I came up with something.

"Because I'd feel too guilty if I walked away."

Stevie nodded slowly. "But he might eat you if you free him. Big,
mean bear, you know, how long has he been in the trap? He's hungry."

"I know, Stevie, I know. I would just feel too guilty." Stevie didn't
say anything for a few seconds. Then he grinned at me.

"Good. That's a good answer." I flushed, suddenly happy. Stevie
reached over to turn on the radio. For a split second the world melted.
I heard a morning report. There was traffic on the Bay Bridge. A

pileup near Berkeley. I pried open my eyes. My arm spastically sought the alarm clock.

Stevie. He snuck up on me sometimes. I sat up in bed. Becky was already gone, off to do a check on the morning shift. I reached over and opened the journal I kept next to my bed. I'd been writing my dreams down on orders from my therapist. Stevie didn't show up much. I felt a pang as I scribbled down the details. I remembered we'd had a conversation about a bear caught in a trap somewhere on the road between Chicago and Tucson twenty-five years ago.

It had been seven years since Stevie killed himself, and seven years since my brain sprang a leak. After Stevie's death, my family had broken—my parents clinging to each other while Jerry disappeared into his Orthodox Jewish community in Brooklyn, and I constantly disappointed them all by not doing "what I was born to do," get married and have a family. In the intervening years, my mom had been stricken with uterine cancer. She had fought it and beaten it twice, but she was a shadow of herself and so was my father, who was devastated by his wife's pain. I had tried to forge my own path, and seven years ago, changed my life. I'd walked away from being an attorney and gone back to the jails hoping to move mountains.

Five years I'd been at it, toiling away in my small corner, fighting and fighting and fighting, trying to get the money for my programs, trying to give the prisoners a chance to become better people. I'd fielded the question hundreds, maybe thousands of times: "Why do you want to help *those* people?" And my answer was always the same. I didn't want to help *those* people, or at least, not just those people. I wanted our community to be safer, I wanted to banish fear and violence, and the only way to do that, it seemed to me, was to work with the people causing the fear and violence, to try to get them to do something different.

I was proud of the changes Marcum, Becky and I had been able to make in San Francisco's jails. We had adult education and high school proficiency classes available for 362 inmates daily. We had addiction programs both in the jails and out in the communities for inmates after their release. Deputy sheriffs came up to me regularly to say that working in County Jail 7 was easier on their psyches, that they were learning something and felt better when they went home at night.

There were inmates like Leroy and Tanya who'd walked away from their demons, walked away from crime and now lived like everybody else, making a paycheck, paying taxes and contributing. But I was bone tired and frustrated. The two days I'd spent reviewing our prisoners' records had depressed me. We were making the jails better for us, and nominally better for the inmates, but increasingly I was beginning to feel like I was missing something, like there was something out in the darkness, like the cliff was coming and I was a big angry bear stuck in the passenger seat needing to escape.

There was a joke we made in the dark moments in the staff room. It happened when we were talking about a prisoner who was doing well in his classes but still fighting in the dorms, and basically a bully. "Look," someone would say, full of sarcasm, "we taught him to read. Let's put up a sign to tell him to stop beating his wife." The joke had always grated on me, but it had begun to feel like an admission of failure. Our jails were full of violent men and none of our programs confronted their violence head-on. O.J. Simpson and the murders of Nicole Simpson and Ron Goldman had just hit the news and it felt like a message. Regardless of his guilt or innocence, it was indisputable that Simpson had beaten his wife and that it had been an ongoing problem. I'd seen the pattern again and again in our inmates. I'd met thousands of these men, and no addiction prevention class or English class in any jail or prison I'd ever seen addressed the issue of a man's violence.

I was frustrated. I was frustrated at work, and also frustrated at home. Becky and I argued nonstop, and it felt connected. The violence I despaired over in the prisoners resonated with me. I wasn't physically violent, but I was an emotional bully just like my dad. When Becky didn't agree with me I could be brutal, screaming and yelling, stomping out of rooms, going completely out of control. I wasn't the same as the men I worked with, but I knew it was still a form of abuse. Becky was a fighter as well, which made for a toxic mix. She would accuse me of being a flirt, I'd accuse her of not being emotionally present. We could build these sparks into giant infernos. The programs at County Jail 7 were the only things that we didn't fight about.

The dream about Stevie distracted me. That morning, I was supposed to be packing a bag and going to Minneapolis for a conference for prison education providers. To tell the truth, I was relieved to be skipping town for a few days.

The cabbie started honking at me. When I finally got outside he glared at me and said, "I'm just about to leave. You keep me waiting so long."

I snarled back, "You want this fucking fare or not, tough guy, 'cause I can call someone else." I slammed the trunk of the car. I knew why I was having the dream. I knew why Stevie was there asking me what I would do about an angry bear. I was the bear.

The conference was one of those burned coffee, plastic pastry, bureaucratic circle jerks where you talk about what you're doing well, you complain about things that never seemed to change, you see some friends you made at the last conference, and you bill it all to the county. My mother, Frieda, would've said, "Well, they meant well," and then fallen silent.

The prison-services community was a ragtag mix of aging hippies who were still fighting the Man, clock-punchers who'd decided that the prison-industrial complex was a dependable paycheck, along with true believers, brilliant fighters and incompetent airheads. This time around, the main thing people were talking about was getting out of the conference and going over to the Mall of America. In the industry exhibits, I sidled up to a table hawking books for convicts. They looked like Dick and Jane stories and I was thinking, what self-respecting convict was going to sit and read this without getting his ass kicked? I began scheming ways to get home.

At lunch on the second day, I sat down with Shannon, a vibrant, bighearted woman who ran programs in the Contra Costa County jails just northeast of San Francisco. We compared notes sometimes. She didn't have many allies in her county. She had to fight for every last scrap and didn't have as extensive a set of programs as we did in San Francisco. But she paid attention to what was new. She asked me what workshop I had attended that morning. Between mouthfuls of rubbery chicken, I told her the guy leading the group on mandatory drug testing seemed like he had dropped two Valiums.

"I know it might sound crazy," Shannon replied, "but I really found my morning session invigorating. You should look at this stuff." Shannon handed over a packet of information. I'd never seen her so excited. I was used to her usual "this is a bunch a of bullshit" response.

"It's about this thing called 'restorative justice,'" Shannon said. "I'd never heard about it. You should read it."

The packet was titled *Understanding Restorative Justice.* The name alone piqued my interest. Nothing I'd seen in the criminal justice system had ever been in the business of "restoring" anything. I'd seen crimes committed, I'd seen people punished, lives and families ruined, but never restoration. The author of the packet (and the person who had given the presentation) was a woman named Kay Pranis. I would later learn that she was considered the mother of restorative justice and had been working to spread its principles for years. I flipped open the packet and read. "Restorative Justice recognizes that crimes hurt everyone: victim, offender and the community and it creates an obligation to make things right. The 3 principles of restorative justice are offender accountability, victim restoration and community involvement to heal the harm caused by crime."

Restorative justice didn't have many real-world examples in the United States. Some jurisdictions were supporting mediation sessions between victims and perpetrators. I'd heard about this. Studies showed that victims wanted to hear their perpetrators express authentice remorse, and just as important, wanted to let that person know how much they'd hurt them. But these kinds of confrontations were delicate and not for everyone and not solely what restorative justice was about. The goal of restorative justice was to heal the victims, for perpetrators to take responsibility for their actions and make meaningful restitution and for governments and communities to be part of the process. There were many ways these principles could be put into practice and they spoke to me on such a visceral level that I packed my bags and immediately went to the airport. I called Marcum to tell him I was coming home early. I had a new program to sell.

Most people, I think, believe that prison or jail should be a horrible experience. People don't think of it as a deterrent so much as just deserts. "They" hurt "us," therefore "we" should hurt "them." For years, politicians have won elections by promising to take away cable television and weight rooms and anything seen to make prison cushy. We have a culture where jokes about prison rape are made out in the open. The prevailing wisdom is that prisoners deserve to be treated like animals; they should fear prison and suffer while they are there. Anyone who has spent time working with prisoners knows this has largely come to pass. What most people don't realize is the consequences of making prisons a living nightmare. Most of the inmates I'd worked with, particularly when I was a law intern, felt punished, but not many of them took responsibility for their crimes, or felt any remorse. Martin Aguerro, the pedophile, the first client I had when I started in 1980, was a case in point. He complained about the squalid treatment and living conditions in jail, he felt wronged, but I never got the sense that he thought about his crimes. In fact, everything about the system of prosecution and defense is set up so that criminals get into a habit of *denying* their responsibility. Every step of the way between the arrest and the trial, people accused of crimes deny everything, or keep silent. It's what their defense attorneys tell them to do. After their trial, if they're convicted, many don't change their mind-set. Why should they? To truly confront what they've done requires confronting the shame and fear and the reality of their situation. Few people choose to do this, because it's difficult. After all, it's hard for noncriminals to take responsibility for doing the wrong thing, much less someone sitting in a prison cell. So criminals blame someone or something else—the cop who caught them, or their lousy upbringing—for their circumstances and spend their time growing angrier and angrier about being treated like an animal. They are usually full of rage when they are released, and less prepared to function as citizens; the predictable products of the monster factory.

But what if that paradigm could be shifted? Restorative justice puts a premium on getting prisoners to confront the harm they've caused, and underscores both their accountability and their potential. Was it possible to bring these principles into our jails? I started writing down ideas on the airplane.

I wanted a new program for the worst men we had locked up, the violent offenders who inflicted the most damage on our communities: the wife beaters, murderers and gangbangers. I modeled it after our SISTER Project. We would create a whole dorm of men brought together to stop their violence. I set the criteria as broadly as possible. I wanted to admit roughly 50 percent domestic violence offenders, and 50 percent random violence offenders, which mimicked the population breakdown in our jails. I didn't care if we got first-time offenders or offenders who had violence in their background, and I didn't care if they volunteered for the program or we told them they had to participate. I wanted to throw the net wide, and collect as many violent men as we could.

If I really started thinking about what I was proposing, I probably would have given up. No one wanted to begin a project with an advisory planning group made up of religious leaders, victims' rights groups, deputies, probation officers, business leaders, someone from the district attorney's office, the police department, housewives, victims of violence, perpetrators of violence, Republicans and Democrats. But that's exactly what I wanted to do. I wanted to bring the Hatfields and the McCoys together to work out their differences. But I knew that if these groups weren't on board at the beginning, than someone could object later on and sink the project.

I was in Marcum's office by the end of the day. He laughed when he saw me steam in. "I see our Sunny has really got something to tell me." I had a terrible poker face, Marcum had a good one, and he gave it to me as I told him my idea.

"Marcum, listen to me, this is it." I handed him the restorative justice handout. "This is the Kabbalah, this is the key to the criminal justice universe." I led him through the packet, the principles of restorative justice, and then to the idea, a dorm full of violent men working to stop their violence. Marcum's eyebrows shot up.

"Schwartz, Schwartz, ya got to slow down with this." I was trying to turn the pages of the packet for him. I wanted to start this yesterday. He voiced some objections, but he didn't say no. I had to hand it to the guy. Most people I knew in criminal justice would have laughed me out of the office. He brought Becky in to sound her out.

"Wow," she said when I finished. "We can do this." I knew she'd like it. It was one of the reasons we were still together. When it came to programs, we almost always saw eye to eye. Still, she was like Marcum, more pragmatic.

"Ya know, Sun," Becky said, "I think we should start with a small group of people, maybe fifteen or twenty." This was exactly what Marcum had said. "I think we should give it a chance to start. No one puts all violent offenders in a single dorm. You know that. That's a recipe for a riot."

I did know that. It was one of the cardinal rules of jail and prison management. No one put violent people together. You spread them across the general population, where you can isolate them and keep a lid on their violent tendencies. But I knew in my gut that we could do it differently. We've changed every other rule in this place, why not this one?

"Come on, Marcum, don't be a pencil dick." Marcum smirked but didn't lose his poker face. "We can't piecemeal this. We have to get the entire dorm invested in dramatic behavior change."

It went on like this, me questioning Marcum's manhood, Marcum offering cautious resistance, Becky laughing in the corner but agreeing with Marcum until finally I had worn them both down.

"Okay, okay, Sunny, I give up. Let's go after a full dorm, but first things first. We need Hennessey. An idea as nuts as this . . . and that's not to say this is a bad idea." Here he winked at me. "An idea like this needs friends. Hennessey is going to blow a gasket if we're not careful."

In order to green-light this, Hennessey was going to have to go way out on a limb. If something went wrong, there would be public outrage, which is never good for a politician who depends on the voters to keep his job.

A week later, Marcum, Hennessey, and I sat down with the sheriff at Liverpool Lil's, a classic San Francisco bar and restaurant. We sat outside, looking out over Presidio Park. A line of tall trees framed our vision, and they were gently swaying in the breeze. I was happy for the peaceful setting. I wound up to it slowly, asking Hennessey to keep an open mind (which he knew was code for "please be ready to take a really big risk"). I gave him the rundown of my experience in Minnesota, how the lightbulb came on, and I showed him the pamphlet. He looked at it for five full minutes before saying anything.

"So, Schwartz, what do you have in mind?"

"I want to start a violence prevention program, and work with violent offenders using the principles of restorative justice. I want to model it after the SISTER Project and the men's addiction program

Roads to Recovery. That means a full dorm of men committed to stopping their violence using a curriculum that we'll design."

Hennessey didn't flip out, God bless him. But he looked wary.

"Gee, Sunny, that's a little risky." He looked at Marcum and said what everyone else had said: "What about riots?"

"There won't be riots, Hennessey," I said, and crossed my fingers. "We will plan this to within an inch of its life. We won't be doing some ding-dong hippie stuff with these guys."

Hennessey asked his follow-up questions, and then fell quiet as he looked at the sky. I could tell that part of him wanted to just say no, and go back to the problems he already had. But I knew Hennessey. I knew that he wanted to shoot for the moon if he could. He wouldn't have let Marcum and me anywhere near a jail if he was just a cautious politician. He still believed in doing the right thing. After what felt like an eternity he finally responded.

"Show me a budget and a working plan when you've got it. I need to be involved in this from start to finish. Tell me again there aren't going to be riots."

"There aren't going to be riots," I replied. In the fifteen years that I'd spent in the criminal justice system, working with prisoners as an advocate, as a lawyer and as an administrator, I was never less sure of a promise I'd made, and had never been more dedicated to making it true. I could see a thin thread stretching from that restaurant overlooking the Presidio back through my life. It wove through each moment of anger and rage, through every fight I had with Becky, through Stevie's suicide, to the moment I was almost attacked in the Queens' Tank, to the first walk I took down Mainline, back through my relationships with my father and my mother and the monster Richard Speck. Violence and rage and fear had given my life its warp and woof. For the first time, it felt like I could reach out and grab that thread, and give it a tug.

That didn't mean I wasn't scared.

CHAPTER 13

1995

Marcum was pacing again. I was sure he was going to cut a groove into the rug around my desk.

"Are you sure we should invite them?" he asked. "I really don't want a war before we even begin."

"Faith, Marcum, you have to have some faith." We had the same conversation every few days. Our first planning meeting was coming up. Marcum told me I was throwing a lit match on a pile of fireworks. The issue was the guest list. I had invited everyone I could think of who had a stake in violence in our communities. This included ex-offenders: Leroy, who was still a preacher and working with at-risk youths, and a former gang member named Hussein who did similar work. Then there were Jean O'Hara and Kathy Lawrence, who were members of Survivors of Murder Victims, a group that fought for families of victims to have a bigger voice in the criminal justice process. Jean and Kathy were also mothers whose children had been murdered. I had also invited Latino activists, African-American goups, gay rights activists, deputy sheriffs, probation officers, a Baptist minister, an Orthodox rabbi and social workers who ran a battered women's shelter. I wanted everyone on the board.

"Just listen, Sunny, we have to have a plan," Marcum went on. "What if Leroy says something about how these prisoners just need a break? What if he goes on a tear about the racist prison system? How do you think the folks from the victims' rights organizations will react? If a former gangbanger says that all these 'poor kids' need is some love and a job, Jean O'Hara might walk out." I sighed. I knew these arguments. I knew I was playing with fire. But what was the alternative? I was wading into one of the most explosive political debates of the last twenty-five years. You had to take chances.

The rules change when you decide to work with violent offenders. I didn't have to be a rocket scientist to know that. I only had to look at the headlines. Back in 1993, twelve-year-old Polly Klaas was abducted from her home in Petaluma, California, and murdered by Richard Allen Davis, a repeat sexual offender who was out on parole. The case was a media event for weeks, blanketing papers across the country. A year later, in 1994, the Klaas case helped convince the California public to vote for Proposition 184, otherwise known as the "Three Strikes and You're Out" law. This law enforced strict sentencing guidelines by which offenders could receive a life sentence after a third felony (regardless of whether or not it was violent). The result was a jump in life sentences for people who had committed relatively minor crimes for their third strike, such as stealing a drill from Sears, or possessing .05 of a gram of heroin, or filling out a false DMV application. In the eighties and nineties, similar tough-on-crime laws had been enacted all across the country. There wasn't room for politicians to enact programs *for* violent offenders unless they were ready to be accused of being weak on crime.

We had been able to get the SISTER Project and Roads up and running in three months and five months, respectively, largely because they were touted as programs for addicts. But with violent offenders the stakes were higher. Sheriff Hennessey would be blamed if our program sparked a riot or if anyone got out and committed murder. In fact, politically speaking, the program was all risk. No headlines would trumpet how many crimes we might avert. But I knew in my heart we had to do it this way, and I believed that I could keep our planning committee meetings civil and successful.

I had the mothers on my side.

After getting the okay from Hennessey, I'd done my homework, searching out all restorative justice projects in the country. The concept itself was thousands of years old. Long before there were courts and laws, communities had come together to police social norms, and figure out ways to "restore" the harm done by people who had caused injury. But as laws developed, particularly in the West, crimes came to be seen as offenses against the "state" rather than the community. In the United States, restorative justice practices had only started to come into vogue in the 1970s. There weren't many places trying to use them. One of the best I'd found was in Genesee County, New York. Genesee County's Sheriff's Office had had a restorative justice program in place since 1981 under which they had pursued alternative forms of punishment beside prison. They had successfully diverted hundreds of criminals into community service, and had set up numerous mediation sessions between perpetrators and their victims.

As part of their program, Genesee County had sought advice from the community on what to do differently. One group of people they'd turned to was mothers whose children had been murdered. I was able to get my hands on a packet of the letters the mothers sent back. They came from many different kinds of women—rich and poor, black and white, college graduates and high school dropouts—but they all spoke in one clear, searing voice. Each mother was writing about the worst thing that had ever happened to her. Every letter was heartbreaking. "My son was murdered by his friend," one letter started:

> Because of that, we lost two young men to violence. My son is dead and buried and will never be here again, and his friend who killed him will forever be in prison and is dead to many. They were "goofing around" and it got out of control. What started out as a joke turned tragic and the madness will never stop until we come together to help bring peace and sanity to our community. I make a plea to the other parents: talk to your children. I make a plea to the police: intervene, set an example. I make a plea to the church: talk to your congregation. Please, we need each other and we need help. Don't let another son or daughter die by another bullet. Please, I do not want company with my tragedy. I beg of you to help.

Every single letter made a similar plea, not for vengeance but for people to come together and make it stop. I was convinced mothers would help me, help me avert a disaster. I was going to read a letter at the beginning of every meeting.

In January 1996, the night before the first meeting of the antiviolence coalition, Becky and I sat at our kitchen table. She was nervous, as Marcum was, that I was courting disaster with the kinds of people I had invited. But that night we just sat there. She wasn't going to fight me now. I smoked a cigarette and she drank a glass of whiskey for her nerves. "We have to do it, Sun. It's going to work" was about the only thing she said.

The antiviolence coalition met the next day at County Jail 7 in a large conference room. Marcum, Becky and I left our offices early to make sure everything was in place. We had coffee, pads of paper, pens and cold sweats.

"Sunny! How are you, my sister!" Leroy bellowed, his voice like a bullhorn. He was one of the first to arrive and he enveloped me in a bone-crushing hug. Soon about forty people were scattered around the room: Japanese and Latino reps from the recovery world, probation officers, cops, even a Chabad rabbi with a black hat and long beard. Deputy Drocco slunk in and gave me a nod. I'd been on him for a month to join the team.

"C'mon, Ricky, I need someone like you," I told him.

"No, babe, you know me, I'm not the meeting type." But that was precisely why I wanted him. Drocco was a natural leader who was respected by the other deputies, a hard-core law-and-order type with a volatile temper who had embraced the new programs of County Jail 7. He was like an old-fashioned coach, a Knute Rockne or Vince Lombardi kind of guy. I'd go down and watch him running a dorm. He had the place under complete control. If an inmate acted up, and it didn't happen often, he barked out, his voice gruff and direct, "Why are you being such a knucklehead? Let's get it together." As soon as the man had calmed down he'd bark out again, "There you go, babe, we all gotta live together." His dorm was calm, well run, and he left no wiggle room for complaining.

I was thrilled he was there. But I was also secretly terrified about how today would go, especially when I saw Jean O'Hara come in. She was a silver-haired grandmother from Pleasanton, California, who had experienced a horrible crime—her daughter and twenty-two-month-old grandson had been murdered by a stranger. She'd gone on to found Survivors of Murder Victims. Pleasanton was about an hour away, and she was one of the last to arrive. She walked in looking nervous and took the last empty seat, which happened to be half occupied by Leroy's bulk. Becky immediately leaned over and asked if we should try to separate them. I shook my head.

"We have to let this play out how it will play out," I whispered back.

With that, I stood up and started the meeting.

"Some of us in this very room have lost loved ones to the most horrific violence," I said. "Some of us in this room have been perpetrators of horrific violence and learned to take responsibility and teach others to stop their violence. But the one thing we have in common is that we all, I hope, want to bring safety back to our homes and our community. That's the goal I have but I know we won't be able to do anything about it unless we stay humble, unless we open our hearts and agree to listen. I want to start by asking all of us to listen. These are the words of a mother."

I read one of the letters. I didn't comment on it, didn't try to put it in context, just let her story sink in. When I finished, I asked everyone for a moment of silence to remember those who have been struck down by violence and to think about why we were there today. People bowed their heads. Leroy and Jean sat quietly next to each other, lost in their own thoughts. There was a sacred hush to the room, one I'd felt sometimes in temple. I felt a deep yearning for connection, for these disparate groups to find common cause and stop the suffering in our communities. I hoped other people felt it, too.

I gave everyone a chance to introduce themselves, and say why he or she had come. Leroy was full of love, and thanked everyone in the Sheriff's Department for their help, but he went on too long. Drocco made me laugh, and cringe a little. "I'm Deputy Richard Drocco, and I'm here because Sunny told me to come. I've been working with inmates for a long, long time. Listen, it's real simple, folks; these guys need to be told what to do, and what they can't do. Some of them are knuckleheads and are never going to change. Some of them I grew up with, and they just need to get a job. These guys don't need to be coddled, they need discipline. I gotta say I'm skeptical . . ." Drocco paused and seemed to be working out what to say. "Let me just say that a lot of these men don't want to change." He sat down. Jean O'Hara stood up next. She looked frail but her voice had power.

"My name is Jean O'Hara. I started an organization called Survivors of Murder Victims. I'm here for my daughter Nancy, and my grandson, little two-year-old Jesse. They were both murdered. I think about them every day, and I've been working to try to honor their memories. They would want me to do this work. I am not sure if this is the place to be but I am willing to listen and see."

Later, during a break, I saw Jean and Leroy speaking softly by the coffee table. Drocco sidled up to me. "That little old lady. I could just cry."

"You okay being here, Ricky?"

"Yeah, Sunny. I wasn't sure, but seeing her . . . she's worth fighting for."

When I gathered folks back in their chairs, I saw Jean give Leroy a motherly pat on the shoulder.

This was the beginning of RSVP, the Resolve to Stop the Violence Project. Hennessey had come up with the name. He loved acronyms. For a while, I thought calling it RSVP sounded too frilly. What are we doing? Inviting the inmates to tea? But the civility implied by the name got to me and so that's what we decided to call it. The general outline of the program stayed the same from the beginning. RSVP would be started in a full dorm, with sixty-two inmates. A variety of group activities developed by the committee would keep the inmates occupied throughout the day.

We met every three weeks for over a year to plan the program. I began each session by reading a letter from a mother. These women kept us humble. Most people stuck with the process. Some did not. Kathy Lawrence, the woman who came with Jean O'Hara from the victims' rights world, never bought into what we were doing. She sat meeting after meeting with her arms crossed, her mouth set into a thin line. In the opening session, she was the first to speak when I asked for comments.

"I don't know if I like it here," Kathy volunteered. "My daughter was murdered and I don't think we should give these offenders anything. I think we should lock them up. Give them as much pain as they have given me. I don't think they can 'recover.' I think they will be lying murderers until the day they die."

I glanced quickly at Leroy, who was sitting behind her, worried he might confront her. But he stayed quiet, giving Kathy her space.

Despite her anger, I didn't see Kathy as the enemy. If anything, she was exactly the kind of person we were trying to serve. I didn't want to give any of the men in our program a free ride, either. But what I think was missing was the realization of what was actually going on in the jails. The men were suffering, sure, but they weren't learning remorse. Their suffering served no purpose except to guarantee the suffering of their next victim.

Most violent offenders got out after nine months, which was the average sentence for assault, the most common violent crime. I'd love to say that locking them up for longer stretches was a solution, but what difference would it make if, when we released them, they went out and committed more crimes? The "throw away the key" argument was never a realistic one anyway. The government couldn't afford it. State budgets across the country were strained by the population already behind bars. Start raising sentences for criminals across the boards and the budgets would collapse. I wanted their time inside to be hard time. I wanted it to be uncomfortable for them. I wanted them to suffer but not in the same way Kathy wanted them to suffer. I wanted them to suffer through remorse, and make changes in their behavior that allowed them to participate in a civilized society.

Kathy stuck with the committee until other obligations caused her to step away. Over the months and years it took to put together the RSVP curriculum, we kept a core team intact. Jean O'Hara took the lead on our victims' rights committee. Deputy sheriffs and probation officers headed up the security and safety component, coming up with the best ways to respond to fights and the dreaded possibility of a riot. Sometimes, I'd shake my head at all the things we were putting together. But the guiding principle was on softening these men rather than hardening them, getting them to feel rather than ignore the pain they'd caused. To do that, they would have to do activities easily derided as "touchy-feely" or San Francisco clichés. We were going to use theater, acupuncture, guided meditation, yoga, with the main activity being various kinds of peer education. I mean, Christ, when were we scheduling the wine and cheese?

But through it all, our diverse group of allies guided the process.

Cops, victims' rights groups and religious leaders, together with social workers, death penalty opponents and prisoner service workers, all realized that making these men truly confront their crimes would take extraordinary measures. Some of the programs looked a little goofy, but we didn't care. We had communities that had been abandoned to violence as their only legacy. We had communities where gang wars and domestic violence were a birthright. We had the men under our custody who were making these communities terrible places to live. We had a chance to change that. In the end, the coalition held together, and we prevailed in creating a program. Jean O'Hara's presence alone reminded us what was at stake. My own memories of Richard Speck and Fred Johnson, the pedophile, reminded me of what was at stake. We all made the choice to try to heal suffering rather than let it fester.

It's ironic, I suppose, that just as RSVP was about to launch, suffering would enter my life, and I too would be forced to make the choice to either try to heal it or let it grow.

I was in another meeting. RSVP was starting three weeks late. Becky was there, and Marcum, as well as a number of new staff people. It was a group with healthy disagreements. Few deputies had given up their fear that there might be riots. Becky, in particular, brought it up fairly regularly, posing the "what if" questions. What if we lost the dorm, what would we do?

In some ways it was an easy question. If we lost the dorm early on, Sheriff Hennessey could lose the next election for coddling violent criminals. I'd lose my job, and I just might lose my faith in humanity. I was certain we wouldn't lose the dorm but . . . what if? These thoughts were shooting me out of bed in the morning, full of anxiety, before the sun came up.

A deputy walked in while we were going over schedules.

"I'm sorry to interrupt, Sunny. There's a Doctor Schwartz on the phone. Says he's your brother and he needs to talk to you."

Marcum and Becky looked up. They both knew that Jerry didn't call me. We almost never spoke. Part of his embrace of Orthodox Judaism meant rejecting me. My lesbianism, my "choice" not to have a traditional family meant that I was just this side of untouchable.

My mind raced as I ran to the phone. I guess Jerry could hear the panic in my voice because the first thing he did was lie. "Everything is okay," he insisted, then quickly got to the news. "But Mom collapsed while she was in the bathroom. Dad couldn't pick her up, an ambulance came and took her to Skokie hospital."

That was all he said. I thanked him for calling and I hung up. I knew my mom was dying. I didn't move for a long time.

It was strange. Here I was in this intense work mode. I had allowed very little to intrude. I was the leader, pushing everyone, running interference at City Hall with the nervous bureaucrats who thought I was creating trouble for the sheriff. I was the one telling everyone it was going to be okay. This was going to be the culmination of my life's work. I didn't have a plan if it failed. I'd bet the house. My sense of self-worth was wrapped up in RSVP, with these violent men, and it was being rolled out in a few days. My mom and I had talked on the phone every once in a while. I talked with my father once in a blue moon, usually when my mother passed me to him. I'd gone home to help my mother the first two times the cancer had struck. Now it had returned, I was sure of it, at the moment that my life's work had reached its culmination. I had to make a choice.

I went back to the meeting, sat down with my colleagues, many of whom were now my friends. Becky reached out and touched me on the shoulder. Tears sprang to my eyes. "I'm sorry, everyone. I can't quite believe this is happening. But my mom is very sick, and I'm going to have to go to Chicago for . . . I don't know how long."

For months, we had all been steeped in the language of healing and reconciliation and restorative justice, so I couldn't have walked into a more supportive room. Marcum leaned over to give me a hug and whispered in my ear. "We've got it, Sunny, you've brought us this far. We can take it from here."

Becky followed me into the hall as I walked out. For all of our fighting, I knew she would step in front of a bullet for RSVP. We hugged and she told me not to worry. I had no fears about the staff's ability to push through the next couple of weeks. They were as dedicated as I was. But I was still afraid.

Would the men respond to the program we'd set up? At the core of everything we were doing were two very simple yet difficult concepts:

accountability and forgiveness. The men who were going to be in our program were almost all victims of trauma in their childhood, trauma that they'd never come to grips with. At the same time, they could barely name the kinds of horrors they'd perpetrated as adults. It was easier for them to feel nothing than to figure out how to own their feelings and take responsibility for what they'd done. We were going to try to teach them how to forgive themselves, and how to seek forgiveness in others. This was unmapped territory for these men, and as I packed up to go home, I realized that it was unmapped territory for me, too. I needed to forgive myself, and I needed to forgive my family and my mother, and I was glad to have every ounce of training I'd received.

I landed in Chicago and took a cab to my parents' house. My father met me at the door, looking pale. His voice kept breaking and trailing off like a weak radio signal. Stevie's suicide had almost destroyed him, and now, with his wife dying, he could barely function. I felt for him but was wary, still fearing his temper and neediness. I sat quietly with him at the kitchen table and thought of Mom. He cried and said cryptically, "Sunny, there are so many would've, should've, could'ves about you kids."

I didn't ask him what he meant. I was betting that he still wished I'd gotten married. I didn't have the stomach to go there with him now.

"Dad, you did the best you could," I told him. "I have a rich life; so do Jerry and Cindy."

I held my dad's hand. Fat tears were rolling down his cheeks, filling in his wrinkles and catching the light. I hadn't realized how old he had become.

My dad mentioned that it was Elul. Elul in the Jewish calendar is the month of repentance in preparation for the High Holidays. It builds through Rosh Hashanah, finally culminating in Yom Kippur, the day of atonement. *Elul* means "search," which felt appropriate, because we were supposed to search our hearts. Tears sprang to my eyes, too.

I didn't feel ready. I felt as if I'd been searching my whole life, trying to find the key so that I could really embrace these people, love my dad and mom and brother unconditionally, despite all our disagreements. I just didn't know if I could do it yet.

My dad had his shofar in the living room leaning against the wall.

A shofar is a hollowed-out ram's horn used in temple. His was about four feet long, made from a gazelle, twisted like a corkscrew. During the month of Elul, the shofar is blown in the temple every weekday after morning services. The sounding of the shofar is a wake-up call, rousing worshippers from their complacency and calling them to repent. When done properly, a shofar blast is a piercing sound, part foghorn and air raid siren. My dad, the jazz trumpet player, had brought a congregation to its feet with his blasts. I asked him to sound it for me. He smiled.

"Sure, Sunny, I would love to." He shuffled to get it. I closed my eyes and thought of him blowing his cornet in our Buick out in front of our house. My father's frustrations and disappointments seemed locked in place. Had I really changed so much? He put the shofar to his lips, tears still staining his checks, and blasted several short notes and a long melancholy one. I could feel his sorrow. He did the best he could. I believed that.

At the hospital, we found Jerry holding my mom's hand. He'd come straight from the airport. She looked up at me. "Hi, Dolly, what took you so long?"

As soon as she called me Dolly, I knew I was home.

My mom was extremely weak, rolling in and out of consciousness. Her cancer had returned and spread and she had days, maybe weeks, to live. Jerry, Cindy, who still lived in town, my dad and I took turns sitting with her. For days, Mom and I didn't talk about much. We just chatted. She'd always had a soft spot for a steamed Chicago Vienna Beef dog with everything and so I'd grab them for lunch. One day, while I was spreading out her dog and fries, she said, "Ya know, Sunny, you're the strong one. You know how to get things done." My heart jumped in my chest. I looked at her closely. I wanted to make sure she was really awake and lucid. She was smiling at me, her eyes shining.

Then she winked at me and said, "Jerry's a *kuni leml.*" *Kuni leml* is Yiddish for fool. My mom used it affectionately. I laughed and my brother, who was sitting just outside the room, laughed as well.

At around six that day, I walked out with Jerry. He had to make a quick trip back to New York for a few days, and I walked him to the car. On the elevator, as the doors shut, I lost it. The accumulation of my mother's suffering finally wrenched my heart open and I started bawling. There was another woman on the elevator. "I'm so sorry," I told the woman. I felt compelled to explain myself. "My mom is so sick and . . ." Another wracking sob cut me short.

She looked at me kindly. "It's okay. I wish I could help. I lost my dad a few years ago." It was a generous response considering I was a train wreck. Jerry stood next to me, looking down, a little awkwardly. He and I had never been that affectionate but in his Orthodox community, physical contact with women, even sisters, was discouraged. The doors rolled open and we walked to the car. I was still crying but had regained some control. At the car, Jerry looked at his shoes. His body was tense, a steel trap. He started to stammer, "Listen, Sunny, I . . ." And then he embraced me.

Through tears he managed to say, "Ma is so special. She's a jewel. I love her so much." Then, after we had both weathered the storm, he let go. He wiped his eyes and I told him to "fly safe." Then I went upstairs to do the night shift.

In Frieda's lucid moments, we talked a little more. We talked about the work I was doing in San Francisco. We talked about the old neighborhood. I told her about going to Laverne Liberty's house to escape my brothers. I told her I wished they'd been better to me. My mother reached out and took my arm. She told me about an *Oprah* show she'd seen recently. She whispered, "Dolly, you have to listen, Oprah says 'we shouldn't hold on to bitterness, it will make us sick.'"

I grabbed my mom's hand. "You know, Ma, I know I've really disappointed you. Who I've chosen to love has disappointed you. I know that. I haven't disappointed me but . . . I just want you to know that I wasn't trying to hurt you—"

"No, Dolly," my mother interrupted, her voice little more than a whisper. Her eyes were shining, looking glassy, but her face was calm. She gave my hand a squeeze. "You didn't disappoint me. You had your wings. You had to fly."

Her words hung in the air. I wanted to dip them in amber and preserve them, hold them to my heart. But the sounds of the hospital intruded—the nurses talking out in the hall, a cart with squeaky wheels going by. My mother closed her eyes and fell asleep. For years,

I'd wanted more from my mom. I wanted her to drop her guard and embrace all of me. I wanted her to look me in the eyes and say, "Ya know, Sunny, you deserved better. I should have stood up for you. I should have insisted on you being treated better." But sitting there with her, I felt okay, maybe for the first time in my life. I smoothed the hair back from her head, and kissed her on the forehead.

Jerry had come back. It had been his night to stay with her and he'd called us at four-thirty in the morning to say it was time. When my dad and I walked in, my mom was gasping for air. I had pictured her going in her sleep, peacefully, but that gasping looked awful. We raised up her bed, which calmed her down a little. I climbed into bed and hugged her. While she struggled to breathe, I held her and told her I loved her.

Finally, she gasped and said, "I love you too, Dolly," and then there were no more breaths. Her body relaxed in my arms. A phrase kept running through my head. I don't know if someone said it or if I made it up. "Love is everything and we can't control anything."

I had finally learned how to forgive.

Shiva for my mom passed in a dream. I wore a conservative black dress, and a long-sleeved white blouse that I'd bought at Loehmann's, a costume as far as I was concerned. Jerry, my dad, Cindy and I sat on the floor. This was the Jewish way. We'd done it for Stevie, too. We were struck down by grief. The room was full of strangers to me—a group of black-suited men came from my parents' temple. Another group came from my brother's temple in Monsey, New York. They'd flown in for the day to pay their respects.

I wondered what my mother would think of all the Orthodox men who came to the house. I knew she'd be happy that Jerry took comfort from them, but she told me more than once, out of earshot from my brother and dad, that she didn't "go for all the extreme stuff." They weren't my mother's people. They wouldn't look at my sister or me. But I was filled with a spirit that was new to me, one that I attributed directly to RSVP even though I hadn't seen a single day of it yet. It was a feeling of acceptance. If these men wanted to sit Shiva for my mother, then they could sit Shiva for my mother. I said my prayers, missed my mother horribly, and, every once in a while allowed myself this thought: *There were no riots.*

The RSVP program started without me. I'd called daily to check in. It began with no fanfare, no major crisis. As I was boarding the plane to go home, I thought of Jean O'Hara, who was going to speak to the inmates in another week. She was leading a phase of the RSVP program called victim impact and she was going to be the first speaker in the dorm. If Jean could feel a shred of humanity for a convict after the loss she'd suffered, feel enough to come and speak to a roomful of them, then who was I to reject my brother and father? I needed to learn how to forgive them.

I arrived home to a San Francisco Shiva with Becky, Marcum and my friends. We sat together and I shared all the pain of losing my mom. A new week began and I vowed to keep my heart open, open to the possibility of change, open to joy and love, even in County Jail 7.

CHAPTER 14

1997

A few weeks after my mother's Shiva, I was sitting in another room of men wearing costumes. Instead of long black coats there were bright orange jumpsuits. Dreadlocks and greasy hair replaced ringlets. I was in the RSVP dorm where sixty violent men were finding their seats in a semicircle of plastic chairs at the front of the dorm.

Gang tattoos snaked up arms and peeked out of T-shirts at necks and forearms. The bigger thugs had ink invading their faces. Latino gangs, in particular, liked to proclaim their affiliations on their cheeks or foreheads. A fat gangbanger sitting a few seats away had *NORTE* written across his cheek. That was one of the more violent gangs in California, and I was hoping he was more poseur than hard-core. I looked at the staff members and the deputy sheriffs positioned around the room. The tension was palpable. We hadn't had riots, but if something were to go wrong, today would be the worst possible day for it.

Jean O'Hara was speaking to the men. She was no wilting flower. She'd given talks to kids at risk before, but this was a different crowd. These were sixty-two of the most violent prisoners in the San Francisco County jail system: gangbangers, wife beaters, pimps and murderers. Jean was giving the first victim impact statement, which we hoped would be an essential pillar of RSVP. It was one of the key additions we made to the curriculum that formed the core of the RSVP program, a curriculum called Manalive.

Manalive was the brainchild of a former community organizer named Hamish Sinclair. I'd first met Hamish in the early 1990s. He looked a little like Ernest Hemingway with an impressive white mane of hair, a booming voice and a thickly lined face. He developed the Manalive curriculum in the 1980s. Manalive was a group therapy program for men who beat their wives but we expanded it so that it applied to any violent offender. Manalive aimed at eradicating men's violent behavior through rigorous self-examination and peer education. I had found Manalive to be head and shoulders above all the other anger management classes at which I'd looked. These anger management classes focused, predictably, on "managing anger," giving men time-outs from their rage, teaching them how to avoid situations that triggered it. When Manalive was successful, men rewired their own emotional minefields, and figured out how to defuse their violent triggers.

The Manalive curriculum teaches that violent men are raised with a "male role belief system" that says they are superior to everyone around them. These male role beliefs say that feelings like shame and sadness show weakness and are to be avoided. Any time men experience these weak emotions, this is a loss of control for them, and their male role belief system insists that they reassert control by any means necessary. This could mean verbal violence or physical violence. Hamish's work in RSVP as well as victim impact has been validated by experts in the field, most notably psychiatrist James Gilligan.

Gilligan's basic theory, based on thirty years of experience working with criminals, echoes Hamish Sinclair's: shame causes violence. Men are taught that feelings of shame are not just uncomfortable, but intolerable, and any experience that produces shame or "loss of respect" must be met with a response. Ask any inmate, particularly any violent inmate, why they are in prison, or why they beat their wife, or why they got into a fight, and you are likely to get a version of this answer: "He/she/they disrespected me," which is then followed by any one of the following: "He got all up in my grill, you know, a man can only take so much." "I didn't want to beat her but what's a man supposed to do? She disrespected me." And finally, "There was no way I could let that pass. I ain't no punk."

RSVP tries to correct this kind of thinking. One of the ways we do this is by creating an environment that requires the men to confront the results of their violence through our victim impact class. Violent men have a diminished capacity to consider their victims' feelings. In fact, they resent and dismiss them. There are many reasons for this. First and foremost, their own childhoods were usually filled with pain and humiliation. This numbs them to feelings of any kind, their own or anyone else's. Then, during their trials, the offenders are kept away from the people they've hurt. This is commonsensical but it perpetuates the criminal's view that their victim is their enemy, whom they have to vanquish in court. In victim impact statements, we try to change that thinking, get the men to feel what they've done, to see that their victims are human beings just like them.

Jean O'Hara had volunteered to try to do it first.

I said a little prayer to myself that we weren't courting disaster by bringing her into this room so early in the program. RSVP had been running for just under a month. Half the men in the dorm had volunteered to enter RSVP. A few were no doubt excited to be in a program that promised to help them, but I wasn't under any illusions. I knew many had volunteered because they thought it might help knock time off their sentences, or make them look good in front of the judge or prosecutor. The Sheriff's Department intake officers had sent the other half to us against their will. Those men, especially, were not happy. Not only did they feel that they'd been sent to the "touchy-feely" jail but also they objected to being classified as violent offenders. On a daily basis, we had interventions with men who refused to participate because they insisted they should not be there. I'd sat in on one of these interventions the day before with Leon, one of our best facilitators. Leon had long hair, gentle eyes and a quiet, disarming voice. He was a former offender with a long record of drug possession, robbery and domestic violence. But he'd conquered his violence and had a razor-sharp instinct about holding other men's feet to the fire.

The inmate with the problem was Jimmy, a drug dealer who was in on a charge of possession with intent to distribute. He was covered in gang tattoos, his neck was like a cinder block, and he had a teardrop inked below his right eye, which can mean that the inmate had killed someone. His record contained no murder charge but it was full of assaults, assaults with a deadly weapon and armed robbery. Leon and I sat him down in an interview room.

"Okay, Jimmy," Leon said. "You've told me five times in group and you've told the deputy sheriff a number of times that you shouldn't be here. I got that right?"

"Man, I been telling you that all week. I got nabbed holding my buddy's coke. I didn't know he even had it. Now you got me with all these dudes talking about my feelings, and you want me to admit I'm violent? You must be crazy."

Leon opened the man's folder and handed over his rap sheet. Jimmy hesitated, scowling at Leon and me, then finally reached out and took the paper.

"That you?" Leon asked.

Jimmy looked down at the sheet for a few seconds. He looked confused. Then he turned sheepish. "Shit, man, is this all me?"

"Yeah," Leon said. "That's all you."

"Well, damn, I guess you got me."

Leon drove the point home. "Can I get an agreement from you that you are a violent man and that you do, in fact, belong here?"

Jimmy scowled again, but finally, through a clenched jaw, relented, "Yeah, I'll agree to that." Most men had never seen their own rap sheet, so Jimmy's reaction wasn't out of the ordinary. But not all men listened to reason as Jimmy had. A few days earlier, during the dorm meeting, I'd watched as half the men rolled their eyes, or sucked their teeth, or folded their arms across their chest, each act a subtle, but potent form of disrespect. It was an uphill climb for these men to get with the program. The system depended on peer support, meaning the inmates who'd been here the longest would help guide the new inmates. But no one had been here longer than three weeks, so no one was a true convert yet.

The men found their seats for Jean's talk, eyeing each other warily. A man scraped his chair up to the semicircle, slung himself into it and folded his arms across his chest, splaying his legs as wide as he could. His every gesture announced that he was annoyed. My jaw tightened. I could feel the defiance and anxiety among the men. We'd supplemented the regular deputy on duty at his post with five other deputy sheriffs. I'd asked Lieutenant Hunsucker and Deputy Drocco to be at the perimeter; both were feared and respected by the inmates. The instructions were clear. Nobody was going to put his head down or slouch in his chair during Jean's talk. No one was even going to clear his throat in a funny way.

I looked over at Becky one last time. The joy and fear of starting RSVP had pushed our own personal bullshit to the background for the time being. We were too scared and excited about RSVP to fight. She gave me a wink and I knew it was time to start.

Bianka, our victim restoration coordinator, gave the introduction. Jean was sitting back with some of the other staff members. She looked as if she had stumbled out of a Norman Rockwell painting. She had walked into the jail this morning with a classic lady's purse draped over her arm. Her hair was short and beauty-shop gray. She just looked too nice to hold the attention of these men.

Bianka wrapped up her remarks: "Jean has come here to talk to you. This is *her* talk. It is not a discussion or a conversation. You will have time to talk later. Right now, it is her time. So give her your full attention and listen." There was scattered applause. Jean stood up and slowly made her way to the center of the semicircle. She was holding a framed picture of a woman and child. She held up the picture as she spoke.

"I would like to introduce you to Nancy and Jesse, my daughter and grandson," Jean said quietly. She took the photo and handed it to the man in front of her. I got a peek at it as it went around. It was one of those drugstore portraits: a mom looking a little glazed grasping a giggly toddler. "Please pass it around the room," Jean asked. "I want everyone to get a look at it. That's a picture of my grandson and my daughter a few months before they were murdered."

The men were fidgety; there was sighing and rocking and shifting in seats. Jean ignored it.

"Early in the morning on January twentieth, nineteen eighty-seven," Jean began, "I woke up from a sound sleep. It was like someone was shaking me but no one was there. I had a terrible feeling. I felt maybe something was wrong with Jesse and my daughter. I felt maybe they needed me. Really, though, I didn't know what it was. I just sensed something was terribly wrong.

"Now, I wasn't someone who put much stock in random feelings. Maybe it was a bad dream I'd had but couldn't remember. Maybe it was an early morning chill. Who knows? I tried to shake it off as I went through the morning. But I couldn't get over the feeling so I finally decided to drop in on Nancy earlier than we'd planned."

The buzz in the room had been dropping as Jean's story began to unfurl. The men were now quieter than I'd ever heard anyone be in a jail. I was scared to breathe, afraid of interrupting. Jean's pain was right there on the surface—the look she had in her eyes, the way she stood, her voice. Most of all, you could see it in her walk. She was taking halting half steps around the circle, as if every fiber in her being resisted telling this story again. But with each short step forward, her story came out. She was mesmerizing.

"Nancy was living in Concord, California, with a man she was very excited about. His name was Paul, and he was good to her, and good to little Jesse, and she had invited her father and me over to meet him for the first time. It was a big deal for Nancy, and for us. Our daughter had never had much luck with men. But she was excited about Paul, and we were excited for her, and for Jesse. Jesse needed a father. He was almost two, and the sweetest little boy, just beginning to put sentences together.

"My husband, Jack, and I were supposed to see them for dinner, but I rushed over early. Jack was still at work, and I dropped by around noon, knocked and knocked, and I got no response. I'd tried calling and got no answer. I'd also tried calling Jesse's babysitter. She'd said that Nancy was supposed to come by that morning to drop off Jesse but she hadn't shown up. Meanwhile, the feeling I had that something was dreadfully wrong just kept growing."

Jean paused here, collecting her thoughts. Her eyes had fogged over. I could picture her standing on those porch steps, fearing what was waiting for her inside. She had stopped moving. Her lip quivered slightly. When she spoke again, she sounded far away. "I called my husband, Jack, at work. I told him to come home, something was terribly wrong with Nancy, I could feel it."

She took another break, and a deep breath, but she was finding her rhythm. Her voice picked up power as the memories tumbled from her.

"I needed to get into the house, I was sure of it. I called Jack at work, and he came home with the extra key and we went back to Nancy's. Jack had put his key in the lock and pushed the door open. We could see two people lying on the living room floor and it looked as though they were watching television, except that there was blood everywhere. A little TV was playing. Jack stepped over and touched Nancy's elbow and said to me, 'She's gone.'"

At that point, Jean turned her focus on the men sitting right in front of her. She stepped forward. Jean's move unnerved the men. They shifted uneasily. "Have any of you lost a loved one to murder?"

She raised her eyes and addressed the question to the whole group. "Has anyone lost a loved one to murder?" A sea of hands went up. Jean made eye contact with a few of the men, nodding at each one.

"Every one of you knows how I feel. I'm sure you do. There are few words to describe the shock and sorrow. I've found that sometimes words just aren't sufficient, you have to tell someone who has been through it themselves." Jean paused again and took a few more half steps back to the center of the circle. Some of my staff had raised their hands, too. My hands stayed in my lap but I was thinking of Stevie.

Jean had bound us together with her question, the criminals and deputies and the staff and the grandmother. We were all united in grief for those we had lost, all our grief now part of her grief.

"The body of my daughter's boyfriend, Paul, was laying next to my daughter. I'd never met him before and here he was dead on the floor in front of me. My husband kept his wits about him, told me to call nine-one-one. So I went straight to the phone and made the call, said get someone here quick, something horrible has happened. My husband, meanwhile, just stepped over both of them. I'm not sure how he got the courage. He ran to the back bedroom to see if he could find our grandson, twenty-two-month-old Jesse. And within probably a minute, he was back and said, 'He's gone, too.'"

Jean's voice remained quiet, but her eyes bore down on the men. "That was the beginning of a nightmare, one that did not end with the arrest of the man who had killed them, one that did not end with his trial. It's a nightmare that hasn't ended.

We would eventually find out that the killer was a man named Richard Goodfellow. He was homeless. He needed money desperately. Paul met him the afternoon before, playing pool, and Paul invited him back to the house to watch TV and have a couple of drinks. Nancy had gone to lay down after putting little Jesse to bed.

We think she was awakened by Jesse crying and heard shouts and fighting between Richard and Paul about a toolbox. We think this because that's what Richard later told the police."

I was struck that Jean called the man by his first name. It felt intimate. It fit with what I'd learned about her in the two years we'd spent on the planning committee. She was a woman of deep principles. She wasn't going to call him a "monster" or an "it." She was going to call him Richard.

"Richard was caught because after the crime, he showed up at his girlfriend's house covered in blood. She eventually turned him in. Richard told the police that Paul had no money and this made him completely lose his temper. I don't know whether he was on drugs or not, I'll never know that. It didn't come out at the trial. The only thing I can think of is that he just went totally crazy and killed Paul. Had Nancy stayed in that bedroom, I think he would have stolen Paul's toolbox, which was the only thing of worth in the apartment, and been on his way. But Jesse woke up. Nancy came out of the bedroom where she was sleeping, saw what was going on. Richard knew she could identify him, he was still in his frenzy, and so he took her. Obviously she must have put up a fight. She had been stabbed in every area of that house because her blood was found everywhere. Just horrible. So, um, and then of course with the baby, that never has made any sense to me . . . never, ever."

Jean faltered for the first time, tears started trickling down her cheeks, and I realized that silently and without any attempt to hide it, most of the men had started crying, too.

"Why Richard had to go and take baby Jesse. That never will make sense, that never will equate. I can't imagine anyone being that . . ." She stopped again and steadied herself. "He had to have had time between murdering Nancy and, we figure, trying to find her car keys, or whatever he was doing. He told the police during his confession that he went in and he slapped the kid a few times and told him to shut up. Jesse had been woken up from a nap and was crying and wouldn't shut up. Richard's answer to that problem was to take him out of his crib, take him through a doorway, where there was light, throw him down on the floor and proceed to stab him fifty-six times."

Some of the men were now shaking, holding their heads in their hands. I had tried to hold back, out of a twisted sense of professional decorum, but then I realized that the point was to feel.

Jean told the men about the trial and Richard Goodfellow's conviction. She said that she had been surprised that the conviction didn't bring her or her husband, Jack, any peace. "We felt that it would all be over with and then we could go back to our lives. And, once we went back to our lives, it would all go away. And it has not, and now we know that it never will.

"The only thing I could do is with everybody I talked to . . ." And here, one after the other, Jean took the hands of each man sitting in the front row. "'Did you hear about Nancy and Jesse?' 'Did you hear what happened to my daughter and my little grandson?' 'Did you hear what happened?'"

Jean was holding a man's hand, one from the group of men she'd approached before, but this time there was no barrier between them. Every man she'd reached out to had taken her hand willingly. Their defenses had come down. She stepped back to the center of the room.

"Gentlemen, Richard took more than three lives that night. Our one remaining daughter, Mary, went into complete denial, and when she comes to visit us, if we start to talk about Nancy, she stands up and leaves. 'I don't wanna hear it,' she says. My husband has never cried because of the loss of Nancy and Jesse. And because he's stuffed all of this pain and he's held it down and held it down and pushed it down— this year, he has had all kinds of surgeries, all kinds of health problems. My coming here and talking to you allows me to take another little piece of it and put it aside. And for that, I thank you.

"I believe that if just one of you men listens, and if one of you can have the courage to change, to give up your violence, then that means another family won't have to go through the pain that my family had to go through, and that we still go through every single day. Thank you, gentlemen, for hearing my story."

Jean O'Hara, the frail, white-haired grandma from Pleasanton, tamed the monsters of County Jail 7. After Jean left, the men were quiet and careful and respectful of one another. They were tender rather than callous and hard. They weren't putting on a show for their lawyers or the judge or the DA in that dorm. They weren't getting any breaks for participating. In that afternoon, they found the ability to share their feelings—their fears, their anger, their sadness and their sense of awe at Jean's courage and civility.

It was a start. I didn't think there would be riots.

CHAPTER 15

1998

Ben Matthews had a swastika inked into his skull. Until his hair grew, he was a walking provocation in the RSVP dorm. Ben was a wiry nineteen-year-old skinhead with a snarl etched onto his lips, not old enough yet to have a beard but he was trying. He was mandated into the RSVP dorm six months after we started. He sat at the edge of his group like a steel trap, waiting for someone to set him off. His eyes were narrow slits, and his foot bounced like a metronome. He'd been a hard-core meth and heroin addict, and he was struggling as both poisons left his system. Every time I saw him, I couldn't take my eyes off the tattoo on his head. It was like he was giving me a permanent "fuck you."

My staff and I had been watching him closely. Every afternoon we met to discuss the most troublesome inmates in the dorm and Ben often topped the list. He had beaten up someone he thought was a homosexual in the Haight, a typical skinhead hate crime. He did it while juiced on a cocktail of meth, heroin and Colt 45 malt liquor. He and a friend had been out looking for trouble. A twenty-five-year-old didn't like his tattoos, told him so, and Ben, in response, pushed him to the ground and had a "boot party" with his head while calling him a "fucking faggot." He kept assaulting him until the cops pulled him off.

Ben had screamed at Earl, RSVP's program manager, during his orientation. "I don't want to be here!" he hollered. "What the fuck is this! I'm not violent. This is war. I'm a soldier against the niggers and the homos. Just let me out of here so I can find my people." Ben made sure to repeat, in case Earl hadn't heard the first time, that he did not belong "in any dorm with niggers, kikes and homos."

Earl, a former wife beater himself, is a block of a man, the kind who looks as if he's recently been inflated, muscles straining at the skin, and largely expressionless except for his eyes. They spark and fire. He listened patiently to Ben's rant until he found an opening.

"Okay, Ben, you're not violent, huh?"

"Hell no!"

"Well, then, why don't you just sit in this dorm and listen and we'll check back with you in, let's say, three weeks and see what you think. If you still feel the same way, we'll see what we can do. Can I get an agreement from you about that?"

Ben squirmed a little. "Whatever, man, but I'm telling you, I just want to go back to a real jail to do straight time. Don't make me sit here with these fuckin' homos. I don't know what I'd do if they looked at me funny, you know."

"Hey, listen," Earl responded, his voice still calm. More than anything, it was important to stay calm with the men. "I need another agreement from you. While you're here, I need you to agree to stop being verbally violent and stop your name calling."

Ben clenched his teeth. Earl told me he thought his teeth might pop.

"Fine," Ben spit back. "That just means I'll never talk, which is fine 'cause I got nothing to say to a room full of niggers."

Earl didn't reply. He had his agreements. That was enough for now. In a normal jail, Ben would have been hooked up with the Aryan Brotherhood, the white supremacist prison gang, within a week. We had gang members in the RSVP population. But they, like everyone else, were too closely supervised to "clique up."

Three other groups of inmates were meeting around the dorm. In one, folded into a similar tough-guy stance like Ben's, was Elroy Franklin. Linebacker-sized, with a thick neck and a belly bursting over his waistband, thirty-one-year-old Elroy had been arrested and charged with assault with a deadly weapon. He'd been waiting in line for movie tickets when he attacked a man he thought was coming on to his girl-friend. The victim was Asian and Elroy had punctuated the beating with racial slurs, calling the man a "motherfucking chink." At his orientation, Elroy had announced to Earl that "I better not be put in a group with no crackers, 'cause I won't hesitate to teach a class on respect." Elroy had mashed his fist into his enormous hand. Earl had rolled his eyes.

Both Elroy and Ben exuded menace, snarling at anyone who came into their space. Elroy almost got into a fight on his second day when he informed a scraggly wife beater to "get out of my chair, honky, or I'll fuck you up." When Ben entered the dorm two weeks after Elroy made his appearance, Earl ruefully reported back to the staff that they were the "Ebony and Ivory of hate."

In six months, we'd had exactly *no* fights in the RSVP dorm. That was an enormous success, considering that everyone thought we'd have riots, and because in a normal dorm, there were, on average, three violent incidents every month. The "old-timers" in the RSVP dorm seemed to be buying into the program.

Manalive was forcing the inmates to look at their presumptions about violence, and the men, it turned out, liked this self-examination. They liked that their intelligence was being respected, liked that they finally had a way to describe their feelings of rage, anger, fear and shame. Manalive came with a specific vocabulary that most of the old-timers had embraced. Inmates were taught that in the male role belief system, they developed their own inner "hit man" who used violence to assert their control over chaotic situations and protect the men from feelings of shame and fear. Men gave their personal hit man names, like "cold-blooded killer," or "silent, impatient bully," or "raging, slick con man." They called the moment when they found themselves about to do violence "fatal peril." The theory was that fatal peril was when your male role belief system was challenged and you called upon your inner hit man to reassert control.

Some men resisted the terminology, and I admit it was esoteric and specialized, but most of the men had embraced it. They liked that they now had tools to assert some control over their violence, that there were options available to them when they felt threatened. They also liked becoming peer educators. In most jails and prisons, there is no way for men to gain respect except by becoming bigger thugs. In the

RSVP dorm, we turned that reality on its head. The more inmates gave up their violent ways, the more respect and authority they received as senior inmate advocates. All the facilitators of the program, in fact, were formerly violent men who had given up their violence. The fact that we had recognized that many of these men craved legitimate respect, socially acceptable respect, and were willing to embrace it was one of the revolutionary aspects of the program, and one of its most successful components.

Now that we'd been running for six months, no longer was every activity an experiment that had to be sold to a hostile crowd. The men knew the schedule and were actively participating. But Elroy and Ben, I believed, would test the progress we'd made. Sheriff Hennessey had been great, but if he faced banner headlines about a race riot in his program facility, our new program might disappear at the next budget meeting.

We had found that the typical initiation period for inmates was three weeks. It usually took them that long to let down their guard. Elroy started to soften somewhere around the two-and-a-half-week mark. In the late afternoon, I'd catch him laughing at the jokes of the older men. His eyes pooled once when another man in his group, a white man, talked about losing his mother to cancer when he was six years old. Elroy had wiped away the tears as soon as they came but this was how things began. Ben, however, couldn't seem to relent. At the end of his second week, he was still a hard, sharp tack.

"Ben has not said a single positive word, and more than that, he's destructive," Leon exclaimed in an afternoon meeting, throwing up his hands. "He can barely hold himself back from calling us all fairy homos for talking about our feelings all the time." Leon was normally a patient man. If he was frustrated, then I knew Ben was a problem.

"Has he actually called anyone that?" I asked.

"No, but he does say over and over that he just wants to go to a normal prison to do straight time," Leon said. "He doesn't want to talk about his feelings. I think he called it, let's see, something totally original. Yeah, I think he called it 'gay.'"

Earl snorted at the joke, then jumped in. "I'm with Leon on this one," Earl said. "Ben's physical presence by itself is a distraction. Those tattoos are awful and he's so wound up the guy is like kryptonite. He's like poison even without saying anything. I can see the other inmates react to him."

"Do you want to bounce him?" I asked. We'd only bounced four guys so far. Two were so addled on drugs they couldn't get with the program. Another went for a month without saying a single word and we ended up sending him to the psych tier. The fourth guy was a gang-banger who, I came to believe, was a true psychopath. He hadn't responded to any form of positive peer pressure, not from the inmates, and not from any of the staff. He stayed defiant, using violent language and threatening the weaker guys in his group on a regular basis. The only contribution he had made was when he talked in group about tor-turing a small dog in his neighborhood. He gave me the creeps. Let's be clear: RSVP wasn't a one-size-fits-all program. We couldn't accom-modate the most extreme monsters, the psychopaths and sociopaths, the serial killers and masochists. Our program required that the men still have some empathy left. Luckily, in my experience, that includes most offenders.

We'd probably cycled through three hundred inmates in that period, so losing four was a good track record. It'd gotten so that most men were either participating in group or staying quiet. If they started causing trouble, we confronted them, and if they couldn't get with the program by the end of week three then we would most likely bounce them. The men we bounced were sent to County Jail 3, where they sat in their cells like animals in a cage. Three of the four guys wrote me later begging to come back.

"I guess I'm not ready to bounce Ben even though I'd love to because it would be easier on my group," Leon said. "But he's not a lost cause yet, though I don't think we can live with the status quo much longer."

In the general population of County Jail 3 or in the prisons like Pel-ican Bay or Folsom, Ben would have been a success. A skinhead who hadn't caused trouble, who hadn't gotten into a fight was a win. Not here. It was not enough for men to sit quietly and stew in their anger or "manage" it. They had to join in, let down their defenses, listen and disclose, and begin to conquer their anger. That's what we expected of them.

At the end of the meeting, I suggested that we confront Ben in an interview room. I wanted a white senior advocate in with Damon, one of our African-American counselors. Senior advocates were inmates who had done enough time in the program to be able to lead discussions and be peer advisors for their fellow inmates. I thought a white inmate allied with a black staff member might shock Ben out of his stubborn stance.

It didn't go well. Damon reported that as soon as he sat down, Ben started to yell. "I am not talking in here with no nigger! Get this motherfucker away from me or I'm gonna lose it." Ben had kicked his chair over and had to be restrained by the deputy sheriff and then isolated. He had behaved like a feral animal backed into a corner.

Ben Matthews was talked about at every staff meeting well beyond his three-week probationary period. He was a riddle. There was a feeling of desperation in his episodes. I got the sense that he was growing exhausted with the effort of being defiant. I saw pain in his eyes, even when he was simmering in group. During breaks he would walk laps around the dorm, his lips moving as if he was talking to himself.

Then, Leon reported a breakthrough. "The dude smiled today, my friends. I saw his teeth. Didn't know he had 'em!"

There hadn't been any triggering event. Something in Ben just cracked. Day by day, his menacing eyes softened. His foot's steady drumbeat slowed and then stopped. I could see him begin to breathe and let down his guard as he realized he wasn't in a place where he had to watch his back every minute of the day. Here he was surrounded by tough-looking men, but they were all talking about their feelings. They were all revealing the ways they had hurt their loved ones and how bad they felt about it. They were supporting one another and challenging one another to talk about things that they were ashamed of. They were learning techniques of listening and communicating that flew in the face of every tough-guy credo he had ever learned. It's difficult to sit in that environment without being affected by it.

A day finally came when Leon reported that Ben had started talking. One minute he was silent, the next he was making agreements, using the language of the group.

"I couldn't believe what happened this morning," Leon reported. "We've got this new guy in the group, this supershort El Salvadoran kid, and he really doesn't know what's going on. He took Ben's pen, and when Ben asked for it back, the guy confronted him. 'Get your own fucking pen!' he told him. And I'm on my feet, and everyone is looking at Ben to see what he would do. And, honest to God, I could've pinched myself. Ben's hands went in front of him, palms up, just like we taught him." Leon was grinning. We taught the men to physically demonstrate the idea of "fatal peril." It was a mnemonic device. When they felt confronted, what we called a "challenge to their male-role belief system," and felt like they might turn to violence, they put their hands out in front of their faces, palms up. The action represented their choice. They could either turn their open hands into fists or put their hands down again. The action forced the men to think before they acted, to actually make the choice not to be violent.

"Ben put it all together," Leon said. "His hands went up and he tells this guy, 'Can I give you some feedback?'" This was the Manalive language, which Ben, unknown to anyone else, had memorized. Leon continued, "So this short kid looked a little stunned. He's only been in here for a day, and he doesn't know what the hell is happening, and he tells Ben, 'Sure.' And Ben, he still has his hands up, says, 'When I saw you take my pen, I was frustrated. I felt hurt. And the way you reacted made me afraid.' I could've hugged Ben right there, I felt so damn proud. Anyway, the new guy didn't know how to react, and Ben kinda lost the thread so I helped him finish. I told the new guy, 'I'd like to make an agreement with you that you respect other people's property and other people's wishes and treat them with respect.' The guy was too stunned to do anything but agree. Ben was breathing and nodding, and the men around him were all clapping him on the back and telling him 'good job.' Deep and amazing work with this kid, I tell you." Leon was laughing. "It's like the minute his hair covered that swastika some sense returned."

The next time I saw Ben, I barely recognized him. He was talking to everyone around him; a motormouth had replaced the silent angry watcher. He was relaxed, his hands rested on his knees. He reached out and touched another inmate on the shoulder, an easy intimacy that was never easy in the joint. He was engaged, eyes soft and smiling. He was a different person.

*   *   *

Leon called for a volunteer for a destruction cycle. The destruction cycle is a central activity in the Manalive curriculum that deconstructs one individual's violent act. It's intended to get men to slow down an act of violence, look at it frame by frame, to understand and, hopefully, conquer it. Often, he had someone in mind. But he was surprised when Ben, tentatively, raised his hand. Leon skeptically raised an eyebrow.

"I'm ready," Ben responded to the unexpressed question and moved his chair to the center of the circle. Two other men took their places at the blackboard behind him. On it they wrote down headings: "Verbal Violence," "Physical Violence," "Emotional Violence" and a few others. They stood at the ready with chalk in their hands.

Ben stared at the ground. The urgency he had had a few minutes earlier now deserted him. His eyes hollowed out as he sat there, his foot started bouncing. Finally, he broke his silence and his voice was like a rock rolling downhill, picking up speed as it went.

"Okay, it was a cold night. I was hanging out in the Haight with one of my boys. We were mixing speed and heroin and shooting up. I fixed myself, then I fixed my buddy."

As Ben talked, one of the men behind him started scribbling on the board, filling in categories. He wrote two entries under "Physical Violence." One was "took drugs," the other was "gave drugs to friend."

"We were bored, I was living on the streets. We decided to go trolling. I told my boy, 'Let's take down some fags.'"

The other man wrote an entry under "Verbal Violence."

"We were hanging out down on Haight Street and this guy was standing near me and noticed my tattoos. He saw the swastika I've got on my head and some of the other white-power ones I've got on my arm. I got into the whole white-power thing back when I was in juvie. I'm a small guy, and I was getting picked on by the Mexicans, they've got the Sureños gang, and they kept beating me up in jail. The only ones who would take me in were the skinheads. They were hooked into the AB [Aryan Brotherhood], and you guys know that meant protection." The men in the circle nodded their agreement. Ben wasn't unique. A minor crime had landed him in a juvenile delinquent facility, where he'd gotten hooked up with a gang, and his crimes had grown worse, eventually turning violent. Many men in the circle could tell similar stories.

"Anyway, that's how I got into it in the first place," Ben continued. "And I started to really believe in the idea of a race war, and feel like, you know, the races had to stick together, 'cause who else is going to protect me?"

There was more frantic writing on the board.

"Anyway, that's when I was living down near Los Angeles. When I got to San Francisco I was deep into it. And I'm out with my buddy and this guy, he starts talking shit to me. And I was practically pro- grammed at that point. No one talks shit to me, and the worst kind of person was someone who was betraying their race. This guy harassing me was a traitor as far as I was concerned. Plus he looked like a fag— I mean, he looked like a homosexual to me. My thinking at the time was if someone like that talks shit to me, they're going to get a beat- down. That's just the way it was. So I pushed him. I gave him a big push, nearly knocked him over."

The two men behind Ben were working nonstop now, filling in various categories. The physical violence section was filling up. Under "Justifications for Violence" were several entries, including "threat to manhood" and "I was programmed for violence."

"So the guy is pissed. He's yelling at me saying something like 'What the hell is wrong with you?' That's when I lost it. I called him a faggot punk. I remember seeing red, my vision becoming narrowed. What do you call it? Almost like tunnel vision, and my mouth filled up with this copper taste and it's almost like I blacked out. I pushed him down and my friend and I started kicking him and kicking him more and more. We were yelling the whole time that he was a faggot punk and 'don't you ever fuck with me again.' I broke his jaw. I broke a few of his ribs. There was blood all over the sidewalk. There was blood on my boots."

Near the end of this story, Ben trailed off until the words caught in his throat. He rubbed his hands up and down on his knees obsessively, and finally found his voice again.

"Someone must have called the cops 'cause a crowd gathered and started yelling at me and pointed me out. Next thing I know I am in the back of a cop car in cuffs." Ben put his head down and slowly shook his head back and forth.

"I was so loaded," he said. "And I was so angry, about everything. I hated my life. I was ashamed of being broke all the damn time, and had been trained to hate all these people. My hit man I call the 'Ruthless Aryan Soldier,' and I was going to take down anyone who betrayed the white race. Now it seems like a dream I had once. Like it's not real."

Finally, Ben looked up. His story was finished, so it was time to move into the second section of the destruction cycle. That's when the other men talked.

"Can I give you feedback?" one inmate asked. Ben folded his arms over his chest.

"Yeah," he said, taking a deep breath.

"Well, when you said you were so loaded that sounded like blaming your violence . . . like you were blaming the drugs for your violence instead of you."

Ben's foot started to bounce. He was working hard to listen and not react. Finally, he put up his hands in supplication, the sign of fatal peril. He held them there for fifteen seconds. The rules of the destruction cycle instructed the men to "listen to feedback with undivided attention, you listen with an open mind, with an open heart, you listen for a kernel of truth, you soften and reflect on the feedback and you don't argue."

Ben gritted his teeth and said, "Thank you. You're right." His foot was still banging away like a jackhammer.

Another man asked if he too could offer feedback. Ben nodded.

"When you said 'I lost it,' that sounded like minimizing . . . like someone else took over for you, like you don't control your hit man, and you weren't in control of your actions."

Ben was getting the hang of it. He nodded vigorously this time.

"I hear you, thanks."

The destruction cycle went on for almost forty-five minutes, with Ben's peers pulling out pieces of his story and categorizing it on the board behind him. The process was painstaking. Each word and action was analyzed. Every excuse that Ben used—that he was "high" when he beat the man up, that he was doing "what he'd been taught," that he'd had to learn violence for "protection"—was talked about and assessed. Any time he tried to disassociate himself from his violence, the other men, or Leon, reminded him that he had chosen to act. It

was the way the men retrained themselves to think about their violence. When men turned around and looked at the board at the end
of the process, many were stunned at how many different kinds of violence they had committed, and the ways that they tried to excuse it.

There was a second side to the destruction cycle. Not only did the
men learn to name their violence and own it, they were also encouraged to name their shame, and own that, too. The men embraced the
pain that Ben had been through in his life. Not only had he talked
about how afraid he was in juvie and how he'd accepted the protection
of the Aryan Brotherhood, Ben had also talked about how his father
had harassed and emotionally abused him and his mom, and that he'd
never gotten over it.

"I'm so sorry that happened to you," Leon had told Ben. "That
shouldn't happen to anyone. No child should have to go through that.
It's not your fault, you know."

"I know, but—"

"There are no buts, Ben," Leon pressed him. "I heard you say you
were sad and scared. Those are real and important emotions. It makes
up our authentic self and when we understand and feel this, we can
learn to intimate instead of violate, you got it?"

"Yeah," Ben exhaled. "I got it." He grabbed his chair and moved
back into the larger group. The men gave it up for him, telling him
"good work, man, thanks for being open." They hugged him, reached
out to pat him on the back. Ben's face was flushed and his hair was wet
with sweat as if he'd run a marathon, but there was nothing tense
about his demeanor. He was relaxed and smiling and human. The rage
I'd grown used to seeing in him, as present and acidic as the tattoos
covering his body, had been put away.

While Ben went through his destruction cycle, Elroy sat in his group
on the other side of the dorm. He had followed a path similar to Ben's,
confronting his demons in the group, confronting the crimes he'd
committed.

He went through a destruction cycle of his own, his voice disap-
pearing in the memories of the man he'd attacked standing in line for
the movies. "This dude made a gesture about my woman," Elroy told

the group. "Like he wanted to hop on her or something. I walked over to him and told him that I would fuck him up if he looked my way again. This little punk ass! He told me to get out of his face. He told me that 'I was tripping' so I hauled off and cracked him. He ended up in the hospital."

Elroy had traveled the emotional gamut during his cycle. When he got angry both legs would splay out and his gigantic arms would clench. When he cried, both legs would fold underneath him, and his eyes would turn to big, bloodshot, watery pools. He was a master at minimizing, saying at first the whole thing was the other guy's fault. "Why did he have to look over at us," and he'd kept himself "controlled." "I had a knife but I didn't use it, I only used my fists!" But revelations assaulted him. He realized as he told the story that the whole reason for the attack—the fact that this guy kept making eyes at his girlfriend—was based on a misguided assumption. "I don't know what the guy was thinking," Elroy said suddenly, a look of confusion playing across his face. "I made it up, I guess. I didn't know what he wanted or what he was doing. Shit, he may not have been doing anything wrong."

"But what if he had?" Earl, who was facilitating the group, had asked. "Would that have made a difference to you."

"Yeah, it would have!" Elroy responded aggressively. But then he caught himself again. "But I guess it shouldn't have."

Once Elroy's defenses fell he, like Ben, was one of the most disciplined participants we had. He sought me out after his fourth month.

"Sunny, I gotta talk at ya for a sec. This place, I just gotta say, this place is the first time I ever had to talk about my feelings and have someone listen."

"I'm glad, Elroy."

"No, you don't get it, Sunny. I've been arrested somewhere like thirty times. I been to a hundred holding cells, had so many damn lawyers I couldn't name a single one, been processed and humiliated so many damn times. But here, this is the first place where I got to work on my problems. The first place!" I'd heard similar things from Latino gangbangers, middle-aged wife beaters and crystal meth dealers. Men like Elroy and Ben told their peers in RSVP what they had never told anyone else. In their excitement they could become euphoric, embracing the group sessions with an almost missionary zeal. It took careful managing, because what they learned on the inside could quickly disappear on the outside, back in their old environments, where they weren't surrounded by positive peer support.

We were just beginning to send our "graduates" out into the world. If we were lucky, we'd get them for six months. Four to five months was the norm. If I'd had my way, we'd get them for two years, because I believed that was how long it took for the program to take hold. This was incredibly difficult work for them, physically and mentally uncomfortable. They had grown up learning how to bury their emotions, learning, as my father and I had, to lash out rather than to feel bad. RSVP was teaching them how to feel, requiring it, and to my never-ending satisfaction, many men were trying.

After Ben and Elroy had been in the dorm for a year, Leon walked into another staff meeting with a big grin on his face. "Guess who's hanging out during their free time?"

Earl and Damon laughed. They already knew. Damon spit it out. "Ebony and Ivory, man, Ben and Elroy are like best friends. That's mighty, Sun. That's mighty."

CHAPTER 16

1999

Deputy Ricky Drocco poked his head into my office. "Sunny, these men down in the dorm are full of crap!"

"What is it this time, Ricky?" I sighed. Drocco was a reality check for me. As RSVP became institutionalized, he was both a believer and a skeptic.

"I'm in *fatal peril,* I'm in *fatal peril,*" Drocco moaned, doing his best exaggeration of a prisoner in group. "I hear these guys go all sincere and boo-hooing during sessions, but you should hear them on the phones."

"What, really? Tell me."

"I just think some of these guys are pulling the wool over your eyes," Drocco said.

"C'mon, Ricky, who do you think is a problem?"

"Argh, Sun, don't worry about it. Forget it, babe, never mind."

"No, Ricky, don't do that. You can't drop a bomb like that and say forget about it. If someone is doing that, you need to call him on it. I need to call him on it. We can't just let it pass."

Drocco shared what he knew with me. I got names, which I passed to the facilitators, and Drocco intervened the next time he heard someone on the phones in the dorm swearing at his partner. It was just one of a thousand small steps. Maintaining RSVP took constant vigilance. No one could slack. The minute you did, jail culture reverted to the lowest common denominator. It reverted to the culture the men brought into the dorms.

We could depend on the criminals resisting the system. They

brought their tribes and hair-trigger tempers. They were always ready to respond to the smallest slight. That was a constant. What was less predictable was maintaining the support of the staff. Deputy sheriffs had to be recruited and trained to embrace RSVP and all the programs of County Jail 7. Rumors were always getting back to me about deputies who thought I was a pillow fluffer, who thought I was wasting my time with the liars who would never change. Becky was critical for maintaining discipline in the ranks of the deputized staff. Whatever problems Becky and I might have had at home, and they were legion, we were always allies at work. The deputies never lost their fear of her and she would bear down like a freight train on anyone who dared step out of line.

None of this was a surprise to me, however. I had come into RSVP with a distrust of deputy sheriffs. What I didn't expect was how much some of them would learn from RSVP, and how much I learned, too.

Three naval midshipmen were sent to County Jail 7. They'd had a one-day furlough to go out in San Francisco. In their twenty-four hours of freedom, they decided to go to the Castro district, beat up a gay man, and put him in the hospital. Something about the sheer stupidity of the crime enraged me and I forced myself to stay away from them. I didn't think I'd be able to keep my emotions in check.

The navy guys were processed into Dorm C, which was a regular program dorm. They were put into college or vocational classes. Because of the nature of their crime, they could have been placed in RSVP, but we didn't have the space.

In the jail we recognized any holiday we could. Many of the men and women came from such terrible educations and knew very little of cultural diversity, so most holidays we celebrated were a way for our teachers to share some history. On Cinco de Mayo, we talked about the Mexicans defeating the French. On Juneteenth, we talked about the Emancipation Proclamation, Abraham Lincoln and the end of slavery. In the last week of June, we talked about Gay Pride Day. And this is where the problems began for our new gay-bashing prisoners.

We were having ITV, Instructional TV, in which we required all prisoners to watch a video and then participate in a discussion with a facilitator. The video we chose that week was a documentary called *The Sharon Kowalski Story*. It told the tragic story of a woman, Kowalski, who was injured in a motorcycle accident and suffered severe brain damage. Kowalski had a lesbian partner whom she'd lived with for years. They'd exchanged rings, bought property together and had intertwined their lives the way any married couple would. But after Kowalski's accident, her parents, with the support of the courts, cut off access to her partner. The movie explored the legal obstacles and inequalities for lesbian and gay couples in American society.

Since the inmates didn't get much television time during the week, they would watch almost anything we put in front of them without much complaint. The navy gay bashers had been in the dorm for about three weeks at this point. They had kept quiet, not distinguishing themselves in the dorm. When the movie started, however, they stood up and turned their backs on the TV and the teachers. Some of the other prisoners followed suit, joining up in a homophobic alliance.

Lieutenant Hunsucker was the supervising officer on duty when the protest occurred. It was his job to deal with the troublemakers while the dorm deputy got everyone else back on schedule. Hunsucker came into my office with a head full of steam.

"Sun, I've got the gay bashers in an empty classroom and I'm about to read them the riot act. I know you're gonna want in on this." He then told me what they'd pulled. I'd resisted dealing with them so far but he was right. I wanted my pound of flesh.

Hunsucker had found ways to infuriate and surprise me. In staff meetings, he was still the first to complain about programs. I found some of the jokes he made to be just this side of Neanderthal. But then he'd rush in, ready to go right at the gay bashers.

He and I walked into the classroom with three sour-looking prisoners. Their haircuts were still military-style buzz cuts. Their legs were splayed, arms were crossed, faces set. Hunsucker started in with a fire-and-brimstone approach.

"This is my jail. I'm the supervisor right now, which means you are under my command. You"—he pointed menacingly at them—"are not going to run things. Now, your hate, and homophobic behavior, will not be tolerated in here and I warn you not to test me. You don't like gay people? That's your pathetic problem. The fact that you had twenty-four hours to have some fun but instead beat up a man because he is gay is stupid and chickenshit. You are not going to play those games here. We will be watching you twenty-four hours a day and one false move and you will be more sorry that you beat that boy up than you ever felt before. You are going to get a real education here. You will learn how to treat all people with respect. That means everyone."

The inmates sat up and listened. Hunsucker was a tough, burly white guy in a uniform, speaking to them like cadets, lecturing them on homophobia, of all things. He could have passed for any of their superior officers. They had to be confused. Their eyes went wide as he hammered at them, and then he turned it over to me. I was enraged. I had walked in with absolutely no sympathy, feeling as disgusted with them as I'd felt about Fred Johnson the pedophile. I wanted to humiliate them and make them squirm. One of them had the name Schwartzkoff,

"Schwartzkoff? Who's Schwartzkoff? Hey, that's similar to my name. Are you Jewish? Do you think we might be related?" I was being childish. "You think you can beat someone up because they're gay? You think your friends should beat you up because you're Jewish?" I looked over at Hunsucker, who was eyeing me skeptically, and I stopped myself. I realized, in an instant, what a remarkable thing we had going. Here was a guy I had once pegged as a homophobic fascist with a badge, trying to build a civil community. Here was Hunsucker, my enemy, doing my job better than I was. I gave up my rant. The guy I was picking on was glaring at me, looking like he wanted to attack. I took a deep breath, and pivoted. "You know, I want to make you squirm the way you made that poor man in the Castro feel fear. I, too, have to control myself to treat you like human beings. If you can't get with a jail program, you will not be able to make it out in the world, a world filled with many different people whether you like it or not. We are giving you an opportunity here to become better people." I looked back at Hunsucker, hoping he would finish it.

"This ain't *Romper Room,*" he concluded. "We aren't about third and fourth chances. We are not going to accept the hate, so you either get with the program now, or your lives get hard. I will make it hard." It was Hunsucker who made the mark with those men. I had given up my authority when I went after one of them. It was that easy to lose it.

The men went back into their dorm. I went back to my office, profoundly thankful. This was becoming a healthier community. These damaged people we brought inside the walls had a chance to take control of their lives and change. They had the chance. Some of them would take it. And they weren't the only ones learning to control their damage. I was learning. Hunsucker was learning. We were all learning each day to make our lives a little richer, a little better. There was a quote I had posted on my wall that I sometimes forgot was there. It was from Egon Bittner, a groundbreaking sociologist who studied the relationship between police and society. He wrote, "The consideration extended to the seemingly undeserving person is not intended for his or her personal benefit, but expresses the moral integrity of the one who extends it. It enhances the dignity of human life, especially in situations where extending it appears to be hopelessly misspent."

Nine months later, the gay bashers were released. I hadn't followed their progress but I recognized them as I drove up to the gate. New releases had the option to take the bus into the city or to walk out the front door. They were walking down the road as I pulled into the parking lot. One of them saw me and walked up to my car. I was a little wary but he smiled nervously and waved. "Ms. Schwartz," he said. "I want you to know, I really learned a lot here and thank you."

I wished him luck and he almost skipped away to the car that was waiting for him.

CHAPTER 17

2000

The deputy flipped the switch. The heavy metal door slid open. I slipped through to soft murmuring. Men were gathered into four groups in front of dry-erase boards. They were talking in hushed tones, and a few were scribbling furiously on the board. Men waited their turn to join the conversation. Except for the county-issue orange, I could be in church, or a lecture hall, anywhere but a jail.

I thought of my first day on Mainline, which is just a random cross-section of criminals, not nearly as hardened as the group we brought together in RSVP. RSVP had the worst our system had to offer. But the difference between Mainline and the RSVP dorm was the difference between chaos and calm. In short, it was the difference between a place where the thugs controlled the culture, and a place that was controlled by all of our better instincts. They might as well have been two different planets.

Each group in RSVP was overseen by a facilitator. Most of the day, veteran inmates led the discussions, and helped control the flow of the day. Ben was facilitating one of the groups, his small, wiry frame folded into a chair off to my left. Elroy was facilitating a group to my right, his bulk engulfing a chair, his hands doing half his talking as he made a point to his group. Both men had been reborn in RSVP and were among our greatest success stories. Ben had spent a year in a postrelease residential treatment center for drug abuse and joined us, after twelve months of training, as a peer educator and facilitator. Elroy had taken a similar journey.

They had ended up becoming dear friends. Ben's mother died

recently and Elroy went with him down to Orange County as he wrapped up his family affairs. I watched them both work for a few minutes. At thirty-two, Elroy was almost ten years older than most of the prisoners, and his imposing physique was offset by a kind face and soothing voice. It rumbled but didn't roar. His size conferred instant respect, and he was also one of our most focused facilitators, never letting standards slip in his group. Ben's nervous energy had moderated. His toe still tapped when he was thinking. He still fidgeted, but it was passion, not anger, that drove him.

A new prisoner was going through a destruction cycle in Ben's group. The man, José, a short Mexican with a long braid down his back, was laughing a little as he told his story.

"So, me and my boys we hang at the corner of Mission and Twenty-second. Oh man, we drink too much." Here he smiled nervously. "We smoke too much, too. For like six months, I don't think I go a day without getting high. And this one night, I go home to get my car keys so we could cruise the hood but my old lady she snatched the car keys outta my hand. So I tell her, 'Bitch, you better not mess with me tonight, I am in no mood for this bullshit.' I was drinking too much and she wouldn't give up the keys. She was like, you know, fighting me for the keys. And I was drunk and I fought back. I was loaded. I barely remember what happened." José wound to a close and looked up.

"What does that mean? You beat her up. What exactly did you do?" Ben asked.

"Man, I dunno, I was pretty wasted," José replied.

"You chose to drink, didn't you?"

"Well, yeah, but . . ."

"You knew you were more violent when you were loaded, right?"

"Sure, man, but everybody I hung out with was drinking." The guy looked put-upon.

"Hey, I'm not picking on you," Ben's tone softened. "But it's important and I want you to recognize the way we talk about our actions, right? The way we talk about them is the way we understand them. Everything we do, at some point, we made a choice to do. If you know you're violent when you drink, then if you drink, you've chosen to be violent, right?"

The men around Ben voiced their agreement. The inmate on the hot seat nodded slowly, letting the idea sink in.

"So tell me what happened after she took your keys," Ben said.

Now the man really began to squirm. "Man, why you want to play me? I just don't remember much, you know."

Ben stayed on him. "Look, that's not gonna fly here. Can I get an agreement from you right now? Can I get an agreement that you will listen as much as you can with an open heart and disclose everything you do remember and know that all of us are violent men. This is the important stuff. You may not remember every detail. But you saw the aftermath, right?" Ben looked at José until he slowly nodded his agreement. "You saw the ambulance come, right? People told you what happened, right? So you tell us that. Tell us the damage that you did. Saying you don't remember is a way we use to avoid responsibility for our actions. If you truly don't remember, you better go learn what you did. The hospital reports will be in your defense attorney's file. There's no excuse for not knowing. Can I get an agreement about that?"

I looked back at the inmate. He was steaming, his eyes were blank, his shoulders tight. But he couldn't escape. His hands slowly came up to show fatal peril. He would have to confront his crimes either today or soon.

On the other side of the room, Elroy was doing the same work in his group. The groups went on all day. RSVP had helped these men. In the first years of the program the evidence had been anecdotal. Men I'd seen come through the jails numerous times I'd realize weren't there anymore. They'd done a hitch in RSVP and I'd hear they had gotten a job driving a bus, or working in an office. But then we got proof that the anecdotes added up to a larger reality. We had sought out Dr. James Gilligan, the violence expert then at Harvard, and he'd agreed to do an evaluation of the program. His study looked at recidivism rates for the RSVP men, and the results were impressive. The simple takeaway from his study was that the more time inmates spent in RSVP, the less likely they were to be rearrested for violent crimes.

Inmates who had participated in RSVP for at least 8 weeks had a rate of arrests for violent crimes per day in the community during their first year

after release from jail that were 46.3% lower than those of the 101 mem-
bers of the control group (p 0.05). For those in RSVP for 12 weeks or
more, the violent crime rearrest rate was 53.1% lower (p 0.05); and those
in for at least 16 weeks had a violent rearrest rate 82.6% lower (p 0.05).
In each of the three pairs of group comparisons, the members of the exper-
imental group who were rearrested spent significantly less time in custody,
and significantly more days in the community before their first arrest (for
either a violent or nonviolent crime), than did those in the control group.*

Gilligan did find that many RSVP graduates were still being sent
back to jail, but most of that was for drug possession instead of violent
crimes. Many men who had gone through RSVP had stopped their
violence. The men who spent longer in RSVP were doing better than
the men who had spent less time. RSVP was helping these men. I had
the hard proof. And, I'm happy to say, RSVP was helping me, too.

After nine years together, after hundreds of fights on old battle-
grounds, Becky and I found something new to fight about—she began
staying out late. She'd never had many of her own friends. She'd
always been a loner. But she'd finally, after many years, made a new
one of her own. The woman was a nurse and had just gone through a
bad breakup after catching her lover in bed with someone else. I
invited her over for Shabbos dinner and she and Becky had hit it off.

Then, over time, Becky slowly grew irritable with me, impatient,
lost behind a newspaper, in front of the television, or just out. She
began going out and not coming home until past midnight. I tried
confronting her. "Come on, Becky, just tell me what's going on."

"There's nothing going on," she'd tell me. "You're imagining it. I
can't believe you would want to start a fight over the first friend I've
had."

When she finally admitted to me that she was having an affair,
some four months after the fact, my heart crumbled. I could not see
straight. I'd been wrecked before, by Stevie, by other women, by my

---

*James Gilligan and Bandy Lee, *The Resolve to Stop the Violence Project: Reducing Violence*
through a Jail-Based Initiative, commissioned report, December 2000.

mother's death, but something about Becky's betrayal brought me to my knees.

In the midst of this, I went to sit in on a Manalive class that we helped run out in the community. Many of our facilitators at County Jail 7 participated in these groups, since they were former violent men themselves. I went to one that Earl facilitated in the basement of San Francisco's Third Baptist Church.

I took my seat as part of the circle. I was the only woman there, and many people knew I was the big mama of RSVP. Some of these men had been inmates in the program. Earl was checking in, going man to man, asking the traditional questions at the beginning of meetings. What's your name? How do you feel? Have you had any moments of fatal peril?

He reached a guy with the build of a construction worker who couldn't answer. He couldn't speak; he put his hands to his face and started breathing hard. Finally, he regained his composure, said his name was Dennis and said he had to talk about what he'd done. His voice was clipped, as if he'd had to bind it in order to make it intelligible.

"My wife is six months pregnant," Dennis said. "She has been cold to me, lately, not talking or giving me anything. I suspected she was cheating on me for a while, but she denied it when I asked her. 'You're fucked up,' she'd say. Once, I was on her for so long she started screaming, 'Get out of my house.' I kept at her, though, more and more. I was calling her a fuckin' whore, telling her she was a piece of dirt, every day I was at her until finally she snapped back.

"She said, 'That's right. I am a whore. I'm sleeping with Roger.' Roger is this asshole she grew up with. My wife, she was real cold. She said, 'Fuck you, and for all I know, it's his baby.' Man . . ." At that moment Dennis's hands went up, indicating fatal peril. Tears were streaming down his face.

"I lost it. I hit her. I knocked her to the ground and kicked her." Dennis started sobbing but kept trying to talk. "I was wrong. I hurt her bad. I might have hurt the baby. I would do anything to turn back time and . . ." He finally couldn't speak anymore. There was a dead silence in the room punctuated by Dennis's sobs.

While Dennis was telling the story, my heart and guts rebelled. I hated him for doing what he had done. I couldn't stop picturing it—a pregnant woman being knocked down, cowering, defenseless, with this big brute standing over her. I hated him. And yet, I felt a shred of pity for the pain he had felt, his feeling of betrayal, and then, all of a sudden, I was overwhelmed. Tears were streaming down my face. I was trying, and failing, to hold back sobs. Before Becky had confessed everything to me, I had felt like the biggest intrusion in her life, like I was a speck on her shoulder that she kept flicking away. I felt like he did. His shame was my shame.

When it came to my turn to speak, I couldn't get the words out. Earl just looked at me with sweet, serious eyes. He wasn't going to bail me out or insist on me talking. He patiently waited until I was ready. Finally, I composed myself enough to look at Dennis and say "Man, I hate you so much for doing that to your wife. And I appreciate that you are trying to look at yourself and working at it so this never happens again. But I hate you for what you did." Dennis looked at me and nodded his head and said nothing. We were both wrecks.

Dennis had reminded me, in the most powerful way possible, that if I didn't figure out how to be okay with what had happened with Becky, I was going down his path. I could either embrace the shame, embarrassment and humiliation, or I could turn it to rage, which would mean I'd never have to deal with these raw feelings.

For once in my life, I had every "justified" reason to go crazy. I wanted to scream, throw Becky's things into the street, slash her tires, lose my marbles. I'd done it to lovers in the past with women who had done nothing wrong. But with Becky, amazingly, I kept the rage in check. I let grief overtake me, and never let it spin out of control. Dennis and RSVP and my own therapy kept reminding me to stay with the hurt but not let it turn violent.

Every morning I would wake up in a puddle, sobbing on my bedroom floor. I felt like I did when my father's temper filled the room, blotting me out. I felt like I did when my mother couldn't stand up for me, when she let my father rage and call me a dreck lesbian. I felt like I did when my brothers left me behind to go play baseball, Stevie yelling, "Get lost, Chubs, no one wants you around." I felt like I did failing the remedial classes, a hopeless loser who didn't deserve love, or happiness. I felt it all. In fact, the only being capable of getting me off the floor was Towby, my beagle, who would drown me in sloppy kisses until I sat up laughing, my misery pushed aside for a minute. I'd pull myself up from my knees, throw coffee down my throat and wander into work a zombie. By the end of the day I'd be alive again. I'd listen to the men of RSVP who would confess to horrible crimes, and admit to shame, and fears and hurts that they had carried for their whole lives, and pledge to do things differently, pledge to get on a better path.

They all were struggling with far greater injuries than mine. Ben's father had abandoned him when he was nine, and rarely reached out to him again. His uncle had molested him. Elroy's mother had been a heroin addict. He'd been abandoned to the foster system when he was twelve. Each of the men they worked with discovered similar shame in their own past and they confronted the pain they caused in their victims. They felt it all together, and I felt it with them.

CHAPTER 18

2000

There was no magic we performed on Ben or the rest of the men in RSVP. There was nothing we did to them that can't be replicated in any other prison or jail. We didn't create new therapeutic techniques. We didn't reinvent the wheel. The list of things we provided for the men was revolutionary simply because almost no one had done what we did in a correctional setting. RSVP can be re-created. It can be re-created in every jail and prison in the country. And it can also fail.

As part of RSVP, we had a program for the victims of RSVP men, which offered counseling and other practical services. It was a core part of our program but we were always scrambling to keep it funded. We let victims know we existed. We did not, as a rule, try to convince them to participate, or try to set up reconciliation meetings between our RSVP men and the victims. It was simply too delicate and depended entirely on the needs and desires of the victim. If a perpetrator wasn't far enough along, if he tried to minimize what he'd done, or excuse it, we risked hurting the victim all over again. We also didn't have the money to do more than we already were. It was a small but important part of the larger program, which ran smoothly until just before Halloween, 2000.

It was Friday morning. Jack-o'-lanterns dotted the halls in the administration wing of County Jail 7. Halloween decorations always gave me the creeps in jail. Demons and ghouls bore too much resemblance to some of the monsters who came through our doors. Before I made it to my office, Leah, one of our administrative assistants, rushed up. Her face was ashen. Leah worked with Bianka in the victims' outreach program, which offered counseling and other help to the victims of RSVP men. Leah could barely speak but managed to say that one of their clients, a domestic violence victim, had been murdered the night before. Neighbors had seen her abusive ex-boyfriend, a man named Tari Ramirez, running from the house with a bloody knife.

"Sunny," Leah said, "Ramirez just spent four months in the RSVP dorm. He was released about three months ago." Her bottom lip was quivering. "What do we do, Sunny, what do we do?"

I lost my balance for a second and sat down heavily in a chair.

I couldn't believe it. Didn't want to believe it. It may sound stupid but I had never prepared for this. We had grown so used to working with the worst monsters the monster factory could produce. I'd grown used to their feeling remorse, taking responsibility for their violence. So many had walked out in better shape than when they'd walked in. This was a sucker punch.

"Leah, what do we know? Are we sure it was one of our guys?"

"Sunny, there were multiple eyewitnesses. People are sure he's the one. I went to get the file as soon as the call came in this morning. Ramirez came to us on a DV charge against Claire Tempongko." *DV* was shorthand for domestic violence. "He was in the RSVP dorm until August, and then was released. He attended the postrelease Manalive classes as well."

"Claire Tempongko, she's the one who was killed?" I asked.

"Yeah." Leah sighed. "They say that last night, Ramirez broke into her home, waited for her and attacked her with a kitchen knife when she came in. Her two kids were right there."

"Oh Jesus, Leah, how old are they?"

"Five and ten."

Later in the morning, I called the entire staff to my office. Everyone knew already. Ben came in looking like he'd been sick to his stomach. The other men who worked in the dorm—Leon, Elroy, Earl and Damon—looked tired. Bianka, Delia and Marcela, our victims' coordinators, had red eyes. There was a feeling of defeat in the room. We'd had only two fights in three years, and each fight was a push and a shove. At the time, that had freaked us out.

"I don't know what to say," I said. "I am devastated like you are. I don't have a speech prepared. I think people should just talk."

There was silence for a long time. Then Ben spoke. "Tari was in my group, I, um, I'm . . . I don't know how I am . . ." Ben's voice trailed off. He was the one who had most recently worked with Ramirez. Ben was running the postrelease Manalive classes for graduates of RSVP. "Ramirez, the guy was like a Boy Scout. He was helpful, he had all the lingo down. He seemed really interested in getting with the program. I guess I missed it."

"Hey," Leon interjected. "You can't blame yourself here. You're doing good work, you know."

"I know Leon, I know," Ben agonized. "But I just can't help but feel this is my fault. I should have known. I'm supposed to be able to see when these guys aren't being straight. I didn't pick it up with this guy at all. What the hell are we doing? Does any of this make sense?" People reached out to support Ben, but we all felt some version of what he was saying.

We went around the room, sharing what we knew, sharing regrets. Earl had had Ramirez in his group in the RSVP dorm. "Ben's right, man. The guy was polite, obedient really. I mean he started out all jacked up, like Ben did, or like me even. You know. He had the 'What the fuck is this? You can't force me to be here' attitude. But he snapped to it real quick."

"Yeah, he did," Ben confirmed. "He used the language. He called other people on their bullshit. I'd sit and wonder sometimes, you know, the subtle clues weren't always right. He seemed like he was parroting the language sometimes. But he was a good liar. I bought it."

Bianka had her own regrets to add. She said she was out in the neighborhoods working with victims. Claire Tempongko had been on her list of clients. "We had an appointment with Claire last week but she canceled. She said she wasn't feeling well. It's not the first time she'd canceled on me but it felt to me like something was wrong. I tried to follow up with her but I never got her on the phone."

Delia remembered meeting Claire from a women's group we had sponsored for survivors of violence. "She sat in the front row. Leon had given a presentation, saying what they were doing with the men. Claire had raised her hand to complain: 'This stuff doesn't work. Tari doesn't take responsibility! He accuses me of being violent!' At the end of the session, I tried to tell her about services, but she'd shrugged them off."

There was only so much to say. My greatest fear had come true. Tari Ramirez had taken the hope of RSVP and subverted it. He had played the system, resisted the peer leadership, and went right back to his abusive ways when he hit the streets. I tried to encourage the staff, telling them we had done what we could to try to help Ramirez and Claire. After Ramirez stopped attending Manalive classes, Ben had done the right thing and called Ramirez's probation officer. Failure to appear was a probation violation, and the PO could have sent Ramirez back to prison, but he didn't.

"You know, we opened the door to a better life for this monster," I said. "Many men have walked through that door. He chose not to."

But the words didn't satisfy. Not even me. We learned more details as the day went on. It turned out that Claire had called the police numerous times after Ramirez was released from our custody to report that he was stalking her. This should have set off alarm bells and sent Ramirez back to prison but the system had failed. Police reports didn't make it to the probation officer. The ones that did weren't followed up on. Claire was murdered. And Tari Ramirez escaped. After two days, he still hadn't been captured.

I called Sheriff Hennessey the day of the murder. I knew it was going to hit the papers.

"Yeah, I heard about it. Killed in front of her children. Just terrible," he said.

"Hennessey, I got to tell you. He spent some time in RSVP. About four months."

"Oh that's terrible, Sunny. You guys all right over there?"

"Yeah, we're shook up, but we're okay."

"Did we do all we could? We make any mistakes?"

"No, Sheriff. He stopped attending classes after his release. We reported him, but he disappeared off of our radar."

He didn't say anything right away. I knew he was relieved to hear it wasn't our fault. I was relieved it wasn't our fault, too. But I was still heartsick and wondering what he would say.

Hennessey finally responded. "Listen, this is a high-risk business. We're not working with altar boys. We're working with violent men. This is a horrible thing that happened, but we have to remember that this is just one of the crimes we weren't able to stop."

There was finger-pointing in the media, a "crisis of conscience," and the blame fell on the police and probation departments. Not on us. There were reforms in the aftermath, overhauls that were long overdue to improve communication between the agencies. Those were good results. But the murder had exposed one of the central problems buried in our criminal justice system, one that my work hasn't begun to touch. There are too many teams working at cross purposes in criminal justice. I was relieved that we weren't to blame for Claire's murder, but just thinking that missed the point. Eighteen years earlier, when I'd tried to find a solution for the release of Fred Johnson, I'd met with a common response from everyone I'd talked to. "It's not my job. You can't save everyone."

I have two responses to that. The first is that the person truly at fault is the perpetrator. Blame ultimately starts and ends there. And so it's a true statement to say that "it's not my fault that this happened." But the second response is that we are either part of a solution or we're not. We either share in its success or failure, or we don't. If we are going to play a role in the life and crime of a community, then all of us, from police to prosecutor to jail worker to ordinary citizen, have to take some stock of what happened to Claire, and what happened to her two children. So the questions, I believe, fall on all of us to answer. How do we stop more children from becoming orphans? How do we stop this cycle of crime? How do we draw a line in the sand and say no more? Men got out of RSVP and renounced their violence but men also got out of RSVP, hit the streets, scored a speedball and went back to sticking up convenience stores. Even an 80 percent reduction in violent rearrests meant that 20 percent were still untouched by what we did. The program "fails" every single day. But that doesn't mean that I didn't get up each day, go into work and search for new ways to make it better, that I didn't fight to make sure no one fell through the cracks, that we wouldn't take our best shot with every single person who came through our doors. This was high risk. After Tari Ramirez killed Claire Tempongko, in RSVP we learned to look at every survivor we worked with as as if they were in a pine box. That was what was at stake.

I talked regularly with our RSVP staff, especially the men who had been violent, about being active in their restorative justice work. What had they done recently to restore the community they'd harmed? In one meeting, I mentioned that I'd received a call from Temple Sinai over in Oakland. They had invited me to come talk to the congregation about our work during their "Peace Seder" on Passover. I wondered whether any of the men wanted to come with me. I asked them to think about it, then we went on to other business.

Ben sought me out in my office a day later.

"Hey, Sunny." He was rubbing his hands together nervously. Usually, he liked to shoot the shit, but today he was like a laser. "Listen, I have something I need to ask you. I've been thinking more and more about what you said in the meeting yesterday about what we can do to give back to the community. I couldn't sleep last night thinking about the synagogue; it seemed right for me and my crimes. But it scares me so much to think about going. What do you think?"

I'd been hoping Ben would think about it. "It's going to be a difficult crowd," I told him. "I've been there a few times and they are a mixed group, a lot of young, active, progressive folks and older folks, too, and some of them are Holocaust survivors. There are going to be a lot of people in that crowd who absolutely despise skinheads, even former ones."

Ben was coiled in the seat across from me. "Sounds scary and good," he told me. "If you think it won't be a problem for the congregation, I am for it, one hundred percent."

I talked to the woman who invited me. She was moved by Ben's story and thought it was worth the risk to have him speak. A month later, on a warm afternoon, Ben and I drove over the Bay Bridge to Temple Sinai in Oakland. Sinai is one of the oldest congregations in the Bay Area. Founded in 1875, it sits in Berkeley's orbit, and for years had been out front putting reading programs in Oakland schools, protesting the war in Vietnam and leading the charge on feminist issues. It is a liberal reform congregation, but that didn't mean I thought Ben would get a loving welcome. I was terrified of how the day would go.

As we drove, Ben was quiet, his hand beating out a rhythm on the armrest. He confessed to me as we parked, "Sunny, I'm scared shit-less." I looked at him. His hair was covering the swastika on his head, and he was wearing a long-sleeve shirt that covered the tattoos on his arms. But how would they see him inside? I'd never been involved in something like this before.

There were about thirty round tables in Temple Sinai's large audi-torium, set and ready for the Passover Seder. I introduced ourselves to the organizer and we found a table with about ten other people. I led the conversation, telling the people what we did, getting the usual oohs and aahs of support. Working with prisoners was a good conver-sation starter. Most people want to know what it's like behind bars. Ben was fidgeting and quiet. Soon the service started.

We drank the wine (Ben abstained) and gave thanks for deliverance from Egypt. The questions were asked—"Why is this night different from every other night?"—by a cute moppet with ringlets tied into ponytails behind her head. Ben's head stayed bowed. We were memo-rializing the Jews' deliverance from slavery to freedom and I was thinking of my deliverance from my relationship with Becky. I imag-ined Ben was thinking of his own victories. He was clean and sober, and had rejected the hate that was suffocating him. I was proud of him, and also worried for him. Sitting at the next table was an elderly cou-ple. I saw tattooed numbers crawling up their arms.

The Seder was nearly over and there was a pause in the service when Temple Sinai's director, a middle-aged woman with a peace but-ton on her lapel, stood for announcements and to introduce us.

I kept my talk short. I told the congregation a little bit about the jails and RSVP and the work we were trying to do. Then I introduced Ben.

"One of my colleagues from the jail who works in the RSVP dorm has come with me, and I want to turn the floor over to him. Some of the things he is going to disclose today are going to be personal, and may be difficult for you to hear. When he's done I want to make sure you know that we will take questions, and take all feedback with an open heart." With that I sat down. Ben sprang from his seat. He was sweating and though he was used to talking in front of crowds, and did it every day in the jails, he fumbled over his words.

"Thank you for having me here," he finally managed to say. He coughed. "I, um, as you might be able to tell, I am very nervous talking to you. Everything I want to share with you is said with a full heart. I work with the men of RSVP as a facilitator. That means I run groups for violent men, directing their conversations, helping with the peer-led therapy, and work one-on-one with them to try to get them to stop their violence. But I also need to share that I was one of them a little over a year ago. Most facilitators in the RSVP dorm were violent men themselves at one time. I was in jail and everything I have done is my fault and my responsibility. I have done some very bad things. For many years, I was a heroin and meth addict, a member of a racist skinhead gang and a thug. I want to share some of my journey with you and will not blame you for hating me." My heart was racing as I watched him turn the corner in his story. I looked around. There was a wariness to the crowd; concerned looks showed themselves at many of the tables. Behind me, someone whispered, "I can't believe they let someone like that in here." My heart skipped.

Ben continued. "I was raised in Orange County. I was a very lonely kid and always wanted to be a part of something. I made some stupid decisions and hooked up with people I thought would look after me. They took me in as part of their family. They were skinheads, and they ate, drank and slept hatred all day long and soon I was doing the same. They made me feel like I was somebody. It was twisted thinking on my part. This skinhead group thought the white race was superior and everyone, especially blacks and Jews, were inferior, thought they were not worth living. Soon I believed it, too. I started believing horrible things about Jewish people, even though my first name, Benjamin, is Jewish. I fueled my hatred with drugs and I became a monster. I hurt a lot of people. I beat up black people, gays and Jewish people in the streets of Van Nuys where I grew up and up here. I was arrested in San Francisco for beating up a random stranger on the street." There were quiet responses all around me. Deep sighs racked the older couple I had noticed earlier. Some of the women I saw looked visibly pained. I checked for the nearest exit in case things turned ugly. I quickly ticked through the ways I could interject to calm an angry crowd. "Come on, folks, let's listen to this man who is now committed to making sure this does not happen again" or "Come on, let's be mensches" or "Yell at me, I invited him" or, worst-case scenario, "Hey, look over there" and then hightail it out the back. But Ben soldiered on.

"But then I was arrested and I never thought I would feel this but it was the best thing to be arrested in San Francisco. I'd been arrested maybe twenty times before but here in San Francisco, they made me go into a dorm, the RSVP dorm, where they taught me how to stop my violence. In RSVP, I was forced to look in the mirror and I didn't like what I saw. I hated what I saw in me. I was ashamed. But RSVP helped me to name it, to accept my shame rather than run from it. Rather than let my shame fuel my violence, I learned to let it be. The work in RSVP helped me be the real man I am today." Ben started tearing up. "I want to tell you how sorry I am for saying horrible things about Jewish people. I want to tell you how sorry I am for trashing a synagogue in San Diego, for yelling out hateful things to people in your community, for assaulting people because I thought they might be Jewish. Part of my recovery process is to try to make restoration to the communities that I've hurt and I want to apologize to you today and say that I will do anything to give back to your community." By this time Ben had lost it. I went over to him and stood next to him. He looked done so I finished for him.

"I want to thank all of you for listening to us and want to open the floor to questions or concerns—" I had more to say but I was interrupted. The congregation began clapping, and they stood up, and started to crowd around Ben and me.

An old man with a thick Eastern European accent took Ben's hand and didn't let go for about five minutes, until he finally said, "I never thought I'd ever see the day when someone who identified with Nazis would say 'I'm sorry.'"

Ben sat down finally, with tears staining his cheeks. The rabbi said the final recitation. I flushed and gave silent thanks and thought of my family. I thought of my mother, my grandmother Bubba, Uncle Henry and Stevie, all dead now. I thought of the raucous Passover meals we had. My father always led the prayers. It was tradition. But my mother always knew the order of events better, always whispered along, filling in the gaps where my father faltered. Someone was read-ing in the large, echoing room at Temple Sinai, but it was the whisper of my mother I heard.

> *And the Lord brought us forth out of Egypt with a strong arm and an outstretched hand, and by great terror, and with signs, and with wonders.*

EPILOGUE

The work in County Jail 7 eventually grew beyond it. And there are many other programs of which I am proud.

We started a charter school for the inmate population, the first of its kind in the country. It was Sheriff Hennessey's idea and I worked with the Republicans in the California leadership to help bring this about. The issue really isn't partisan. I haven't met a Democrat or Republican who hasn't responded to the idea that what we need to do with prisoners is get them to hold a mirror up to their behavior and their lives, not get them to kneel on pebbles. The first step in holding up that mirror is getting the prisoners a basic education.

I'm proud of getting to walk out onto the San Francisco Giants' diamond every year for Strike Out Violence Day. Back in 1996, I received a call from the new general manager of the team, Brian Sabean. At first I thought it was a prank call from a buddy who was as big a baseball nut as I was. But after a few embarrassing minutes, I finally started to listen. Brian said he'd heard about RSVP. His team had a policy of 100 percent player participation in a community cause, and he was wondering if the Giants could get involved in our work. Later, in his office, as I tried hard not to revert to teenybop questions about players' personal habits, I told him about sitting in the bleachers of Wrigley Field as a teenager, marveling at the combined energy of the fans. I wondered what would happen if we could get those fans thinking about violence in their homes and community. The sheriff, Larry Baer, Brian Sabean and I agreed to devote a day at the ballpark to raising awareness, and a year later, Strike Out Violence Day was born.

The event was the first of its kind in the country, where a major-league sports team, a law enforcement agency and a national domestic violence agency collaborated to educate fans on resources to stop violence. It included a pregame ceremony where ex-offenders, victims of violence and community leaders stood together to promote a peaceful society. To date we are in our tenth year, and close to 500,000 fans later, we have successfully married a compelling public awareness day with America's favorite pastime—baseball.

I'm also proud of being Trisha Meili's pitching coach. Trisha Meili became notorious as the Central Park jogger who was beaten, raped and left for dead in New York in 1989. In 2003, she wrote a book about her attack and recovery and revealed her identity. That year I invited her to throw out the first pitch at Strike Out Violence Day. Trisha also agreed to give a victim impact statement to the men of RSVP. We stood in the parking lot of County Jail 7 practicing her fastball. She had a pretty good arm.

Her presentation to the men of RSVP was phenomenal. She talked about her recovery, how she felt blessed not to remember the details of the attack, how she had to learn how to be a person again: how to speak, how to write, how to add and subtract. It was the first time she'd met with violent offenders. It was the first time she'd come close to the kind of men who had hurt her.

One of our inmates stood up during her question-and-answer period and confessed that he had raped someone. He said it was the first time he had ever told anyone this and that he would never have the opportunity to say he was sorry to his victim but that he was sorry for what had been done to Trisha. Trisha blanched as the man spoke, her face a riot of emotions. But when he was through she accepted his apology. On the ride to the ballpark she told me she was heartened. She felt that if just one of the men were changed by what she'd said, then she had hope. At the ballpark, she threw a fastball down the middle into the catcher's mitt while the crowd roared.

On the flip side of all that hope, of course, is the reality facing many of the people we are working with. The inmates in the San Francisco jails are the dregs of society, and disappointment and failure are our daily companions. Tari Ramirez was on the run for five years before he was apprehended in Mexico. He was extradited in 2006. Some people in my office went to his first evidentiary hearing. Claire Tempongko's family was there, their faces drawn and tight, having to see, just like everyone else in that room, the bloody evidence photos, the gruesome record of Claire's last moments. As I write this, Tari Ramirez is preparing to go on trial. I fully expect him to be convicted and do time, but nothing that happens now will undo the damage he has done. He will always be an example of the limits of our program. Anyone in the RSVP dorm has the potential to be like Tari Ramirez. Every year we have men leave the program whose transformations feel profound but who revert to their old ways when they hit the streets. The only test for men in RSVP is whether they can carry their transformation to the streets, and resist the pull of their old culture, their old habits, and become good men. Even some of our greatest success stories have fallen.

Ben faltered. He got lost in alcohol and had to step away from the jails, found a job managing a café and got back on track. Elroy, sadly, didn't make it. One day, we found out he was a deadbeat dad, not making his child support payments. Soon I heard from people on the street that he was using. His eyes narrowed when I called him to my office and asked him if he'd been smoking weed. His face became hard like his old convict mug shot—blank, tough, a look of provocation. He asked if I was going to fire him. I asked him if he would agree to take a drug test.

"Sunny, there's gonna be no trouble. *No trouble,* I tell you, because I'm clean as a whistle. I promise you that."

Elroy tested positive for marijuana. His job was to teach other men to be honest and accountable and he had stopped making payments to his child, and he lied to me. I had to fire him. I called him every few weeks to check up on him, but he slipped away, consumed by shame, never able to be honest with me. In 2006 he came back to the jails, this time as a prisoner on a drug possession charge. I took some solace in the fact that it wasn't for a violent offense.

The kind of men who come to RSVP are the reason so many people are sickened by the criminal justice system. They are the reason the American people have institutionalized a no-tolerance policy toward criminals. These men are the dirtbags who beat their wives, who start the gang wars, who shoot innocent children in the street over turf, who are addicted to drugs and rob and beat up people to support their habit,

and keep coming back to jail over and over again. You have to know that
you will often fail.

The word I use most with my staff is *humility*. I remind us all to stay
humble, to know that the men we work with often come from the second, third and fourth generation of incarcerated men. Those men
have inherited violence, substance abuse and the absence of personal
responsibility like a birthright. We know how profoundly difficult it is
to break these patterns, and that failure with some of the men is not
just a possibility, it is a daily expectation that carries the promise of profound tragedy. I also know, having had to struggle to maintain the programs every year, how hard it is to convince lawmakers, and voters,
that the betterment of criminals is worth spending money on. Voters
have been happy to spend money on jails and prisons, but not on anything to keep these men out of jail.

I haven't talked much about money yet. The fights I've had to try
to get each of our programs funded could fill their own book, though
I'm not sure anyone would read it. They are mind-numbing tales of
bureaucratic logjams and Solomonic decision making. I have often
been given the choice: Do you want reading or domestic violence prevention this year? You've only got money for one. Programs usually
are the last thought in a perpetually cash-strapped criminal justice system. My approach has always been not to make the choice. We find the
money for the programs elsewhere—from grants, from local funders,
from wherever we can get it. But money is only part of the battle. Programs are about leadership. If the leadership wants a workout room
for correctional officers rather than a parenting class then that's what
happens. In San Francisco County, I've been lucky to work with Sheriff Michael Hennessey. His even-keeled approach and dedication to
the principle of programs has been steadfast. He knows that these men
and women will be making a round-trip to prison after their release if
we don't do something.

But the challenge is for all of us, not just for me or for Sheriff Hennessey in our small corner of San Francisco. What if all the juvenile
and adult correctional facilities in the country were set up to address
the problems and deficiencies of our criminal class from day one of
lock up? What kind of society would we be if we made sure each prisoner received the therapy, education and peer pressure pushing him to

do the right thing so that when he's released, he can grow up and get a job and stop terrorizing us. If that happened we could stop the violence and stop building prisons. I believe violent people have to be taken out of circulation. But it need not be a permanent removal if we stop sending them to monster factories and instead direct them to places that invest in their success.

The approach and principles I have described are biblical. You hurt someone, you take responsibility. You give back to the person and community that you harmed. There is nothing innovative about that idea. This is basic human decency, what I call being tough *and* smart on crime. And it works. Former Harvard professor and violence expert Dr. James Gilligan, who studied our program, found dramatic reductions in violent rearrests after just four months in RSVP. Four months can change behavior! This is revolutionary, and it didn't take an arm and a leg to do it. A healthy budget for RSVP, which includes postrelease programs such as job training, therapy, life skills and housing (critical to the program's effectiveness) is forty-four dollars per prisoner per day on top of the ninety-six dollars we now spend in San Francisco County to house and feed them. The money actually saved by society in court costs and medical bills and everything related to crime, not to mention the reduction of trauma for generations, would be astronomical. This isn't a money issue; it's a perception issue. What is needed is leadership.

In 2008, Westchester County in New York initiated RSVP East. County Executive Andrew Spano, his right-hand man Larry Schwartz and Commissioner Rocco Pozzi, like Sheriff Hennessey, took the risk of importing the full RSVP program into their jails, the only other institution in the country to do so. In Valhalla Jail, as in County Jail 7, they have a dorm filled with violent offenders. I was on the floor the first week of the program with forty-four monsters, who were tough, tattooed and snarling. Within days they had abandoned their hard exteriors and started to learn how to be accountable for their actions, and talk with their hearts and their minds. When it began, the Westchester folks had the same reservations we'd had in San Francisco: Does it work? Can we keep correctional workers safe? Is it worth it? How do we pay for it? But they committed to the program seeing the need to stop the cycle of violence.

We've won awards for RSVP. The most notable is probably the

Innovations in American Government Awards from Harvard University. They call it the Oscars for government public service. But while it's wonderful to be recognized, it pains me that our approach should be considered innovative. I think it should be as common as court time. If I've done my job right, after reading this book, hopefully you will think so, too.

I have a two-year-old named Ella. There is too much to tell about how I came to be a mother in a loving relationship with a beautiful, brilliant woman whom I adore, who is tough on me, and kind and generous. Recovery from the habits of my childhood is an everyday activity, but my partner, Lauren, keeps me honest. I promised Ella, our daughter, when she was born that wherever she went, I would always be there for her. And I asked only two things of her: that she please love baseball and never vote for bullies. So far, she's embraced our season tickets to the Giants, and she has another sixteen years before she can vote.

Jerry called me the other day. He invited Lauren, Ella and me to come for a visit. His sixteen-year-old daughter got on the phone and said, "Ella is my cousin, so when can we meet her?" I was delightfully floored. His four children are all grown. I have met them all, and they are sweet and beautiful. It's taken twenty-five years for my brother and me to get to this point, but we aren't locked into the roles we had as children. He has broken from his shell, and I have broken from mine. People can change, hard-core criminals, aloof older brothers and loud-mouthed sisters alike. Looking back now, I can see he was struggling with the challenge our family posed, same as I was. He had his own way of dealing, which sometimes left me out. My child, I hope, will know what it is to have a loving extended family and to understand the true meaning of being a mensch.

Lauren and I take turns taking care of Ella during the week. On one of my days with her, we were at the park and she took off running. Before I could stop her she'd run right up to a homeless guy splayed on a bench. My stomach clenched. Primal fear took over as my little girl approached a guy who was unkempt and smelly and damp and was probably mentally ill. Ella's hand went to his knee. She smiled, gurgled out a Hi. I finally caught up and put my arms around her. "I'm sorry," I blurted. The man looked at me and smiled. "That's okay. It's not every day I'm touched by an angel."

Here I was about to snatch my kid away without a second thought after spending twenty-five years convincing others not to judge people at face value. And he surprised me with his humanity! And you know what? I get it. I completely understand the objections and utter impatience people have with criminals. They have hurt us, our pocketbooks, our souls. I too can fall into a fearful us-versus-them mind-set, and feel I would want to kill anyone who hurt my child. I get it.

But what do we want to do about that anger? We spend more than 10 billion dollars a year in California, thirty-four thousand dollars per inmate per year to incarcerate criminals. California has about 312,000 people behind bars. Around 280,000 of them will eventually be released. Across the country, there are over 2 million criminals in jails or prisons. This year alone, 650,000 criminals will be released nationwide. Most of the places where these men and women are held are monster factories. The prisoners have nothing to do, they stew and rage and whine until they are released. I've sometimes been called a radical and a prison abolitionist. In some ways, it's true. I am both of those things. I do want to abolish *traditional* incarceration, but not all incarceration. I want to expect more of the men and women who are supposedly repaying their debt to society. The only way to do this is to challenge them to learn, to strive, to become better citizens. I also firmly believe there are some people who are beyond our help who should probably never again see the light of day. Tari Ramirez is probably one of them. But the 650,000 people who aren't psychopathic killers and will be released into our communities this year need something better than monster factories, and so do we.

I still have dreams as I wander the halls of the jails I've patrolled for a quarter of a century. These prisoners are different from the ones I first met here in the 1980s. They seem more violent, less capable of empathy. But their stories of desperation, of failure, of violence, are the same. So is their potential. Whether we want to admit it or not, our fate is tied to them because, like it or not, they will be released into our communities at some point. We have the tools to help them join us as partners, as allies, as citizens, and not enemies. In my dreams, we start to use these tools, bring them into every prison in the country, not just into my jail in San Francisco. In my dreams, we remake the monster factories into engines of accountability rather than instruments of retribution and despair. And I know in my heart that we can make these dreams real, if only we have the courage to dream them together.

ACKNOWLEDGMENTS

My gratitude is boundless.

I want to first thank Michael Hennessey, our sheriff, the mensch, who for over twenty-eight years has given me the freedom to grow and create and take wonderful chances for the citizens of San Francisco. If every sheriff was like Hennessey, the world would be a safer and more decent place.

This book is about my life and in no way do I want to convey that I did this work alone. On the contrary, many people are responsible for the programs described in this book. I want to acknowledge the contributions of those individuals who were instrumental in conceiving and running these programs. To Leo Bruen, Erik Camberos, Muin Daly, Deputy Richard Drocco, Tijanna Eaton, Marcela Espino, Lieutenant Desiree Felix, Deputy Sheila Frazier, Delia Ginorio, Elyse Graham, Sergeant Dean Gross, Siddiq Jihad, Floyd Johnson, Lazanius Johnson, Dr. Martin Jones, George Jurand, Bhavani Kludt, Maureen Lees, Karen Levine, Leslie Levitas, Lieutenant Robby Limacher, Ramona Massey, Joanne McAllister, Jean O'Hara, Bianka Ramirez, Captain Tom Redmond, Lieutenant Richard Ridgeway, Jerry Scoggins, Roberto Varea, Reverend Billy Ware and countless other deputy sheriffs and civilian staff. They have renewed my faith in humanity and have given the San Francisco Sheriff's Department the ability to turn a small corner of the monster factory into a place of change, hope and accountability. To the Honorable Leslie Katz, for being the first elected official to get RSVP funded.

To Becky Benoit and Michael Marcum for your gutsy leadership. Without you RSVP would have remained just a good idea.

To Hamish Sinclair, who pioneered Manalive and has trained

thousands of men to unlearn the male-role belief system that fuels their violence.

To Ruth Morgan and Community Works West for not taking no for an answer and insisting that expressive arts be part of RSVP. She recognized that men develop empathy through theater exercises and group work, things that also give survivors and victims a dignified voice.

To those who came before me in this work, especially Ray Towbis, who is the pioneer of prisoner programs in San Francisco. He was the first civilian allowed in the San Francisco jails to work with convicts. He taught us how to question authority. He redefined the word *chutzpah*. Thank you, Ray. May you always watch over the castaways.

To the survivors of violence, may you always walk with your heads held high and continue to gain the courage to love and to live as fully integrated and self-determined human beings.

To the ex-offenders who have had the courage to look at themselves in the mirror and say, "I was wrong, I am accountable, I am sorry; I will stop my violence for your sake, for my sake, and for the sake of our communities."

To Deborah Mitchell and Mark Rosenthal for smart and compassionate therapy.

To my amazing agent, Priscilla Gilman, who never ceases to astound me with her heartfelt intelligence, empathy and advocacy for what is right and just. I remain amazed at your ability to immediately understand the importance of this work.

To Alexis Gargagliano, our gracious and phenomenal editor who understands matters of the heart and mind. Thank you for your skills in getting this "call to action book" edited so people truly understand.

To David Boodell, my co-writer, who must be a lesbian Jew trapped inside a heterosexual Catholic man's body. You have transformed my words and life into something that has exceeded my dreams. Liesl, thank you for supporting such a beautiful and talented man.

To my family: Cindy, who taught me the power of sharing and the beauty of art and music; Jerry, who made me popcorn and watched *Gunsmoke* with me on Saturday nights; my mother, Frieda, who saw the goodness in everyone; my father, Seymour, who brought crazy, passionate music and spontaneity into my life.

To Stevie, even though I still ache for you, I forgive you for leaving without saying good-bye. I am so sorry for your pain. Thank you for teaching me about survival and that mean curveball.

To Steve and Merilee Obstbaum, who have taught me the true meaning of family. I am forever grateful for your generosity, care and advocacy. Papa Steve, I will always remember your serious talks, urging me to write about my work. You set this off!

To my beloved Lauren, your beauty, honesty and brilliance knock me off my feet daily. Reality with you is the best fantasy I have ever had. No joke, this book would not be possible if not for you.

Finally, to our Ella Frieda, whose extraordinary spirit already shines brightly everywhere she goes. May our work make the world a safer and more compassionate place to live for you and all children. Beautiful Ella, may you always walk tall and be proud of who you are.

Here's to the peaceful revolution.

RESOURCES

The resources and books listed below are either directly related to and pro-
vided guidance for the programs described in this book or are national
resources to get help.

Al-Anon
  www.al-anon.org

Alcoholics Anonymous
  www. alcoholics-anonymous.org

Community Works West
  www.community-works-ca.org/

Family Violence Prevention Fund
  www.endabuse.org

San Francisco Sheriff's Department Five Keys Charter School
  www.fivekeyscharter.org

Manalive
  www.manaliveinternational.org

Narcotics Anonymous
  www.na.org

Restorative Justice Online
  www.restorativejustice.org

University of Minnesota Restorative Justice
at the School of Social Work
   www.rjp.umn.edu

San Francisco Sheriff's Department
Resolve to Stop the Violence Project (RSVP)
   www.resolvetostoptheviolence.org

Bazemore, Gordon and Mara Schiff. *Juvenile Justice Reform and Restorative Justice: Building Theory and Policy from Practice*. Portland, Oregon: Willan Publishing, 2005.

Gilligan, James, MD. *Preventing Violence*. New York: Thames & Hudson, 2001.

Gilligan, James, MD. *Violence: Reflections on a National Epidemic*. New York: Vintage, 1997.

Pranis, Kay. *The Little Book of Circle Processes: A New/Old Approach to Peacemaking*. Intercourse, Pennsylvania: Good Books, 2005.

Zehr, Howard. *The Little Book of Restorative Justice*. Intercourse, Pennsylvania: Good Books, 2002.

ABOUT THE AUTHORS

Sunny Schwartz is a nationally recognized expert in criminal justice reform and a twenty-seven-year veteran of the criminal justice system who has devoted her career to reforming traditional incarceration, well characterized by the stereotype of "idle and wasted downtime." Ms. Schwartz speaks nationally about the establishment of the Resolve to Stop the Violence Project (RSVP), an internationally recognized, award-winning restorative justice program that brings together traditionally opposing groups in order to confront comprehensively the costs of violence. Ms. Schwartz and the RSVP method of stopping crime have been featured on national television, including *The Oprah Winfrey Show,* the Discovery Channel, PBS and *Larry King Live,* and earned the prestigious Innovations in American Government Award, sponsored by the Ash Institute at Harvard University's Kennedy School of Government.

David Boodell is a writer and documentary filmmaker living in Los Angeles. Like Sunny, he grew up in Chicago, but while she was at Wrigley, he was in the Comiskey Park bleachers rooting for the White Sox. He got his start with National Public Radio working for a Chicago arts and current affairs show and then began working in television as a writer, producer and supervising producer for nonfiction television on A&E, the History Channel, Discovery and other networks. His most recent film is *Facing Life: The Retrial of Evan Zimmerman.* This is his first book.